MW01247179

CLINICAL NEUROSURGERY

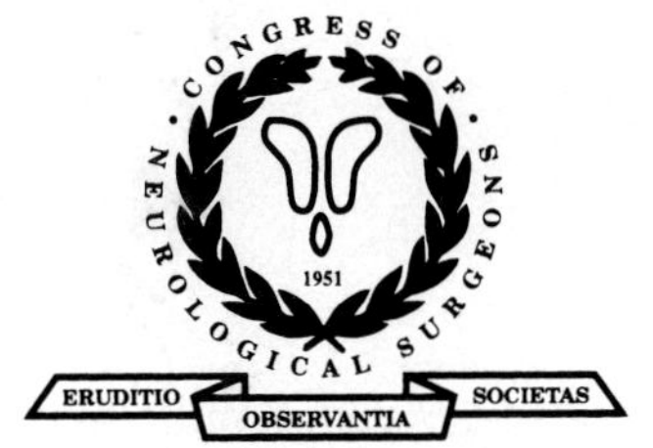

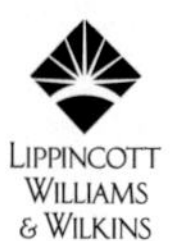

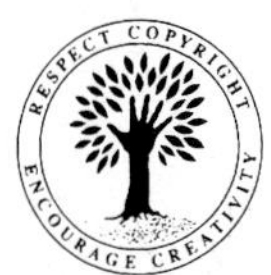

Accurate indications, adverse reactions, and dosage schedules for drugs are provided in this book, but it is possible that they may have changed. The reader is urged to review the package information data of the manufacturer of the medications mentioned.

Printed in the United States of America
(ISBN 0-7817-5072-5)

CLINICAL NEUROSURGERY

Volume 50

Proceedings

OF THE

CONGRESS OF NEUROLOGICAL SURGEONS

Philadelphia, Pennsylvania
2002

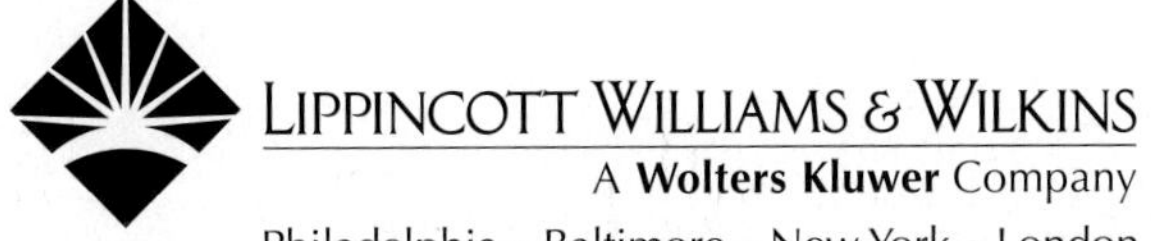

Preface

DISCOVERY • LEADERSHIP • FREEDOM

The 52nd Annual Meeting of the Congress of Neurological Surgeons was held in Philadelphia, Pennsylvania, at the Pennsylvania Convention Center from September 21–September 26, 2002. *Clinical Neurosurgery*, Volume 50, represents the official compendium of the platform presentations from the meeting. As stated by Stephen M. Papadopoulos, President of the Congress of Neurological Surgeons, "The theme, *Discovery • Leadership • Freedom*, not only reflects the city and the historic role of our Nation's forefathers, but clearly embodies the essential elements of modern neurosurgery." The 52nd Annual Meeting of the CNS was the first fully digital meeting in the history of neurosurgery. The contents of the entire meeting, as well as other useful information such as the CNS Membership directory, Philadelphia city guide, and Epocrates pharmacopoeia software, were contained on Palm Pilot i705s, which were distributed to every medical registrant.

The Annual Meeting Chair, Richard G. Ellenbogen, Scientific Program Co-Chairs, Joel D. MacDonald and Nelson M. Oyesiku, and the entire committee designed a meeting with exceptional scientific content and innovative educational programs. In addition to the outstanding presentations during the first three General Scientific Sessions (Discovery, Leadership, and Freedom to Expand the Neurosurgeon's Domain), the fourth GSS provided a thorough discussion of the current medical liability crisis. Highlights of the meeting included Dr. Papadopoulos's Presidential Address and the three presentations by this year's Honored Guest, Dr. Volker K.H. Sonntag. Dr. Sonntag offered insight into the evolution of the spine specialist, the future of spine surgery, and the neurosurgeon as a mentor and student. Wonderful Special Lectures were delivered by the Third Annual Walter E. Dandy Orator, scientist and conservationist Jane Goodall, Ph.D.; Chairman of the Board of the Institute for Genomic Research and President of Celera Genomics, J. Craig Ventner Ph.D.; eBay President and CEO, Meg Whitman; Emeritus Special Lecturer, Bennett M. Stein, M.D.; and Vice Chief of Staff of the Army, General John M. Keane.

In addition to the Presidential Address, Honored Guest Lectures, and General Scientific Session papers, this year's *Clinical Neurosurgery* includes an additional section compiling the excellent manuscripts from the recipients of the various CNS and Joint Section Resident and Young Investigator Awards. The Editorial Board would like to thank all of the General Scientific Session speakers and Resident/Young Investigator Awardees for their timely manuscript submissions. Current CNS President Mark Hadley deserves special credit for succeeding in manuscript recruitment when all conventional communication tactics had failed. We would also like to thank Christine Arnold at Lippincott Williams & Wilkins for her invaluable publishing assistance and patience. Lastly, special kudos to Ruchey Sharma at Columbia University for her editorial and administrative help.

We look forward to seeing you in October, in Denver, Colorado for the 53rd Annual Meeting.

Guy M. McKhann II, M.D.
Editor-in-Chief

Editorial Board
Charles S. Cobbs, M.D.
E. Sander Connolly, Jr., M.D.
Murat Gunel, M.D.

Honored Guests

1952—Professor Herbert Olivecrona, Stockholm, Sweden
1953—Sir Geoffrey Jefferson, Manchester, England
1954—Dr. Kenneth G. McKenzie, Toronto, Canada
1955—Dr. Carl W. Rand, Los Angeles, California
1956—Dr. Wilder G. Penfield, Montreal, Canada
1957—Dr. Francis C. Grant, Philadelphia, Pennsylvania
1958—Dr. A. Earl Walker, Baltimore, Maryland
1959—Dr. William J. German, New Haven, Connecticut
1960—Dr. Paul C. Bucy, Chicago, Illinois
1961—Professor Eduard A. V. Busch, Copenhagen, Denmark
1962—Dr. Bronson S. Ray, New York, New York
1963—Dr. James L. Poppen, Boston, Massachusetts
1964—Dr. Edgar A. Kahn, Ann Arbor, Michigan
1965—Dr. James C. White, Boston, Massachusetts
1966—Dr. Hugh A. Kravenbühl, Zurich, Switzerland
1967—Dr. W. James Gardner, Cleveland, Ohio
1968—Professor Normal M. Dott, Edinburgh, Scotland
1969—Dr. Wallace B. Hamby, Cleveland, Ohio
1970—Dr. Barnes Woodhall, Durham, North Carolina
1971—Dr. Elisha S. Gurdjian, Detroit, Michigan
1972—Dr. Francis Murphey, Memphis, Tennessee
1973—Dr. Henry G. Schwartz, St. Louis, Missouri
1974—Dr. Guy L. Odom, Durham, North Carolina
1975—Dr. William A. Sweet, Boston, Massachusetts
1976—Dr. Lyle A. French, Minneapolis, Minnesota
1977—Dr. Richard C. Schneider, Ann Arbor, Michigan
1978—Dr. Charles G. Drake, London, Ontario, Canada
1979—Dr. Frank H. Mayfield, Cincinnati, Ohio
1980—Dr. Eben Alexander, Jr., Winston-Salem, North Carolina
1981—Dr. J. Garber Galbraith, Birmingham, Alabama
1982—Dr. Keiji Sano, Tokyo, Japan
1983—Dr. C. Miller Fisher, Boston, Massachusetts
1984—Dr. Hugo V. Rizzoli, Washington, DC
Dr. Walter E. Dandy (posthumously), Baltimore, Maryland
1985—Dr. Sidney Goldring, St. Louis, Missouri
1986—Dr. M. Gazi Yasargil, Zurich, Switzerland
1987—Dr. Thomas W. Langiftt, Philadelphia, Pennsylvania
1988—Professor Lindsay Symon, London, England
1989—Dr. Thoralf M. Sundt, Jr., Rochester, Minnesota

1990—Dr. Charles Byron Wilson, San Francisco, California
1991—Dr. Bennett M. Stein, New York, New York
1992—Dr. Robert G. Ojemann, Boston, Massachusetts
1993—Dr. Albert L. Rhoton, Jr., Gainesville, Florida
1994—Dr. Robert F. Spetzler, Phoenix, Arizona
1995—Dr. John A. Jane, Charlottesville, Virginia
1996—Dr. Peter J. Jannetta, Pittsburgh, Pennsylvania
1997—Dr. Nicholas T. Zervas, Boston, Massachusetts
1998—Dr. John M. Tew, Cincinnati, Ohio
1999—Dr. Duke S. Samson, Dallas, Texas
2000—Dr. Edward R. Laws, Charlottesville, Virginia
2001—Dr. Michael L. J. Apuzzo, Los Angeles, California
2002—Dr. Volker K. H. Sonntag

Officers of the Congress of Neurological Surgeons 2002

STEPHEN M. PAPADOPOULOS, M.D.,
President

MARK N. HADLEY, M.D.,
President-Elect

VINCENT C. TRAYNELIS, M.D.,
Vice President

GERALD E. RODTS, JR., M.D.,
Secretary

PAUL J. CAMARATA, M.D.
Treasurer

ISSAM A. AWAD, M.D.,
Past President

EXECUTIVE COMMITTEE

P. DAVID ADELSON, M.D.
CHRISTOPHER C. GETCH, M.D.
JOEL D. MACDONALD, M.D.
DANIEL K. RESNICK, M.D.
B. GREGORY THOMPSON, JR., M.D.
CHRISTOPHER E. WOLFLA, M.D.
ANTHONY L. ASHER, M.D.
RICHARD G. ELLENBOGEN, M.D.
ISABELLE M. GERMANO, M.D.
DAVID F. JIMENEZ, M.D.
DOUGLAS S. KONDZIOLKA, M.D.
MICHAEL L. LEVY, M.D.
KARIN MURASZKO, M.D.
NELSON M. OYESIKU, M.D.
BEVERLY C. WALTERS, M.D.

Editors-in-Chief
Clinical Neurosurgery

Volume	*Date*	*Editor-in-Chief*
1	1953	Raymond K. Thompson, M.D.
2	1954	Raymond K. Thompson, M.D. & Ira J. Jackson, M.D.
3	1955	Raymond K. Thomspon, M.D. & Ira J. Jackson, M.D.
4	1956	Ira J. Jackson, M.D.
5	1957	Robert G. Fisher, M.D.
6	1958	Robert G. Fisher, M.D.
7	1959	Robert G. Fisher, M.D.
8	1960	William H. Mosberg, Jr., M.D.
9	1961	William H. Mosberg, Jr., M.D.
10	1962	William H. Mosberg, Jr., M.D.
11	1963	John Shillito, Jr., M.D., & William H. Mosberg, Jr., M.D.
12	1964	John Shillito, Jr., M.D.
13	1965	John Shillito, Jr., M.D.
14	1966	Robert G. Ojemann, M.D. & John Shillito, Jr., M.D.
15	1967	Robert G. Ojemann, M.D.
16	1968	Robert G. Ojemann, M.D.
17	1969	Robert G. Ojemann, M.D.
18	1970	George T. Tindall, M.D.
19	1971	George T. Tindall, M.D.
20	1972	Robert H. Wilkins, M.D.
21	1973	Robert H. Wilkins, M.D.
22	1974	Robert H. Wilkins, M.D.
23	1975	Ellis B. Keener, M.D.
24	1976	Ellis B. Keener, M.D.
25	1977	Ellis B. Keener, M.D.
26	1978	Peter W. Carmel, M.D.
27	1979	Peter W. Carmel, M.D.
28	1980	Peter W. Carmel, M.D.
29	1981	Martin H. Weiss, M.D.
30	1982	Martin H. Weiss, M.D.
31	1983	Martin H. Weiss, M.D.
32	1984	John R. Little, M.D.
33	1985	John R. Little, M.D.
34	1986	John R. Little, M.D.
35	1987	Peter McL. Black, M.D., Ph.D.
36	1988	Peter McL. Black, M.D., Ph.D.

37	1989	Peter McL. Black, M.D., Ph.D.
38	1990	Warren R. Selman, M.D.
39	1991	Warren R. Selman, M.D.
40	1992	Warren R. Selman, M.D.
41	1993	Christopher M. Loftus, M.D.
42	1994	Christopher M. Loftus, M.D.
43	1995	Christopher M. Loftus, M.D.
44	1996	M. Sean Grady, M.D.
45	1997	M. Sean Grady, M.D.
46	1998	M. Sean Grady, M.D.
47	1999	Matthew A. Howard III, M.D.
48	2000	Matthew A. Howard III, M.D.
49	2001	Matthew A. Howard III, M.D.
50	2002	Guy M. McKhann II, M.D.

Contributors

Aytac Akbasak, M.D.
Surgical Neurology Branch
National Institute of Neurological Disorders and Stroke
National Institutes of Health
Bethesda, Maryland

Michael L.J. Apuzzo, M.D.
Edwin M. Todd, M.D./Trent H. Wells Jr. Professor of Neurological Surgery
And Radiation Oncology, Biology and Physics
Department of Neurological Surgery
Keck School of Medicine, University of Southern California
Los Angeles, California

Allan J. Belzberg, M.D., F.R.C.S.C
Department of Neurosurgery
Johns Hopkins University
Laurel, Maryland

Edward C. Benzel, M.D.
Chairman, Spine Institute
Vice Chairman, Department of Neurosurgery
Residency Program Director, Department of Neurosurgery
Cleveland Clinic Foundation
Cleveland, Ohio

Antonio Bernardo, M.D.
Division of Neurological Surgery
Barrow Neurological Institute
St. Joseph's Hospital and Medical Center
Phoenix, Arizona

R. Hunt Bobo, M.D.
Surgical Neurology Branch
National Institute of Neurological Disorders and Stroke
National Institutes of Health
Bethesda, Maryland

Steven Brown, Ph.D.
Research Imaging Center
University of Texas Health Science Center
San Antonio, Texas

Richard D. Bucholz, M.D., F.A.C.S.
K.R. Smith Endowed Chair in Neurosurgery
Saint Louis University School of Medicine
Saint Louis, Missouri

Kim J. Burchiel, M.D., F.A.C.S.
John Raaf Professor and Chairman
Neurological Surgery
Oregon Health & Science University
Portland, Oregon

Indro Chakrabarti, M.D.
Resident
Neurosurgery
Keck School of Medicine
University of Southern California
Los Angeles, California

Dongwoo John Chang, M.D., F.R.C.S.C.
Division of Neurological Surgery
The Ohio State University
Columbus, Ohio

Lun Chen, M.D.
Department of Neurosurgery
Johns Hopkins University
Laurel, Maryland

Richard E. Clatterbuck, M.D., Ph.D.
Division of Neurological Surgery
Barrow Neurological Institute
St. Joseph's Hospital and Medical Center
Phoenix, Arizona

Daniel J. Curry, M.D.
Associate Professor of Surgery
Department of Surgery
The University of Chicago
Chicago, Illinois

Stephen Dodd, Ph.D.
Research Imaging Center
University of Texas Health Science Center
San Antonio, Texas

Michael J. Dorsi, B.A.
Department of Neurosurgery
Johns Hopkins University
Laurel, Maryland

Robert D. Ecker, M.D.
Department of Neurological Surgery
Mayo Clinic and Foundation
Rochester, Minnesota

Richard G. Fessler, M.D., Ph.D.
John Harper Seeley Professor and Chief
Neurosurgery
University of Chicago
Chicago, Illinois

John C. Flickinger, M.D., F.A.C.R.
Professor
Radiation Oncology
University of Pittsburgh
Pittsburgh, Pennsylvania

Peter T. Fox, M.D.
Research Imaging Center
University of Texas Health Science Center
San Antonio, Texas

David M. Frim, M.D., Ph.D.
Associate Professor of Surgery
Department of Surgery
The University of Chicago
Chicago, IL

Steven Giannotta, M.D.
Professor
Neurosurgery
Keck School of Medicine
University of Southern California
Los Angeles, California

Thomas Goffman, M.D.
Radiation Oncology Branch
National Cancer Institute
National Institutes of Health
Bethesda, Maryland

Nitin Gogate, M.D.
Surgical Neurology Branch
National Institute of Neurological Disorders and Stroke
National Institutes of Health
Bethesda, Maryland

Lee R. Guterman, Ph.D., M.D.
Assistant Professor
Neurosurgery
School of Medicine and Biomedical Sciences, University at Buffalo
State University of New York
Buffalo, New York

Mark N. Hadley, M.D.
Professor of Neurosurgery
University of Alabama
Birmingham, Alabama

L. Nelson Hopkins, M.D.
Professor and Chairman
Neurosurgery and Radiology
School of Medicine and Biomedical Sciences
University at Buffalo
State University of New York
Buffalo, New York

Jay U. Howington, M.D.
Assistant Instructor
Clinical Neurosurgery
School of Medicine and Biomedical Sciences
University at Buffalo
State University of New York
Buffalo, New York

Janis Ingham, Ph.D.
Department of Speech and Hearing Sciences
University of California, Santa Barbara
and

Research Imaging Center
University of Texas Health Science Center
San Antonio, Texas

Roger Ingham, Ph.D.
Department of Speech and Hearing Sciences
University of California, Santa Barbara
and
Research Imaging Center
University of Texas Health Science Center
San Antonio, Texas

Un J. Kang, M.D., Ph.D.
Associate Professor of Surgery
Department of Surgery
The University of Chicago
Chicago, Illinois

Douglas Kondziolka, M.D.,M.Sc., F.R.C.S.C., F.A.C.S.
Professor and Vice-Chairman
Department of Neurological Surgery
University of Pittsburgh
Pittsburgh, Pennsylvania

Jack L. Lancaster, Ph.D.
Research Imaging Center
University of Texas Health Science Center
San Antonio, Texas

Rafael C. Lee, M.D.
Professor of Surgery
Department of Surgery
The University of Chicago
Chicago, Illinois

Mario Liotti, M.D.
Research Imaging Center
University of Texas Health Science Center
San Antonio, Texas

Russell R. Lonser, M.D.
Surgical Neurology Branch
National Institute of Neurological Disorders and Stroke
National Institutes of Health
Bethesda, Maryland

L. Dade Lunsford, M.D., F.A.C.S.
Professor and Chairman
Department of Neurological Surgery
University of Pittsburgh
Pittsburgh, Pennsylvania

Joseph R. Madsen, M.D.
Associate Professor of Surgery
The Children's Hospital Boston
Harvard Medical School
Boston, Massachusetts

Cameron G. McDougall, M.D.
Division of Neurological Surgery
Barrow Neurological Institute
St. Joseph's Hospital and Medical Center
Phoenix, Arizona

Lee McDurmont
Manager, Data Services
Department of Surgery
Saint Louis University
Saint Louis, Missouri

Richard A. Meyer, M.S.
Department of Neurosurgery and the Applied Physics Laboratory
Johns Hopkins University
Laurel, Maryland

Shalini Narayana, Ph.D.
Research Imaging Center
University of Texas Health Science Center
San Antonio, Texas

Tung T. Nguyen, M.D.
Surgical Neurology Branch
National Institute of Neurological Disorders and Stroke
National Institutes of Health
Bethesda, Maryland

Eric W. Nottmeier, M.D.
Division of Neurological Surgery
Barrow Neurological Institute
St. Joseph's Hospital and Medical Center
Phoenix, Arizona

Edward H. Oldfield, M.D.
Surgical Neurology Branch
National Institute of Neurological Disorders and Stroke
National Institutes of Health
Bethesda, Maryland

Jeffery J. Olson, M.D.
Surgical Neurology Branch
National Institute of Neurological Disorders and Stroke
National Institutes of Health
Bethesda, Maryland

Stephen L. Ondra, M.D.
Associate Professor of Neurological Surgery
Northwestern University
Chicago, Illinois

Svetlana D. Pack, Ph.D.
Surgical Neurology Branch
National Institute of Neurological Disorders and Stroke
National Institutes of Health
Bethesda, Maryland

Stephen M. Papadopoulos, M.D.
Department of Neurological Surgery
Barrow Neurological Institute
Phoenix, Arizona
and
Adjunct Associate Professor
Department of Neurological Surgery
University of Michigan
Ann Arbor, Michigan

David G. Piepgras, M.D.
Chair, The American Board of Neurological Surgery
Department of Neurologic Surgery
Mayo Clinic
Rochester, Minnesota

Esther Pogatzki, Ph.D.
Department of Neurosurgery
Johns Hopkins University
Laurel, Maryland

Bruce E. Pollock, M.D.
Division of Radiation Oncology
Mayo Clinic and Foundation
Rochester, Minnesota

Faheem A. Sandhu, M.D.
Spinal Fellow
Neurosurgery
University of Chicago
Chicago, Illinois

R. Michael Scott, M.D.
Professor of Surgery
The Children's Hospital Boston
Harvard Medical School
Boston, Massachusetts

Frederick A. Simeone, M.D.
Professor
Neurosurgery
Drexel University College of Medicine
Philadelphia, Pennsylvania

Volker K.H. Sonntag, M.D.
Division of Neurological Surgery
Barrow Neurological Institute
St. Joseph's Hospital and Medical Center
Phoenix, Arizona

Robert F. Spetzler, M.D.
Division of Neurological Surgery
Barrow Neurological Institute
St. Joseph's Hospital and Medical Center
Phoenix, Arizona

Nitin Tandon, M.D.
Center for Neurosurgical Sciences and Research Imaging Center
University of Texas Health Science Center
San Antonio, Texas

Nicholas Theodore, M.D.
Division of Neurological Surgery
Naval Medical Center San Diego
San Diego, California

Vincent C. Traynelis, M.D.
Department of Neurosurgery
The University of Iowa
Iowa City, Iowa

Alex B. Valadka, M.D.
Associate Professor
Department of Neurosurgery, Baylor College of Medicine
Chief of Neurosurgery, Ben Taub General Hospital
Houston, Texas

Dennis G. Vollmer, M.D.
Center for Neurosurgical Sciences
University of Texas Health Science Center
San Antonio, Texas

Alexander O. Vortmeyer, M.D.
Surgical Neurology Branch
National Institute of Neurological Disorders and Stroke
National Institutes of Health
Bethesda, Maryland

Stuart Walbridge, B.S.
Surgical Neurology Branch
National Institute of Neurological Disorders and Stroke
National Institutes of Health
Bethesda, Maryland

Beverly C. Walters, M.D.
Clinical Professor
Neurosurgery
New York University
New York, New York

David A. Wright, Ph.D.
Research Associate
Department of Surgery
The University of Chicago
Chicago, Illinois

Zhengping Zhuang, M.D., Ph.D.
Surgical Neurology Branch
National Institute of Neurological Disorders and Stroke
National Institutes of Health
Bethesda, Maryland

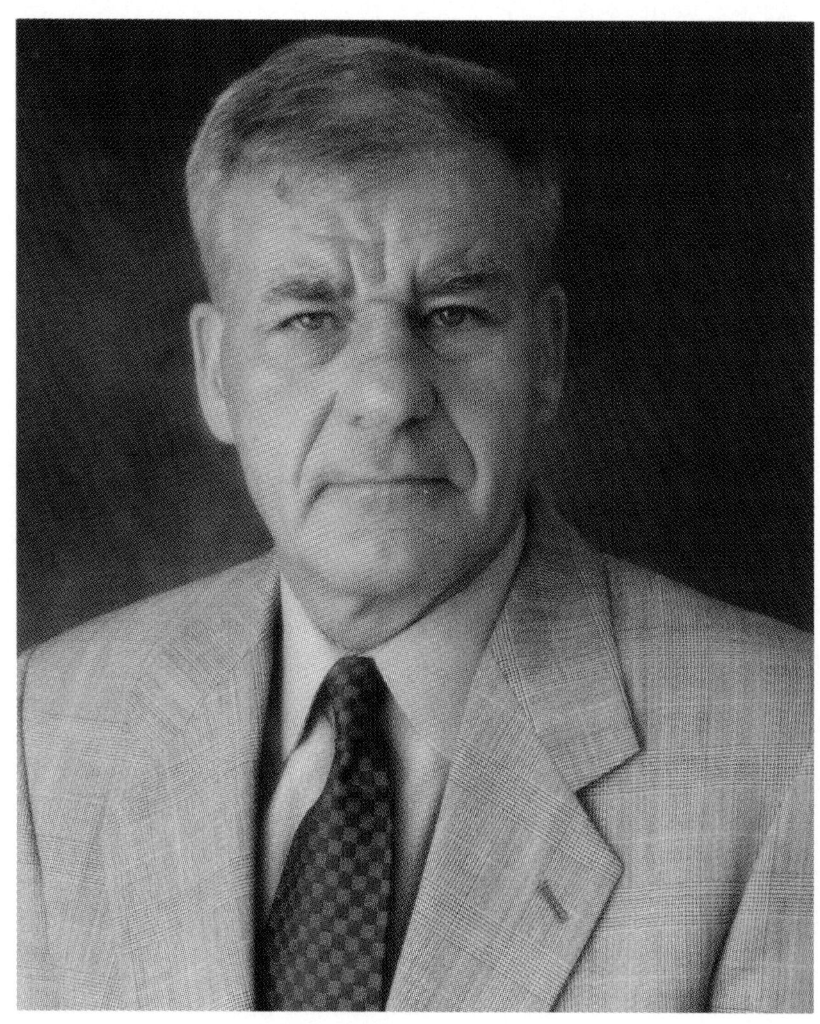

Volker K.H. Sonntag, M.D.

Biography

Volker K.H. Sonntag, M.D., was born November 23, 1944, in Graundenz, Germany, to Heinz Sonntag and Gisela (née) Albrecht. His family immigrated to America in 1957 and settled in Arizona (where he was amazed to discover that oranges grew on trees), and he subsequently continued his education. He attended Arizona State University in Tempe, AZ, from 1963 to 1967, receiving a Bachelor of Arts degree in Chemistry, *summa cum laude.* From 1967 to 1971, he attended the University of Arizona School of Medicine. He served as President of his graduating class and completed his internship there in 1972. In 1972, Dr. Sonntag moved to Tufts–New England Medical Center Hospital in Boston, MA, where he trained as one of the first residents under Bennett M. Stein, M.D., Professor and Chairman, Department of Neurosurgery. He completed his residency in 1977.

Dr. Sonntag then practiced in Youngstown, OH, for a year before moving to Phoenix, AZ, to practice neurosurgery in 1978. In 1983, he joined the Barrow Neurological Institute (BNI), where he has since remained. At the BNI, Dr. Sonntag has served as Vice-Chairman of the Division of Neurological Surgery and as Chairman of the Spine Section since 1984, as Director of the Spine Fellowship Program since 1988, and as Director of the Residency Program since 1995. In 2000, he assumed the endowed Alumni Chair for Spine Research at the BNI. In 1985, he was appointed Clinical Associate Professor of Surgery at the University of Arizona in Tucson, AZ. In 1989, he was promoted to Professor of Clinical Surgery.

Dr. Sonntag has received many awards for his contributions to teaching and mentoring of young neurosurgeons, an aspect of his career to which he has a strong personal commitment. At the BNI, he has received the Teacher of the Year Award seven times. In 2000, he was chosen as Mentor of the Millennium by his residents. He was also chosen as the Honored Guest for Lifetime Leadership and Mentoring to Young Neurosurgeons by the American Association of Neurological Surgeons Young Neurosurgeons Committee. The Volker K.H. Sonntag Fund for research was established by the North American Spine Society in 2001 as its first named fund. In 1999, the Joint Section on Disorders of the Spine and Peripheral Nerves established the Volker Sonntag Fellowship Award to encourage clinical research.

Dr. Sonntag has also received many other honors for his community service, research, and outstanding achievements. In 1981, he was elected as an honorary alumnus of Alpha Omega Alpha for his outstanding accomplishments for the Class of 1971. In 1982, he was elected as a Fellow to the American College of Surgeons. In 1987, he received the University of Arizona College of Medicine Alumni Medal (Outstanding Graduate for the last 20 years). He was a member of the *Think First* National Board between 1994 and 1998, testifying to his strong commitment to the prevention of spinal cord injuries. In 1999, he received the Meritorious Service Award from the Joint Section on Disorders of the Spine and Peripheral Nerves.

Through laboratory and clinical research, Dr. Sonntag has devoted his career to improving our understanding of spinal disorders, especially cervical and upper cervical spine disorders. His academic output has been prolific. He has written more than 60 chapters for important neurosurgical texts and more than 200 articles for refereed and nonrefereed journals. He is the co-editor of four major textbooks: *Principles of Spinal Surgery, Essentials of the Spine, Surgical Treatment of Discogenic Diseases of the Spine,* and *Surgery of the Craniovertebral Junction.* Currently, he is serving as a Section Editor of the spine volume for the newest edition of *Youman's Neurological Surgery,* which is still in press. That his surgical and scientific expertise is highly esteemed by his peers is further evidenced by the 11 editorial boards on which he is currently serving, including journals such as *Neurosurgery* (Principal Reviewer), *Journal of Neurosurgery, Acta Neurochirurgica,* and *Spine*. He is also highly sought as a speaker and has given more than 600 presentations at institutions, professional meetings, and universities around the world. He has been invited as a Visiting Professor to more than 40 institutions. Despite his academic, teaching, and clinical obligations, Dr. Sonntag has been an active member and leader in many professional neurosurgical and spine societies throughout his career, holding more than 20 professional memberships. He has been a member of the Congress of Neurological Surgeons since 1980, serving on about a dozen committees over the years. Notably, he was a member of the Executive Committee from 1985 to 1993. Since 1982, he has been a member of the American Association of Neurological Surgeons and presently is serving as this organization's Vice President. In 1992–1993, Dr. Sonntag served as the Chairman for the Joint Section on Disorders of the Spine and Peripheral Nerves. He also has served as the President of the North American Spine Society (2000–2001) and of the Rocky Mountain Neurosurgical Society (1991–1992). He is a member of the Neurosurgical Society of America and was elected to the Society of Neurological Surgeons in 1991, serving as the Chair of the Membership Committee in 1993–1994. In 1995, he was elected to the Academy of Neurological Surgeons. In 1998, he became a Director of the American Board of Neurological Surgeons and is currently Chair of the Recertification Committee.

Above all, Dr. Sonntag is devoted to his family. He has been married to his wife, Lynne, a pediatric nurse practitioner, since 1974. They have three children: Ailssa, who graduated from the University of California–Los Angeles in 2000 with a degree in communications (*summa cum laude*); Christopher, who is in his second year at Arizona State University; and Stephen, who is in the fifth grade. He is an accomplished medical philatelist and avid *aficionado* of vintage comedic cinema. In his spare time, Dr. Sonntag also enjoys coaching soccer (for the 13th straight year) and jogging.

Bibliography

REFEREED JOURNALS

Total Refereed Manuscripts (131)

PUBLISHED 2002 (1)

Guest J, Eleraky MA, Apostolides PJ, Dickman CA, Sonntag VKH: Traumatic central cord syndrome: Results of surgical management. J Neurosurg (Spine 1) 97:19–26, 2002.

PUBLISHED 2001 (7)

Adams M, Crawford N, Chamberlain R, Sonntag VKH, Dickman CA: Biomechanical comparison of anterior cervical plating and combined anterior/lateral mass plating. The Spine Journal 1(3):166–170, 2001.

Cagli S, Crawford NR, Sonntag VKH, Dickman CA: Biomechanics of Grade I degenerative lumbar spondylolisthesis. Part 2: Treatment with threaded interbody cages/dowels and pedicle screw. J Neurosurg 94(1 Suppl):51–60, 2001.

Chen TY, Crawford NR, Sonntag VKH, Dickman CA: Biomechanical effects of progressive anterior cervical decompression. Spine 26(1): 6–14, 2001.

Crawford NR, Cagli SC, Sonntag VKH, Dickman CA: Biomechanics of Grade I degenerative lumbar spondylolisthesis. Part 1: In vitro model. J Neurosurg 94(1 Suppl):45–50, 2001.

Sawin PD, Dickman CA, Crawford NR, Melton MS, Bichard WD, Sonntag VKH: The effects of dexamethasone on bone fusion in an experimental model of posterolateral lumbar spinal arthrodesis. J Neurosurg 94(1 Suppl):76–81, 2001.

Schievink W, Wijdicks E, Meyer F, Sonntag VKH: Spontaneous intracranial hypotension mimicking aneurysmal subarachnoid hemorrhage: Neurosurgery 48(3):513–517, 2001.

Sonntag VKH, Han PP, Vishteh AG: Anterior cervical discectomy. Neurosurgery 49:909–912, 2001.

PUBLISHED 2000 (2)

Eleraky MA, Theodore N, Adams M, Rekate HL, Sonntag VKH: Pediatric cervical spine injuries: Report of 102 cases and review of the literature. J Neurosurg 92(1 Suppl):12–17, 2000.

Theodore N, Sonntag VKH: Spinal surgery: The past century and the next. Neurosurgery 46(4):767–777, 2000.

PUBLISHED 1999 (7)

Eleraky MA, Llanos C, Sonntag VKH: Cervical corpectomy: Report of 185 cases and review of the literature. J Neurosurg 90(1 Suppl):35–41, 1999.

Fehlings M, Rao S, Tator C, Skaf G, Arnold P, Benzel E, Dickman C, Cuddy B, Green B, Hitchon P, Northrup B, Sonntag VKH, Wagner F, Wilberger J: The optimal radiologic method for assessing spinal canal compromise and cord compression in patients with cervical spinal cord injury: Part II: Results of a multicenter study. Spine 24(6):605–615, 1999.

Hurlbert RJ, Theodore N, Drabier JB, Magwood AM, Sonntag VKH: A prospective randomized double-blind controlled trial to evaluate the efficacy of an analgesic epidural paste following lumbar decompressive surgery. J Neurosurg 90(4 Suppl):191–197, 1999.

Rekate HL, Theodore N, Sonntag VKH et al: Pediatric spine and spinal cord trauma. State of the art for the third millennium. Childs Nerv Syst 15:743–750, 1999.

Sonntag VKH, Detwiler PW, Porter RW: Neurological surgery. J Am Coll Surg 188(2):161–170, 1999.

Sonntag VKH, Dickman CA (Topic Editors): Thoracic spine. Neurosurgical Focus 6 Article 5, 1999.

Vishteh AG, Crawford NR, Melton MS, Spetzler RF, Sonntag VKH, Dickman CA: Stability of the craniovertebral junction after unilateral occipital condyle resection: A biomechanical study. J Neurosurg 90(1 Suppl):91–98, 1999.

PUBLISHED 1998 (14)

Apostolides PA, Karahalios DG, Yapp RA, Sonntag VKH: Use of the BendMeister rod bender for occipitocervical fusion: Technical note. Neurosurgery 43(2):389–390, 1998.

Bracken MB, Shepard MJ, Theodore RH, Holford TR, Leo-Summers L, Aldrich EF, Fazi M, Fehlings M, Herr DL, Hitchon PW, Marshall LF, Nockels RP, Pascale V, Perot PL Jr, Piepmeier J, Sonntag VKH, Wagner F, Wilberger JE, Winn HR, Young W: Methylprednisolone or tirilazad mesylate administration after acute spinal cord injury 1-year follow up. Results of the Third National Acute Spinal Cord Injury Randomized Controlled Trial. J Neurosurg 89:699–706, 1998.

Chen TY, Dickman CA, Eleraky M, Sonntag VKH: The role of decompression for acute incomplete cervical spinal cord injury in cervical spondylosis. Spine 23(22):2398–2403, 1998.

Detwiler PW, Porter RW, Harrington TR, Sonntag VKH, Spetzler RF: Vascular decompression of a vertebral artery loop producing cervical radiculopathy. J Neurosurg 89:485–488, 1998.

Dickman CA, Sonntag VKH: Posterior C1-C2 transarticular screw fixation for atlantoaxial arthrodesis. Neurosurgery 43(2):275–280, 1998.

Eleraky MA, Apostolides PJ, Dickman CA, Sonntag VKH: Herniated thoracic discs mimic cardiac disease: Three case reports. Acta Neurochir 140(7):643–646, 1998.

Eleraky M, Masferrer R, Sonntag VKH: Posterior atlantoaxial facet screw fixation in rheumatoid arthritis. J Neurosurg 89(8):8–12, 1998.

Greene KA, Gorman WF, Sonntag VKH: Gentle cervical hyperextension causing quadriplegia in an older man with symptomatic cervical spondylosis. J Am Geriatr Soc 46(2):208–209, 1998.

Levi AD, Choi WG, Keller PJ, Heiserman JE, Sonntag VKH, Dickman CA: The radiographic and imaging characteristics of porous tantalum implants within the human cervical spine. Spine 23(11):1245–1251, 1998.

Levi AD, Sonntag VKH: Management of posttraumatic syringomyelia using an expansile duraplasty: A case report. Spine 23(1):128–132, 1998.

Masferrer R, Gomez C, Karahalios DG, Sonntag VKH: Efficacy of pedicle screw fixation in the treatment of spinal instability and failed back surgery: A 5-year review. J Neurosurg 89(3):371–377, 1998.

Naderi S, Crawford Neil, Song GS, Sonntag VKH, Dickman CA: Biomechanical comparison of C1-C2 posterior fixations. Cable, graft, and screw combinations. Spine 23(18):1946–1956, 1998.

Porchet F, Sonntag VKH, Vrodos N: Cervical amyloidoma of C2. A case report and review of the literature. Spine 23(1):133–138, 1998.

Vishteh AG, Schievink WI, Baskin JJ, Sonntag VKH: Cervical bone spur presenting with spontaneous intracranial hypotension. Case Report. J Neurosurg 89(3):483–484, 1998.

PUBLISHED 1997 (11)

Apostolides PJ, Theodore N, Karahalios DG, Sonntag VKH: Triple anterior screw fixation of an acute combination atlas-axis fracture. Case Report. J Neurosurg 87:96–99, 1997.

Bracken MB, Shepard MJ, Theodore RH, Leo-Summers L, Aldrich EF, Fazi M, Fehlings M, Herr DL, Hitchon PW, Marshall LF, Nockels RP, Pascale V, Perot RP Jr, Piepmeier J, Sonntag VKH, Wagner F, Wilberger JE, Winn HR, Young W: Administration of methylprednisolone for 24 or 48 hours or tirilazad mesylate for 48 hours in the treatment of acute spinal cord injury. Results of the Third National Acute Spinal Cord Injury Randomized Controlled Trial. JAMA 277(20):1597–1604, 1997.

Broc GG, Crawford NR, Sonntag VKH, Dickman CA: Biomechanical effects of transthoracic microdiscectomy. Spine 22(6):605–612, 1997.

Kick SA, Sonntag VKH, Spetzler RF: Neurosurgery at the Barrow Neurological Institute. Neurosurgery 41(4):930–937, 1997.

Levi AD, Dickman CA, Sonntag VKH: Management of postoperative infections after spinal instrumentation. J Neurosurg 86:975–980, 1997.

Levi AD, Sonntag VK, Dickman CA, Mather J, Li RH, Cordoba SC, Bichard B, Berens M: The role of cultured Schwann cell grafts in the repair of gaps within the peripheral nervous system of primates. Exp Neurol 143:25–36, 1997.

Ronderos JF, Jacobowitz R, Sonntag VKH, Crawford NR, Dickman CA: Comparative pull-out strength of tapped and untapped pilot holes for bicortical anterior cervical screws. Spine 22(2):167–170, 1997.

Song GS, Theodore N, Dickman CA, Sonntag VKH: Unilateral posterior atlantoaxial transarticular screw fixation. J Neurosurg 87(6): 851–855, 1997.

Sonntag VKH: Neurosurgical spine fellowships: The Phoenix model. Acta Neurochir (Wien) 69:130–134, 1997.

Sonntag VKH: Point of view. Spine (22)12:1318, 1997.

Westmark RM, Westmark KD, Sonntag VKH: Disappearing cervical disc. J Neurosurg 86:289–290, 1997.

PUBLISHED 1996 (6)

Apostolides PJ, Dickman CA, Golfinos JG, Papadopoulos SM, Sonntag VKH: Threaded Steinmann pin fusion of the craniovertebral vertebral junction. Spine 21(14):1630–1637, 1996.

Dickman CA, Greene KA, Sonntag VKH: Injuries involving transverse atlantal ligament: Classification and treatment guidelines based upon experience with 39 injuries. Neurosurgery 38:44–50, 1996.

Dickman CA, Rosenthal D, Karahalios DG, Paramore CG, Mican CA, Apostolides PJ, Lorenz R, Sonntag VKH: Thoracic vertebrectomy and reconstruction using a microsurgical thoracoscopic approach. Neurosurgery 38:279–293, 1996.

Paramore CG, Dickman CA, Sonntag VKH: Radiographic and clinical follow-up review of Caspar plates in 49 patients. J Neurosurg 84: 957–961, 1996.

Paramore CG, Dickman C, Sonntag VKH: The anatomical suitability of the C1-2 complex for transarticular screw fixation. J Neurosurg 85:221–224, 1996.

Sonntag VKH, Klara P: Controversy in spine care. Is fusion necessary after anterior cervical discectomy? Spine 21(9):1111–1113, 1996.

PUBLISHED 1995 (12)

Boden SD, Andersson GBJ, Fraser RD, Garfin SR, Goel VK, Hanley EN Jr, Katz JN, Pope MH, Sonntag VKH: Selection of the optimal procedure to achieve lumbar spinal fusion. Introduction. 1995 Focus Issue Meeting on Fusion. Spine 20(24 Suppl):166S, 1995.

Boden SD, Sumner DR, Andersson GBJ, Fraser RD, Garfin SR, Goel VK, Hanley EN Jr, Katz JN, Pope MH, Sonntag VKH, Spratt KF, Zeblick TA: Biologic issues in lumbar spinal fusion. Introduction. 1995 Focus Issue Meeting on Fusion. Spine 20(24 Suppl):100S–101S, 1995.

Dickman CA, Crawford NR, Brantley AGU, Sonntag VKH: Biomechanical effects of transoral odontoidectomy. Neurosurgery 36:1146–1152, 1995.

Dickman CA, Foley KT, Sonntag VKH, Smith MM: Cannulated screws for odontoid screw fixation and atlantoaxial transarticular screw fixation. J Neurosurg 83:1095–1100, 1995.

Dickman CA, Sonntag VKH: Surgical management of atlantoaxial nonunions. J Neurosurg 83:248–253, 1995.

Garfin SR, Spratt KF, Andersson GBJ, Boden SD, Fraser RD, Soel VK, Hanley EN Jr, Katz JN, Pope MH, Sonntag VKH: Use of internal fixation instrumentation. Introduction. 1995 Focus Issue Meeting on Fusion. Spine 20(24 Suppl):154S–156S, 1995.

Katz JN, Spratt KF, Andersson GBJ, Boden SD, Fraser RD, Garfin SR, Goel VK, Hanley EN Jr, Pope MH, Sonntag VKH, Sumner DR, Zdeblick TA: Epidemiology. Introduction. 1995 Focus Issue Meeting on Fusion. Spine 20(24 Suppl):76S–77S, 1995.

Lawton MT, Porter RW, Heiserman JE, Jacobowitz R, Sonntag VKH, Dickman CA: Surgical management of spinal epidural hematoma: Relationship between surgical timing and neurological outcome. J Neurosurg 83:1–7, 1995.

Pope MH, Goel VK, Sumner DR, Andersson BJ, Boden SD, Fraser RD, Garfin SR, Hanley EN Jr, Katz JN, Sonntag VKH, Spratt KF: Biomechanics. Introduction. 1995 Focus Issue Meeting on Fusion. Spine 20(24 Suppl):84S, 1995.

Sonntag VKH, Marciano FF: Is fusion indicated for lumbar spinal disorders? Spine 10(24 Suppl):138S–142S, 1995.

Tominaga T, Dickman CA, Sonntag VKH, Coons S: Comparative anatomy of the baboon and the human cervical spine. Spine 20(2): 131–137, 1995.

Zeblick TA, Hanley EN Jr, Sonntag VKH, Andersson GBJ, Boden SD, Fraser RD, Garfin SR, Goel VK, Katz JN, Pope MH: Indications for lumbar spinal fusion. Introduction. 1995 Focus Issue Meeting on Fusion. Spine 20(24 Suppl):124S–125S, 1995.

PUBLISHED 1994 (5)

Dickman CA, Crawford NR, Tominaga T, Brantley AGU, Coons S, Sonntag VKH: Morphology and kinematics of the baboon upper cervical spine: A model of the atlantoaxial complex. Spine 19(22):2518–2523, 1994.

Golfinos JG, Dickman CA, Zabramski JM, Sonntag VKH, Spetzler RF: Repair of vertebral artery injury during anterior cervical decompression. Spine 19(22):2552–2556, 1994.

Greene KA, Dickman CA, Marciano FF, Drabier J, Drayer BP, Sonntag VKH: Transverse atlantal ligament disruption associated with odontoid fractures. Spine 19(20):2307–2314, 1994.

Herman JM, Sonntag VKH: Cervical corpectomy and plate fixation for postlaminectomy kyphosis. J Neurosurg 80(6):963–970, 1994

Levy DI, Sonntag VKH: Titanium dural clip testing. Technical note. J Neurosurg 81:947–949, 1994.

PUBLISHED 1993 (5)

Dickman CA, Papadopoulos SM, Sonntag VKH, Spetzler RF, Rekate HL, Drabier J: Traumatic occipitoatlantal dislocations. J Spinal Disord 6(4):300–313, 1993.

Dickman CA, Zabramski JM, Rekate HL, Sonntag VKH: Epitome: Spinal cord injuries in children without radiographic abnormalities. West J Med 158(1):67–68, 1993.

Khayata M, Sonntag VKH, Spetzler RF: The intraoperative applications of the Diasonics 900 mobile neuroimaging system. Neurosurgery 32(5):869–870, 1993.

Mamourian AC, Dickman CA, Drayer BP, Sonntag VKH: Spinal epidural abscess: Three cases following spinal epidural injection demonstrated with magnetic resonance imaging. Anesthesiology 78(1):204–207, 1993.

Marcotte P, Dickman CA, Sonntag VKH, Karahalios DG, Drabier J: Posterior atlantoaxial facet screw fixation. J Neurosurg 79:234–237, 1993.

PUBLISHED 1992 (4)

Bracken MB, Shepard MJ, Collins WF Jr, Holford TR, Baskin DS, Eisenberg HM, Flamm E, Leo-Summers L, Maroon JC, Marshall LF, Perot PL Jr, Piepmeier J, Sonntag VKH, et al: Methylprednisolone or naloxone treatment after acute spinal cord injury: 1-year follow-up data: Results of the Second National Acute Spinal Cord Injury Study. J Neurosurg 76:23–31, 1992.

Hadley MN, Fitzpatrick BC, Sonntag VKH, Browner CM: Facet fracture-dislocation injuries of the cervical spine. Neurosurgery 30:661–666, 1992.

Pappas CTE, Harrington T, Sonntag VKH: Outcome analysis in 654 surgically treated lumbar disc herniations. Neurosurgery 30(6):862–866, 1992.

Tuite GF, Papadopoulos SM, Sonntag VKH: Caspar plate fixation for the treatment of complex hangman's fractures. Neurosurgery 30:761–765, 1992.

PUBLISHED 1991 (9)

Bailes JE, Hadley MN, Quigley MR, Sonntag VKH, Cerullo LJ: Management of athletic injuries of the cervical spine and spinal cord. Neurosurgery 29(4):491–497, 1991.

Dickman CA, Mamourian A, Sonntag VKH, Drayer BP: Magnetic resonance imaging of the transverse atlantal ligament for the evaluation of atlantoaxial instability. J Neurosurg 75:221–227, 1991.

Dickman CA, Sonntag VKH, Papadopoulos ST, Hadley MN: The interspinous method of posterior atlantoaxial arthrodesis. J Neurosurg 74:190–198, 1991.

Dickman CA, Zabramski JM, Hadley MN, Rekate HL, Sonntag VKH: Pediatric spinal cord injury without radiographic abnormalities: Report of 26 cases and review of the literature. J Spinal Disord 4(3):296–305, 1991.

Herman JM, Sonntag VKH: Diving accidents: Mechanism of injury and treatment of the patient. Crit Care Nurs Clin N Am 3(2):331–337, 1991.

Papadopoulos SM, Dickman CA, Sonntag VKH: Atlantoaxial stabilization in rheumatoid arthritis. J Neurosurg 74(1):1–7, 1991.

Papadopoulos SM, Dickman CA, Sonntag VKH, Rekate HL, Spetzler RF: Traumatic atlantooccipital dislocation with survival. Neurosurgery 28(4):574–579, 1991.

Pappas CTE, Gibson AR, Sonntag VKH: Decussation of hind-limb and fore-limb fibers in the monkey corticospinal tract: Relevance to cruciate paralysis. J Neurosurg 75:935–940, 1991.

Sonntag VKH, Douglas RA: Management of cervical spinal cord trauma. J Neurotrauma 9(Suppl 1):S385–S396, 1991.

PUBLISHED 1990 (5)

Bracken MB, Shepard MJ, Collins WF, Holford TR, Young W, Baskin DS, Eisenberg HM, Flamm E, Leo-Summers L, Maroon J, Marshall LF, Perot PL, Piepmeier J, Sonntag VKH, Wagner FC, Wilberger JE, Winn HR: A randomized, controlled trial of methylprednisolone or naloxone in the treatment of acute spinal cord injuries: Results of the Second National Acute Spinal Cord Injury Study. N Engl J Med 322:1405–1411, 1990.

Dickman CA, Hadley MN, Pappas CTE, Sonntag VKH, Geisler FH: Cruciate paralysis: A clinical and radiographic analysis of injuries to the cervicomedullary junction. J Neurosurg 73:850–858, 1990.

Dickman CA, Shedd SA, Spetzler RF, Shetter AG, Sonntag VKH: Spinal epidural hematoma associated with epidural anesthesia: Complications of systemic heparinization in patients receiving peripheral vascular thrombolytic therapy. Anesthesiology 72:947–950, 1990.

Liu SS, Williams KD, Drayer BP, Spetzler RF, Sonntag VKH: Synovial cysts of the lumbosacral spine: Diagnosis by MR imaging. AJR Am J Roentgenol 154:163–166, 1990.

Sonntag VKH, Douglas RA: Management of spinal cord trauma. Neurosurg Clin N Am 1(3):729–750, 1990.

PUBLISHED 1989 (7)

Dickman CA, Hadley MN, Browner CM, Sonntag VKH: Neurosurgical management of acute atlas-axis combination fractures. A review of 25 cases. J Neurosurg 70:45–49, 1989.

Dickman CA, Rekate HL, Sonntag VKH, Zabramski JM: Pediatric spinal trauma: Vertebral column and spinal cord injuries in children. Pediatr Neurosci 15:237–255, 1989.

Hadley MN, Dickman CA, Browner CM, Sonntag VKH: Acute axis fractures: A review of 229 cases. J Neurosurg 71:642–647, 1989.

Hadley MN, Sonntag VKH, Rekate HL, Murphy A: The infant whiplash-shake injury syndrome: A clinical and pathological study. Neurosurgery 24(4):536–540, 1989.

Hadley MN, Spetzler RF, Sonntag VKH: The transoral approach to the superior cervical spine. A review of 53 cases of extradural cervicomedullary compression. J Neurosurg 71:16–23, 1989.

Liu SS, Johnson PC, Sonntag VKH: Meningioangiomatosis: A case report. Surg Neurol 31:376–380, 1989.

Liu SS, Williams KD, Drayer BP, Spetzler RF, Sonntag VKH: Synovial cysts of the lumbosacral spine: Diagnosis by MR imaging. AJNR Am J Neuroradiol 10:1239–1242, 1989.

PUBLISHED 1988 (8)

Dickman CA, Sonntag VKH, Johnson PC, Medina M: Amyloidoma of the cervical spine: A case report. Neurosurgery 22(2):419–422, 1988.

Dickman CA, Zabramski JM, Sonntag VKH, Coons S: Myelopathy due to epidural varicose veins of the cervicothoracic junction: Case report. J Neurosurg 69:940–941, 1988.

Hadley MN, Browner CM, Liu SS, Sonntag VKH: New subtype of acute odontoid fractures (Type IIA). Neurosurgery 22(1):67–71, 1988.

Hadley MN, Dickman CA, Browner CM, Sonntag VKH: Acute traumatic atlas fractures: Management and long-term outcome. Neurosurgery 23(1):31–35, 1988.

Hadley MN, Martin NA, Spetzler RF, Sonntag VKH, Johnson PC: Comparative transoral dural closure techniques: A canine model. Neurosurgery 22(2):392–397, 1988.

Hadley MN, Zabramski JM, Browner CM, Rekate H, Sonntag VKH: Pediatric spinal trauma: Review of 122 cases of spinal cord and vertebral column injuries. J Neurosurg 68:18–24, 1988.

Pappas CTE, Johnson PC, Sonntag VKH: Signet-ring cell lymphoma of the central nervous system. Case report. J Neurosurg 69:789–792, 1988.

Sonntag VKH, Hadley MN, Dickman CA, Browner CM: Atlas fractures: Treatment and long-term results. Acta Neurochir (Suppl) 43: 63–68, 1988.

PUBLISHED 1987 (2)

Browner C, Hadley MN, Sonntag VKH, Mattingly LG: Halo immobilization brace care: An innovative approach. J Neurosci Nurs 19(1):24–29, 1987.

Hadley MN, Sonntag VKH, Amos MR, Hodak JA, Lopez LJ: Three-dimensional computed tomography in the diagnosis of vertebral column pathological conditions. Neurosurgery 21(2):186–192, 1987.

PUBLISHED 1986 (3)

Hadley MN, Sonntag VKH, Grahm TW, Masferrer R, Browner C: Axis fractures resulting from motor vehicle accidents. The need for occupant restraints. Spine 11(9):861–864, 1986.

Hadley MN, Sonntag VKH, Pittman HW: Suprascapular nerve entrapment: A report of seven cases. J Neurosurg 64:843–848, 1986.

Marano SR, Calica AB, Sonntag VKH: Bilateral upper extremity paralysis (Bell's cruciate paralysis) from a gunshot wound to the cervicomedullary junction. Neurosurgery 18(5):642–644, 1986.

PUBLISHED 1985 (4)

Bloomfield SM, Sonntag VKH: Delayed cerebral vasospasm after uncomplicated operation on an unruptured aneurysm: Case report. Neurosurgery 17:792–796, 1985.

Hadley MN, Browner C, Sonntag VKH: Axis fractures: A comprehensive review of management and treatment in 107 cases (Mayfield Award). Neurosurgery 17:281–290, 1985.

Marano SR, Fischer DW, Gaines C, Sonntag VKH: Anatomical study of the superficial temporal artery. Neurosurgery 16:786–790, 1985.

Nehls DG, Sonntag VKH, Murphy AR, Johnson PC, Waggener JD: Fibroblastic tumor of the abducens nerve. Case report. J Neurosurg 62:296–299, 1985.

PUBLISHED 1984 (2)

Marano SR, Sonntag VKH, Spetzler RF: Planum sphenoidale meningioma mimicking pituitary apoplexy: A case report. Neurosurgery 15:859–862, 1984.

Sonntag VKH: Unusual presentations of lumbar stenosis. Ariz Med 41:228–234, 1984.

PUBLISHED 1983 (1)

Sonntag VKH, Plenge KL, Balis MS, Raudzens P, Hodak JA, Clark RJ, Waggener JD: Surgical treatment of an abscess in a Rathke's cleft cyst. Surg Neurol 20:152–256, 1983.

PUBLISHED 1982 (2)

Demakas JJ, Sonntag VKH, Kaplan AM, Kelley JJ, Waggener JD: Surgical management of pineal area tumors in early childhood. Surg Neurol 18:435–440, 1982.

Sonntag VKH: The early management of cervical spine injuries. Ariz Med 39:644–647, 1982.

PUBLISHED 1981 (4)

Sonntag VKH: Trans-sphenoidal hypophysectomy for intractable cancer pain. Ariz Med 38:23–25, 1981.

Sonntag VKH: Management of bilateral locked facets of the cervical spine. Neurosurgery 8:150–152, 1981.

Sonntag VKH, Kelley JJ: Adult shunt ascites. Ariz Med 38:182–184, 1981.

Sonntag VKH, Waggener JD, Kaplan AM: Surgical removal of a hemangioma of the pineal region in a four week old infant. Neurosurgery 8:586–588, 1981.

PUBLISHED 1980 (1)

Sonntag VKH, Waggener JD: Congenital dermoid cyst of the anterior fontanel in a Mexican-American. Surg Neurol 13:371–373, 1980.

PUBLISHED 1979 (1)

Plenge KL, Sonntag VKH: Chronic subdural hematoma causing "transient ischemic attacks" in a young woman. Ann Neurol 6:279, 1979.

PUBLISHED (2)

Sonntag VKH: Acute subdural hematoma with a lucid interval. JAMA 240:2284–2285, 1978.

Sonntag VKH, Stein BM: Intracerebral Ewing's sarcoma: Case report. Neurosurgery 2:55–57, 1978.

PUBLISHED 1977 (3)

Scott RM, Sonntag VKH, Wilcox LM, Adelman L, Rockel T: Visual loss from opticochiasmatic arachnoiditis after tuberculous meningitis: Case report. J Neurosurg 46:524–526, 1977.

Sonntag VKH, Steiner S, Stein BM: Neurosurgery and the physician assistant: Surg Neurol 8:207–208, 1977.

Sonntag VKH, Yuan R, Stein BM: Giant intracranial aneurysms: A review of 13 cases. Surg Neurol 8:81–84, 1977.

PUBLISHED 1976 (1)

Cummings J, Sonntag VKH, Scott RM: Ascites complicating ventriculo-peritoneal shunting in an adult. Surg Neurol 6:135–136, 1976.

PUBLISHED 1974 (1)

Sonntag VKH, Stein BM: Arteriopathic complications during treatment of subarachnoid hemorrhage with epsilon-aminocaproic acid. J Neurosurg 40:480–485, 1974.

PUBLISHED 1970 (1)

Sonntag VKH: Effects of L-dopa on five patients with Parkinsonism. Ariz Med 27:96–98, 1970.

NONREFEREED JOURNALS

Total Nonrefereed Journals (90)

Adams M, Sonntag VKH: Surgical treatment of metastatic cervical spine disease. Contemp Neurosurg 23(5):1–6, 2001.

Bartolomei J, Henn JS, Lemole GM, Lynch J, Dickman CA, Sonntag VKH: Application of frameless stereotaxy to spinal surgery. BNI Quarterly 17(1):35–40, 2001.

Henn JS, Deshmukh V, Sonntag VKH: Resection of vertebral osteoid osteoma with frameless stereotactic assistance: Case report. BNI Quarterly 17(1):41–43, 2001.

Lemole GM Jr, Henn JS, Zabramski JM, Sonntag VKH: The management of cranial and spinal CSF leaks. BNI Quarterly 17(4):4–13, 2001.

Theodore N, Partovi S, Walker M, Sava P, Sonntag VKH: Preoperative helical CT angiography for C1-2 transarticular screw placement: A new technique. BNI Quarterly 17(3):49–52, 2001.

Theodore N, Sonntag VKH: Decision making in degenerative cervical spine surgery. Clin Neurosurg 48:260–276, 2001.

Theodore N, Vishteh AG, Baskin JJ, Sonntag VKH: Titanium mesh cage interbody fusion in the thoracolumbar spine. Techniques in Neurosurgery 7(2):119–126, 2001.

Cherny WB, Sonntag VKH: Myelomeningocele repair. BNI Quarterly 16(4):11–14, 2000

Detwiler PW, Porter RW, Han PP, Karahalios DG, Masferrer R, Sonntag VKH: Surgical treatment of lumbar spondylolisthesis. Advances and Technical Standards in Neurosurgery 26:331–343, 2000.

Lemole GM, Theodore N, Sonntag VKH: Progressive spondylosis. BNI Quarterly 16(1):33–34, 2000.

Porter RW, Detwiler PW, Lawton MT, Sonntag VKH, Dickman CD: Postoperative spinal epidural hematomas: Longitudinal review of 12,000 spinal operations. BNI Quarterly 16(1):10–17, 2000.

Feiz-Erfan I, Detwiler PW, Porter RW, Sonntag VKH, Spetzler RF: Ondine's curse. BNI Quarterly 14(2):15–17, 1999.

Detwiler PW, Porter RW, Clark R, Sonntag VKH: Nonsurgical treatment of a cervical epidural abscess. BNI Quarterly 15(2):26–27, 1999.

Levi A, Sonntag VKH, Dickman CD: Management of postoperative infections after spinal surgery. Techniques in Neurosurgery 5(4):274–281, 1999.

Naderi S, Crawford NR, Melton MS, Sonntag VKH, Dickman CA: Biomechanical analysis of cranial settling after transoral odontoidectomy. BNI Quarterly 15(3):4–10, 1999.

Vishteh AG, Baskin JJ, Sonntag VKH: Controversy in operative techniques for cervical spondylosis discectomy: Autograft versus allograft versus no graft. Techniques of Neurosurgery 5(2):146–152, 1999.

Vishteh AG, Feiz-Erfan I, Sonntag VKH: Type I modic changes associated with acquired lumbar spondylolisthesis after L4-5 microdiscectomy. BNI Quarterly 15(4):26–27, 1999.

Apostolides PJ, Karahalios DG, Sonntag VKH: Technique of occipitocervical fusion with a threaded Steinmann pin. Operative Techniques in Neurosurgery 1(2):63–66, 1998.

Apostolides, PJ, Karahalios DG, Sonntag VKH: Technique of posterior atlantoaxial arthrodesis with transarticular facet screw fixation and interspinous wiring. Operative Techniques in Neurosurgery 1(2):67–71, 1998.

Apostolides PJ, Vishteh AG, Sonntag VKH: Technique of transoral odontoidectomy. Operative Techniques in Neurosurgery 1(2):58–62, 1998.

Baskin JJ, Vishteh AG, Dickman CA, Sonntag VKH: Techniques of anterior cervical plating. Operative Techniques in Neurosurgery 1(2):90–102, 1998.

Cagli S, Dickman CA, Sonntag VKH: Ossification of posterior longitudinal ligament in the cervical spine: Clinical manifestations and surgical treatment. Neuro-Orthopedics 24:1–12, 1998.

Detwiler PW, Porter RW, Sonntag VKH, Dickman CA: Laparoscopic anterior lumbar interbody fusion. Contemp Neurosurg 20(25):1–6, 1998.

Detwiler PW, Porter RW, Marciano FF, Dickman CA, Sonntag VKH: Lumbar spine fusion with and without instrumentation. Operative Techniques in Neurosurgery 1(3):142–150, 1998.

Detwiler PW, Porter RW, Dickman CA, Sonntag VKH: Lumbar spine interbody fusion with use of synthetic implants. Operative Techniques in Neurosurgery 1(3):113–119, 1998.

Detwiler PW, Porter RW, Sonntag VKH: Facet-sparing lumbar laminectomy. Operative Techniques in Neurosurgery 1(3):120–125, 1998.

Eoh W, Eleraky M, Sonntag VKH: Surgical management of cervical spine metastases: A retrospective study. Neuro-Orthopedics 25:27–37, 1998.

Eleraky MA, Baskin JJ, Sonntag VKH: Elongating a bone graft for corpectomy: Technical note. BNI Quarterly 14(4):12–13, 1998.

Karahalios DG, Apostolides PJ, Geldmacher TR, Sonntag VKH: Image-guided spinal surgery. Operative Techniques in Neurosurgery 1(3):104–112, 1998.

Karahalios DG, Apostolides PJ, Sonntag VKH: Technique of pedicle screw fixation of the lumbosacral spine. Operative Techniques in Neurosurgery 1(3):134–141, 1998.

Naderi S, Detwiler D, Sonntag VKH: Degenerative spondylolisthesis: When to fuse? Crit Rev Neurosurgery 8:217–220, 1998.

Sawin PD, Sonntag VKH: Techniques of posterior subaxial cervical fusion. Operative Techniques in Neurosurgery 1(2):72–83, 1998.

Sonntag VKH (guest editor): Introduction. Operative techniques of the cervical spine. Operative Techniques in Neurosurgery 1(2):57, 1998.

Sonntag VKH (guest editor): Introduction. Operative techniques of the thoracolumbar spine. Operative Techniques in Neurosurgery 1(3): 103, 1998.

Vishteh AG, Apostolides PJ, Karahalios DG, Sonntag VKH: Technique of anterolateral thoracolumbar plating. Operative Techniques in Neurosurgery 1(3):126–133, 1998.

Vishteh AG, Baskin JJ, Sonntag VKH: Techniques of cervical discectomy with and without fusion. Operative Techniques in Neurosurgery 1(2):84–89, 1998.

Vishteh AG, Sonntag VKH, Apostolides PJ, Dickman CA: Anterolateral thoracic and lumbar screw plate fixation. Neuro-Orthopedics 23:29–44, 1998.

Baskin JJ, Vishteh AG, Theodore N, Sonntag VKH: Posterior cervical screw arthrodesis. Crit Rev Neurosurg (7) 2:89–98, 1997.

Dickman CA, Sonntag VKH, Russell J: The laparoscopic approach for instrumentation and fusion of the lumbar spine. BNI Quarterly 12(3):26–36, 1997.

Karahalios D, Apostolides P, Sonntag VKH: Degenerative lumbar spinal instability: Technical aspects of operative treatment. Clin Neurosurg 44:109–135, 1997.

Konstantinou D, Levi A, Sonntag VKH, Dickman CA: Odontoid screw fixation: BNI Quarterly 3(2): 14–19, 1997.

Sonntag VKH, Naderi S: The current role of CT myelography and myelography in neurosurgical practice. Crit Rev Neurosurg 7(1):24–28, 1997.

Apostolides PJ, Vishteh AG, Dickman CA, Koopot R, Sonntag VKH: Anterior surgical approaches to the cervicothoracic spine. Techniques in Neurosurgery 1(4):230–239, 1996.

Karahalios DG, Apostolides PJ, Sonntag VKH: Stabilization and fusion techniques for atlantoaxial instability. Crit Rev Neurosurg 6:13–19, 1996.

Pappas CTE, Sonntag VKH: Surgical management of the thoracic herniated disc. Techniques in Neurosurgery 1(4):257–260, 1996.

Ronderos JF, Sonntag VKH: Approaches to the thoracic spine. Techniques in Neurosurgery 1(4):222–229, 1996.

Sonntag VKH: Illustrative case. Techniques in Neurosurgery 1(4):218–221, 1996.

Vardiman AB, Sonntag VKH, Dickman CA: Thoracic spine instrumentation Techniques in Neurosurgery 1(4):240–256, 1996.

Westmark R, Sonntag VKH: Complications of thoracic spine surgery. Techniques in Neurosurgery 1(4):290–295, 1996.

Dickman CA, Ronderos JF, Sonntag VKH: Stabilization of the craniovertebral junction in rheumatoid arthritis. Part I: Pathophysiology, diagnosis, and surgical criteria. Contemp Neurosurg 17(11):1–6, 1995.

Dickman CA, Ronderos JF, Sonntag VKH: Stabilization junction in rheumatoid arthritis. Part II: Surgical techniques. Contemp Neurosurg 17(12):1–6, 1995.

Flores A, Sonntag VKH, Dickman CA: Idiopathic spinal epidural lipomatosis: Report of two cases and review of the literature. BNI Quarterly 11(3):22–25, 1995.

Marciano FF, Greene KA, Apostolides PH, Dickman CA, Sonntag VKH: Pharmacologic management of spinal cord injury: A review of the literature. BNI Quarterly 11(2):2–11, 1995.

Paramore CG, Sonntag VKH: Advances in spinal instrumentation. Jpn J Neurosurg 4(2):111–120, 1995.

Greene KA, Marciano FF, Sonntag VKH: Pharmacological strategies in the treatment of spinal cord injuries: A critical review. Crit Rev Neurosurg 4:254–264, 1994.

Pappas CTE, Sonntag VKH: Lumbar stenosis in the elderly. Neurosurgery Quarterly 4(2):102–112, 1994.

Sonntag VKH, Dickman CA: Craniocervical stabilization. Clin Neurosurg 40:243–272, 1994.

Sonntag VKH, Herman JM, Spetzler RF: Intramedullary tumors in adults: Recent surgical experience with 54 patients. Spinal Surgery 8:152–159, 1994.

Dickman CA, Crawford NR, Brantley AGU, Sonntag VKH, Koeneman JR: In vitro cervical spine biomechanical testing. BNI Quarterly 9(4):17–26, 1993.

Dickman CA, Sonntag VKH: Wire fixation for the cervical spine: Biomechanical principles and surgical techniques. BNI Quarterly 9(4): 2–16, 1993.

Dickman CA, Sonntag VKH, Marcotte PJ: Techniques of screw fixation of the cervical spine. BNI Quarterly 9(4):27–39, 1993.

Hadley MN, Sonntag VKH: Cervical disc herniations: The anterior approach to symptomatic interspace pathology. Neurosurg Clin North Am 1(4):45–52, 1993.

Dickman CA, Douglas RA, Sonntag VKH: Occipitocervical fusion: Posterior stabilization of the craniovertebral junction and upper cervical spine. BNI Quarterly 6(2):2–14, 1992.

Dickman CA, Sonntag VKH, Marcotte PJ: Techniques of screw fixation of the cervical spine. BNI Quarterly 8(2):9–26, 1992.

Sonntag VKH: Early surgery urged for at-risk craniocervical junction patients. Neuroscience Forum 2(2):10–13, 1992.

Sonntag VKH, Herman JM: Reoperation of the cervical spine for degenerative disease and tumor. Clin Neurosurg 39:244–269, 1992.

Sonntag VKH, Douglas RA: Management of cervical spinal cord trauma. Neurosurgical Quarterly 9(Suppl 1):S385–S396, 1992.

Baldwin HZ, Rekate HL, Sonntag VKH: Diagnosis, surgical management, and outcome of the adult tethered cord syndrome. BNI Quarterly 7(4):16–22, 1991.

Cherny WB, Sonntag VKH, Douglas RA: Lateral mass posterior plating and facet fusion for cervical spine instability. BNI Quarterly 7(2): 2–11, 1991.

Sonntag VKH, Kalfas I: Innovative cervical fusion and instrumentation techniques. Clin Neurosurg 37:636–660, 1991.

Spetzler RF, Dickman CA, Sonntag VKH: The transoral approach to the anterior cervical spine. Contemp Neurosurg 13(9):1–6, 1991.

Douglas RA, Baldwin HZ, Johnson PC, Sonntag VKH, Spetzler RF: Recurrent spinal angioblastic meningioma of the hemangiopericytic type: A case report. BNI Quarterly 6(4):13–20, 1990.

Hadley MN, Branch CL, Geisler FH, Sonntag VKH: Expert exchange: Management of cervical spine instability. Perspectives in Neurological Surgery 1:45–75, 1990.

Papadopoulos SM, Sonntag VKH: Caspar plate instrumentation. Perspectives in Neurological Surgery 1(1):87–92, 1990.

Sonntag VKH, Douglas RA: Management of spinal cord trauma. Neurosurg Clin North Am 1(3):729–750, 1990.

Sonntag VKH, Hadley MN: Surgical approaches to the thoracolumbar spine. Clin Neurosurg 36:168–185, 1990.

Dickman CA, Harrington TR, Sonntag VKH, Drayer BP, Bird CR: Magnetic resonance imaging in the diagnosis of disk space infection. BNI Quarterly 5(2):14–18, 1989.

Hadley MN, Browner CM, Dickman CA, Sonntag VKH: Compression fractures of the thoracolumbar junction: A treatment algorithm based on 110 cases. BNI Quarterly 5(3):10–19, 1989.

Hadley MN, Sonntag VKH, Rekate H: Pediatric vertebral column and spinal cord injuries. Contemp Neurosurg 10(13):1–6, 1988.

Pappas CTE, Rigamonti D, Sonntag VKH, White WL, Carter LP: Herniated thoracic discs. BNI Quarterly 4(1):7–11, 1988.

Rigamonti D, Sonntag VKH, Shetter AG, Spetzler RF: Trigeminal schwannomas. BNI Quarterly 4(3):9–14, 1988.

Sonntag VKH, Hadley MN: Nonoperative management of cervical spine injuries. Clin Neurosurg 34:630–649, 1988.

Hadley MN, Sonntag VKH: Acute axis fractures. Contemp Neurosurg 9(2):1–6, 1987.

Sonntag VKH: Neuroscientists on stamps. BNI Quarterly 3(3):29–34, 1987.

Zabramski JM, Hadley MN, Browner CM, Rekate H, Sonntag VKH: Pediatric spinal cord and vertebral column injuries. BNI Quarterly 2(2):11–17, 1986.

Bloomfield SM, Sonntag VKH, Spetzler RF: Pineal region lesions. BNI Quarterly 1(3):10–23, 1985.

Hadley MN, Browner C, Sonntag VKH: Miscellaneous fractures of the second cervical vertebra. BNI Quarterly 1(4):34–39, 1985.

Masferrer R, Hadley M, Bloomfield SM, Spetzler RF, Sonntag VKH: Transoral microsurgery resection of the odontoid process. BNI Quarterly 1(3):34–40, 1985.

Nehls DG, Spetzler RF, Shetter AG, Sonntag VKH: Application of new technology in the treatment of cerebellopontine angle tumors. Clin Neurosurg 32:223–241, 1985.

Sonntag VKH: History of spinal cord surgery. BNI Quarterly 1(3):41–47, 1985.

BOOKS EDITED

Sonntag VKH, Vollmer F: Spine. In Winn HR (Editor-in-Chief), Sonntag VKH (section ed): Youman's Neurological Surgery, 5th ed, Philadelphia, W. B. Saunders, in press.

Dickman CA, Spetzler RF, Sonntag VKH (eds): Surgery of the Craniovertebral Junction. New York: Thieme, 1998.

Menezes AH, Sonntag VKH (eds), Benzel EC, McCormick P, Papadopoulos SM (section eds): Principles of Spinal Surgery. New York: McGraw-Hill, 1996.

Weinstein JN, Rydevik BL, Sonntag VKH (eds): Essentials of the Spine. New York: Raven Press, 1995.

Sonntag VKH: The high pressure of several substituted naphthalenes over copper-chromium oxide and raney nickel catalyst (thesis). Tempe, Arizona State University, 1967.

CHAPTERS

Total Book Chapters (75)

IN PRESS (40)

Baskin JJ, Dickman CA, Sonntag VKH: Occipitocervical fusion. In Winn HR (ed): Youmans Neurological Surgery, 5th ed, Philadelphia: W. B. Saunders.

Baskin JJ, Vishteh AG, Dickman CA, Sonntag VKH: Anterior cervical instrumentation. In Winn HR (ed): Youmans Neurological Surgery, 5th ed, Philadelphia: W. B. Saunders.

Bartolomei J, Lynch J, Spetzler RF, Sonntag VKH: Thoracic stabilization: Anterior, lateral, and posterior. In Aminoff MJ, Daroff RB (eds): Encyclopedia of Neurological Sciences, San Diego, CA: Academic Press.

Bartolomei J, Lynch J, Spetzler RF, Sonntag VKH: Conus medullaris syndrome. In Aminoff MJ, Daroff RB (eds): Encyclopedia of Neurological Sciences, San Diego, CA: Academic Press.

Bartolomei J, Sonntag VKH: Anterior approach including cervical corpectomy (degenerative). In Winn HR (ed): Youmans Neurological Surgery, 5th ed, Philadelphia: W. B. Saunders.

Bartolomei J, Spetzler RF, Sonntag VKH: Brain herniation and surgical management. In Aminoff MJ, Daroff RB (eds): Encyclopedia of Neurological Sciences, San Diego, CA: Academic Press.

Detwiler PW, Porter RW, Sonntag VKH: Lumbar spinal stenosis: Part A. Laminectomy without fusion. In Zdeblick TA, Anderson P, Stillerman C, Benzel ED (eds): Controversies in Spine Surgery. St. Louis: Quality Medical.

Elder W, Sonntag VKH: Cervical spine stabilization. In Aminoff MJ, Daroff RB (eds): Encyclopedia of Neurological Sciences, San Diego, CA: Academic Press.

Feiz-Efran I, Javedan S, Sonntag VKH: Lumbar radiculopathy. In Aminoff MJ, Daroff RB (eds): Encyclopedia of Neurological Sciences, San Diego, CA: Academic Press.

Gerber M, Sonntag VKH: Lumbar stenosis. In Aminoff MJ, Daroff RB (eds): Encyclopedia of Neurological Sciences, San Diego, CA: Academic Press.

Gerber M, Sonntag VKH: Trauma (overview). In Aminoff MJ, Daroff RB (eds): Encyclopedia of Neurological Sciences, San Diego, CA: Academic Press.

Gerber M, Sonntag VKH: Neurogenic claudication and cauda equina syndrome. In Aminoff MJ, Daroff RB (eds): Encyclopedia of Neurological Sciences, San Diego, CA: Academic Press.

Gerber M, Vishteh AG, Baskin JJ, Dickman CA, Sonntag VKH: Fractures of the axis. In Batjer, Loftus, Ondra (eds): Textbook of Neurological Surgery, New York: Lippincott Williams & Wilkins.

Guest JD, Sonntag VKH: Biological strategies of CNS repair. In Winn HR (ed): Youmans Neurological Surgery, 5th ed, Philadelphia: W. B. Saunders.

Henn JS, Elder WJ, Lemole GM Jr, Sonntag VKH: Techniques and indications for bone graft harvest. In Papadopoulos SM and Cervical Spine Study Group (eds): Manual of Cervical Spine Internal Fixation, Ann Arbor, MI.

Henn JS, Henn DM, Sonntag VKH: Laminectomy. In Aminoff MJ, Daroff RB (eds): Encyclopedia of Neurological Sciences, San Diego, CA: Academic Press.

Henn JS, Lemole GM Jr, Apostolides PJ, Sonntag VKH: Occipitocervical fusion with a threaded rod and braided cables. In Papadopoulos SM and Cervical Spine Study Group (eds): Manual of Cervical Spine Internal Fixation, Ann Arbor, MI.

Henn JS, Lemole GM Jr, Sonntag VKH: Laminoplasty. In Aminoff MJ, Daroff RB (eds): Encyclopedia of Neurological Sciences, San Diego, CA: Academic Press.

Nottmeier EW, Ames C, Sonntag VKH: Spinal cord tumors, treatment of. In Aminoff MJ, Daroff RB (eds): Encyclopedia of Neurological Sciences, San Diego, CA: Academic Press.

Nottmeier EW, Ames C, Sonntag VKH: Spondylosis. In Aminoff MJ,

Daroff RB (eds): Encyclopedia of Neurological Sciences, San Diego, CA: Academic Press.

Paramore C, Theodore N, Sonntag VKH: Upper cervical and craniocervical decompression. In Benzel E (ed): Spine Surgery: Techniques, Complication Avoidance and Management. Philadelphia: W. B. Saunders.

Paramore C, Theodore N, Sonntag VKH: Cervical spondylosis with minimal myelopathy: To decompress or not to decompress. Spine Surgery: Techniques, Complication Avoidance and Management. Philadelphia: W. B. Saunders.

Ponce FA, Han PP, Sonntag VKH: Cervical radiculopathy. In Aminoff MJ, Daroff RB (eds): Encyclopedia of Neurological Sciences, San Diego, CA: Academic Press.

Sonntag VKH: Cervical laminectomy. Section: Syringomyelia. In Kempe's Operative Neurosurgery, 2nd ed. Philadelphia: Current Medicine.

Sonntag VKH: Cervical laminectomy. Section: Trauma. In Kempe's Operative Neurosurgery, 2nd ed. Philadelphia: Current Medicine.

Sonntag VKH: Cervical radiculoneuropathy: Section: Posterior approach—keyhole. In Kempe's Operative Neurosurgery, 2nd ed. Philadelphia: Current Medicine.

Sonntag VKH: Anterior cervical discectomy and fusion-cervical radiculoneuropathy. In Kempe's Operative Neurosurgery, 2nd ed. Philadelphia: Current Medicine.

Sonntag VKH: Cervical radiculopathy. Section: Anterior cervical plating. In Kempe's Operative Neurosurgery, 2nd ed. Philadelphia: Current Medicine.

Sonntag VKH: Lumbar stenosis. In Kempe's Operative Neurosurgery, 2nd ed. Philadelphia: Current Medicine.

Sonntag VKH: Spondylolisthesis. In Kempe's Operative Neurosurgery, 2nd ed. Philadelphia: Current Medicine.

Sonntag VKH: Retroperitoneal approach. In Kempe's Operative Neurosurgery, 2nd ed. Philadelphia: Current Medicine.

Sonntag VKH: Intramedullary spinal cord tumor. Ependymoma. In Kempe's Operative Neurosurgery, 2nd ed. Philadelphia: Current Medicine.

Sonntag VKH: Intradural extramedullary tumor. Thoracic meningiomas. In Kempe's Operative Neurosurgery, 2nd ed. Philadelphia: Current Medicine.

Sonntag VKH: Cauda equina conus medullaris. Ependymoma. In Kempe's Operative Neurosurgery, 2nd ed. Philadelphia: Current Medicine.

Sonntag VKH: Cervical laminectomy. Section: Posterior cervical fusion technique. Lateral mass. In Kempe's Operative Neurosurgery, 2nd ed. Philadelphia: Current Medicine.

Sonntag VKH: Lumbar radiculopathy. Section: Herniated intervertebral disc. Microdiscectomy. In Kempe's Operative Neurosurgery, 2nd ed. Philadelphia: Current Medicine.

Sonntag VKH: Cervical cordotomy. In Kempe's Operative Neurosurgery, 2nd ed. Philadelphia: Current Medicine.

Sonntag VKH: Intra- and extradural tumor. Dumbbell schwannoma. In Kempe's Operative Neurosurgery, 2nd ed. Philadelphia: Current Medicine.

Theodore N, Sonntag VKH: Spinal cord injury without radiographic abnormality. In Aminoff MJ, Daroff RB (eds): Encyclopedia of Neurological Sciences, San Diego, CA: Academic Press.

Zubay G, Dickman CA, Sonntag VKH: Basic principles of spinal internal fixation. In Winn HR (ed): Youmans Neurological Surgery, 5th ed, Philadelphia: W. B. Saunders.

PUBLISHED (35)

Lemole GM Jr, Bartolomei J, Henn JS, Sonntag VKH: Thoracic fractures. In Vaccaro A (ed): Fractures of the Cervical, Thoracic, and Lumbar Spine. New York: Marcel Dekker, 2002, pp 405–437.

Porter RW, Sonntag VKH: Primary spinal cord disorders. In Fardon D, Garfin S (eds): Orthopaedic Knowledge Update—Spine 2, Rosemont, IL: American Academy of Orthopaedic Surgeons, 2001, pp 401–410.

Apostolides PJ, Vishteh AG, Sonntag VKH: The technique of transoral odontoidectomy. In Mayer HM (ed): Minimally Invasive Spine Surgery (A Surgical Manual). Berlin-Heidelberg: Springer-Verlag, 2000, pp 11–16.

Baskin JJ, Sawin PD, Dickman CA, Sonntag VKH: Surgical techniques for stabilization of the subaxial cervical spine. In Schmidek H (ed): Operative Neurosurgical Techniques, 4th ed. Philadelphia: W.B. Saunders, 2000, pp 2075–2104.

Detwiler PW, Porter RW, Han PP, Karahalios D, Masferrer R, Sonntag VKH: Surgical treatment of lumbar spondylolisthesis. In Cohadon et al. (eds): Advances and Technical Standards in Neurosurgery. New York: Springer-Verlag, 2000, pp 331–346.

Guest JD, Sonntag VKH: Patient selection and timing of surgical intervention. In Benzel EC, Tator CH (eds): Contemporary Management of Spinal Cord Injury: From Impact to Rehabilitation. Park Ridge, IL: American Association of Neurological Surgeons, 2000, pp 1–14.

Theodore N, Sonntag VKH: Spinal surgery from the Eisenhower years to the third millennium. In Barrow DL, Kondziolka D, Laws E, Traynelis V (eds): Fifty Years of Neurosurgery: The Golden Anniversary of the Congress of Neurological Surgeons. Baltimore: Lippincott Williams & Wilkins, 2000, pp 277–291.

Theodore N, Sonntag VKH: Spinal instrumentation as implanted neural prosthesis. In Maciunas RJ (ed): Neural Prosthesis. Park Ridge, IL: American Association of Neurological Surgeons, 2000, pp 1–7.

Baskin JJ, Greene KA, Vishteh AG, Sonntag VKH: Operative treatment of unstable hangman's fractures. In Zdeblick T, Benzel E, Anderson PA, Stillerman CB (eds): Controversies in Spine Surgery. Surgical Treatment and Medical Management. St. Louis: Quality Medical, 1999, pp 71–83.

Crawford N, Dickman C, Sonntag VKH: Principles of spinal biomechanics. In Crockard A, Haywood R, Hoff J (eds): Neurosurgery. The Scientific Basis of Clinical Practice. Oxford: Blackwell Science Ltd, 1999, pp 1073–1092.

Levi ADO, Sonntag VKH: Neurosurgical procedures in spine trauma. In Capen D, Haye W (eds): Comprehensive Management of Spine Trauma. St. Louis: C.V. Mosby, 1998, pp 331–344.

Sonntag VKH: Standard specification for cranial traction tongs and halo external spinal immobilization devices. Annual Book of ASTM Standards Section 13 Volume 13.01. West Conshohocken, PA: ASTM International, 1998, pp 1268–1277.

Hurlbert RJ, Sonntag VKH: Anterior cervical spine stabilization with the Codman Locking Plate System. In Rengachary SS, Wilkins RH (eds): Neurosurgical Operative Color Atlas. Park Ridge, IL: American Association of Neurological Surgery, 1997, pp 157–165.

Vishteh AG, Baskin JJ, Shen AC, Sonntag VKH: Decompression and stabilization of spinal metastases. In Maciunas RJ (ed): Advanced Techniques in Central Nervous System Metastases. Park Ridge, IL: American Association of Neurological Surgery, 1997, pp 233–243.

Ronderos JF, Dickman CA, Sonntag VKH: Posterior instrumentation of the cervical spine. In Youmans J (ed): Neurological Surgery, 4th ed, Volume 3, Trauma. Benign Spine Lesions. Philadelphia: W.B. Saunders, 1995, pp 2297–2314.

Sonntag VKH, Dickman CA: Occipitocervical and high cervical fusion. In Wilkins RH, Rengachary SS (eds): Neurosurgery, 2nd ed. New York: McGraw-Hill, 1995, pp 327–337.

Sonntag VKH, Dickman CA: Occipitocervical instrumentation. In Hitchon PW, Traynelis VC, Rengachary S (eds): Techniques in Spinal Fusion and Stabilization. New York: Thieme, 1994, pp 107–116.

Sonntag VKH, Francis PM: Patient selection and timing of surgery. In Benzel EC, Tator CH (eds): Contemporary Management of Spinal Cord Injury. Park Ridge, IL: American Association of Neurological Surgery, 1994, pp 97–108.

Sonntag VKH, Marcotte P: Deformity correction and maintenance of alignment. In Benzel EC (ed): Spinal Instrumentation. Park Ridge, IL: American Association of Neurological Surgery, 1994, pp 211–223.

Dickman CA, Sonntag VKH: Surgical techniques for the stabilization of the cervical spine. In Schmidek HH, Sweet WH (eds): Operative Neurosurgical Techniques, 3rd ed. Philadelphia: W.B. Saunders, 1993, pp 1849–1874.

Dickman CA, Sonntag VKH: The intensive care management of spinal cord injury. In Andrews BT (ed): Neurosurgical Intensive Care. New York: McGraw-Hill, 1993, pp 243–249.

Sonntag VKH, Dickman CA: Cervical spine fusion. In Salcman M (ed): Annual of Neurosurgery. Philadelphia: Current Medicine, 1993, pp 13.1–13.20.

Sonntag VKH, Dickman CA: Operative management of occipitocervical and atlantoaxial instability. In Holtzman RN, McCormick PC, Farcy JPC (eds): Contemporary Perspectives in Neurosurgery. Spinal Instability. New York: Springer-Verlag, 1993, pp 255–294.

Sonntag VKH, Dickman CA: Treatment of upper cervical spine injuries. In Rhea GL (ed): Spinal Trauma: Current Evaluation and Management. Park Ridge, IL: American Association of Neurological Surgery, 1993, pp 25–74.

Sonntag VKH, Francis P: Controversies in spinal cord syndromes. In Garfin SR, Northrup B (eds): Surgery for Spinal Cord Injuries. New York: Raven Press, 1993, pp 15–31.

Sonntag VKH, Marcotte PJ: Neurogenic claudication. In Carter LP, Spetzler RF (eds): Neurovascular Surgery. New York: McGraw-Hill, 1993, pp 1241–1250.

Sonntag VKH, Dickman CA: Pediatric spinal cord injury. In Piepmeier JM (ed): The Outcome Following Traumatic Spinal Cord Injury. Mount Kisco, New York: Futura, 1992, pp 139–171.

Sonntag VKH, Hadley MN: Management of cervical spine facet fracture-dislocations. In Camins MB, O'Leary PF (eds): Disorders of the Cervical Spine. Baltimore: Williams & Wilkins, 1992, pp 459–464.

Sonntag VKH, Herman JM: Spinal neoplasms. In Little JR, Awad IA (eds): Reoperative Neurosurgery. Baltimore: Williams & Wilkins, 1992, pp 129–154.

Sonntag VKH, Marciano FF: Spinal cord trauma: Better prognoses with new pharmacological procedures? In Peter K, Lawin P, Bern T (eds): Intensivmedizin 1992. 13. Internationales Symposium Uber Aktuelle Probleme der Not Fallmedizin Und Intensivtherapie, Munchen. Stuttgart, Thieme-Verlag, 1992, pp 166–170.

Sonntag VKH, Hadley MN: Management of upper cervical spine instability. In Wilkins RH, Rengachary SS (eds): Neurosurgery Update II. New York: McGraw-Hill, 1991, pp 222–233.

Sonntag VKH, Hadley MN: Traumatic upper cervical spinal instability. In Cooper PR (ed) Management of Posttraumatic Spinal Instability. Park Ridge, IL: American Association of Neurological Surgeons, 1991, pp 222–223.

Sonntag VKH, Hadley MN: Management of nonodontoid upper cervical spine injuries. In Cooper P (ed): Management of Posttraumatic Spinal Instability. Park Ridge, IL: American Association of Neurological Surgery, 1990, pp 99–110.

Sonntag VKH, Hadley MN, Spetzler RF: The transoral-transclival approach to the upper cervical spine. In Sundaresan SN, Schmidek HH, Schiller AL, Rosenthal DI (eds): Tumors of the Spine: Diagnosis and Clinical Management. Philadelphia: W.B. Saunders, 1990, pp 319–328.

Sonntag VKH, Hadley MN: Treatment of thoracolumbar spine injuries. In Pitts LH, Wagner F (eds): Craniospinal Trauma. New York: Thieme, 1989, pp 186–196.

Contents

CHAPTER

1

2002 Congress of Neurological Surgeons Presidential Address

STEPHEN M. PAPADOPOULOS, M.D.

One year ago, I stood before you on this stage and was handed the gavel by Dr. Issam Awad. Being elected as the President of the Congress of Neurological Surgeons has been an extraordinary honor. The year has been filled with a number of challenges, and I hope that I have led this organization, on behalf of our membership, to a higher pursuit of its goals and mission.

One of my most difficult challenges has been the task of writing this Presidential Address. In fact, one of my first thoughts as I learned of my nomination was "Oh, my God, I have to give a Presidential Address!" I have learned to be in my comfort zone, giving talks about neurosurgical techniques, spinal surgery, image-guided surgery . . . all seemingly "natural."

I have been fortunate to have the phenomenal support of a very talented and committed group of neurosurgeons on the CNS Executive Committee in addition to a host of others, volunteering their time, effort, intellect, and energy throughout the year.

Most importantly, I have a family—Penny, my wife, and three boys, Michael, Matthew, and Marcus—that bring light into my life and have supported me in all of my endeavors.

I remember a number of years ago, as a young member of the CNS Executive Committee, reviewing a then-updated version of the CNS Mission Statement. We struggled to capture the essence of the mission of our organization and our profession.

I had planned to read the text of that mission statement to you, but following the advice of my oratory critics, Penny and Michael, who thought it would be far to dry for the beginning of an address; I have put it up on the screen (*Fig. 1.1*).

> The Congress of Neurological Surgeons exists for the purpose of promoting the public welfare through the advancement of neurosurgery, by a commitment to **excellence in education**, and by dedication to research and scientific knowledge. The Congress of

Congress of Neurological Surgeons
"Mission Statement"

"The Congress of Neurological Surgeons exists for the purpose of promoting the public welfare through the advancement of neurosurgery, by a commitment to **excellence in education**, and by dedication to research and scientific knowledge. The Congress of Neurological Surgeons maintains the vitality of our learned profession through the **altruistic volunteer efforts** of its members and the development of **leadership in service** to the public, to our colleagues in other disciplines, and to the special needs of our fellow neurosurgeons throughout the world and at every stage of their professional lives."

FIG. 1.1 The Congress of Neurological Surgeons Mission Statement.

> Neurological Surgeons maintains the vitality of our learned profession through the **altruistic volunteer efforts** of its members and the development of **leadership in service** to the public, to our colleagues in other disciplines, and to the special needs of our fellow neurosurgeons throughout the world and at every stage of their professional lives.

Some important themes permeate this statement: excellence in education, altruistic volunteer efforts, and leadership in service.

The neurosurgical specialty represents a small group of individuals. Our unique drive, work ethic, and goal orientation are evident at even a young age. Our specialty is vibrant and intellectually complex. We are inherently competitive, yet compassion is at the soul of our nature. Of the 210 million adults in the United States, a bit over 180 million have completed high school, 50 million have completed college, 800,000 have completed medical school, and only 4,300 practice the specialty of neurosurgery. We represent about 1 out of 50,000 adults in the United States. We are an elite group. We are the "chosen" in a sense. We all have God-given talents and abilities that not all people enjoy. We have been given the intellectual and technical tools necessary to be neurosurgeons, to be part of the "Queen of Surgical Specialties."

We have each, however, chosen and pursued this profession by free will. We have freely chosen to work hard, to hone our skills, to continually educate ourselves, to provide our patients with the highest possible level of care that our abilities allow.

We are leaders.

We chose to be leaders (*Fig. 1.2*).

Harold Greneen wrote of leadership: "Leadership cannot really be taught, it can only be learned."

John Kotter said: "Leaders establish the vision for the future and set the strategy for getting there."

And Martin Luther King, Jr.: "A genuine leader is not a searcher of consensus, but a molder of consensus."

We must be prepared for the call to leadership when it is sought for and achieved and when it is merely thrust upon us. This never became so clear to me as it was a year ago, when I became President of the Congress of Neurological Surgeons. Suddenly, the weight of leadership was upon my shoulders; some said this was a position I sought to achieve; yet leadership brings unexpected challenges and equally unexpected rewards.

President George W. Bush sought leadership. He strategized to achieve it, and he fought for it, relentlessly. The perhaps unanticipated "call" occurred on September 11, 2001. A new, unexpected, unrehearsed, unprecedented level of leadership was called for. Our president has embraced the call, demonstrating a quality of leadership many doubted he fully possessed. Even the president's fiercest critics have voiced support and admiration for his skills, tenacity, and commitment. Perhaps President Bush's greatest ability is his ability to recognize talented leaders, empower them, and surround himself with them.

In 1993, a small group of opportunistic lawyers specializing in product liability litigation led an organized effort against medical device

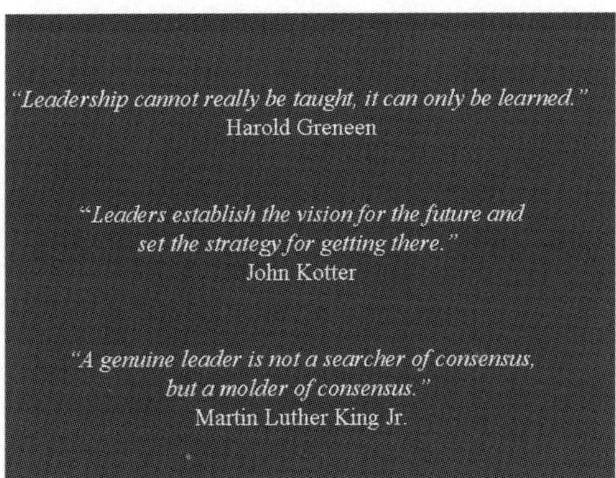

FIG. 1.2 Leadership.

manufacturers, the U. S. Food and Drug Administration, the CNS, other medical organizations, and even individual surgeons in the now-famous pedicle screw lawsuits. Organized neurosurgery spent over 1 million dollars in defense of these suits. Corporations spent several hundred million dollars. Ron Pickard, then CEO of Sofamor Danek, was called to a new kind of leadership unfamiliar to a businessman with a phenomenal record of success in the corporate world. Mr. Pickard organized an industry consortium to fight the accusations brought forth by the litigants. In 1996, he wrote a letter to orthopedic and neurosurgeons: "We will not be intimidated and will not be coerced. We hope you will join with us as we continue to fight against extortion and for the advance of medical science and the care of patients." Mr. Pickard was a tenacious leader of the fight, refusing to give in, almost losing his own company, crushed by the weight of escalating defense costs in the process. The rest is history. The CNS, many individual surgeons, and more importantly, our patients owe a great deal to the leadership of this individual, found in the seemingly unlikely ranks of corporate America. Mr. Pickard was also receptive to the call, prepared, and he, too, instinctively embraced it without hesitation.

Clergy describe the call as exactly that: a call, a divine directive. Michael Lindvall, the pastor of Brick Presbyterian Church in New York City described it to me like this: "The call is that intersection at which one's God-given talents and abilities meet the needs of society." In fact, he goes on to say that a central tenant of Judeo-Christian theology is the assertion of moral obligation for each of us to use our given talents to the good of mankind.

The call to leadership has been, and should always be, answered by each and every one of us. We must look beyond the traditional roles of leadership. We all must be receptive, prepared, and instinctively embrace it without hesitation.

We are altruistic volunteers.

We chose this role also.

Even the most elite are called to service (*Fig. 1.3*).

Shirley Chisholm wrote: "Service is the rent that you pay for room on this earth."

Albert Einstein: "There is no greater satisfaction for a just and well-meaning person than the knowledge that he has devoted his best energies to the service of a good cause."

And again from Martin Luther King, Jr.: "That's your definition of greatness . . . It means that everybody can be great. Because everybody can serve. You don't have to have a college degree to serve. You don't have to make your subject and your verb agree to serve . . . You

"Service is the rent that you pay for room on this earth."
Shirley Chisholm

"There is no greater satisfaction for a just and well meaning person then the knowledge that he has devoted his best energies to the service of a good cause."
Albert Einstein

"That's your definition of greatness.....It means that everybody can be great. Because everybody can serve. You don't have to have a college degree to serve. You don't have to make your subject and your verb agree to serve....You don't have to know the second theory of thermodynamics in Physics to serve. You only need a heart full of grace. A soul generated by love. And you can be that servant."
Martin Luther King Jr.

FIG. 1.3 Service.

don't have to know the second theory of thermodynamics in physics to serve. You only need a heart full of grace. A soul generated by love. And you can be that servant."

As President of the United States, Jimmy Carter was deeply committed to social justice and basic human rights. In addition to promoting peace and human rights through the nonprofit Carter Center in Atlanta, he and his wife, Rosalyn, have led the Jimmy Carter Work Project for Habitat for Humanity International for 1 week each year. Their involvement with Habitat for Humanity began when the former president led a work group to New York City to help renovate a six-story building with 19 families in need of decent, affordable shelter. That experience planted the seed, and the Jimmy Carter Work Project has been an internationally recognized event ever since. Habitat for Humanity will build 1,000 houses in 18 countries.

President Carter deftly evades recognition for his tireless service. "We have become small players in an exciting global effort to alleviate the curse of homelessness," Carter said. "With our many new friends, we have worked to raise funds, to publicize the good work of Habitat, to recruit other volunteers, to visit overseas projects and even build a few houses."

Albert Schweitzer was a brilliant theologian and musician, but it was his service as a medical missionary that brought Schweitzer's name and his values to the attention of the entire world. After receiving his medical degree from the University of Strasbourg, he established a hospital in Lambarene Gabon, an impoverished republic in Africa. Winner of the 1952 Nobel Peace Prize for his efforts to create a "brotherhood of nations," he contributed the prize money to building a village for lepers.

Service is at the soul of the Hippocratic oath and an obligation for all of us blessed and entrusted with the ability to care for others.

We are educators.

We are teachers and mentors.

We are role models.

Since the days of Hippocrates, physicians have been teachers and mentors. Education is central to our discipline, amongst ourselves, our children, our patients.

Some of us choose to teach in formal settings, such as in universities, medical schools, and residency training programs.

Karin Murasko, Chief of Pediatric Neurosurgery at the University of Michigan, has dedicated her life to teaching. She has trained scores of young neurosurgical residents in the art and science of pediatric neurosurgery. Each year, she also leads a medical team, including those same neurosurgical residents, on an annual trip to Guatemala, fittingly dubbed "Project Shunt." Over the years, she and her team have treated hundreds of children with hydrocephalus and spinal dysraphism who otherwise have no access to modern medical care. Yes, Karin is a teacher in the classical sense, but she is also a mentor, a mentor of character, a mentor of compassion, and a mentor of giving of one's self.

Some of us choose to be mentors in church, on the soccer fields, in scouting, and a variety of settings and places.

It is central to our profession. It is our obligation.

Our foremost obligation, however, may be the education of ourselves. We, more than any others, must be open to the opportunities of learning. We must embrace new knowledge. We must embrace innovation.

I recently read a sermon by Michael Lindvall entitled "Believing Is Seeing." He describes a cartoon that appeared in *The New Yorker* a few months ago: "It pictured a line of church-goers being greeted by the minister as they file out the front door after Sunday services. One of them, hat in hand, is shaking hands with the pastor. The caption has him saying to the minister: 'So I'll have to believe it to see it?' " The cartoonist, of course, refers to what many call the spiritual road of faith; one must first make the "leap of faith"—the believing—to begin the walk down the road and discover its bounty—the seeing. The experience is hidden from those who will not risk the spiritual road. The road itself is the teacher, and if you never take it, there is, of course, nothing to be seen.

This is true for so many "risks" in life. Parenting, education, career choice, one's first neurosurgical operative procedure, all require an initial a "leap of faith" to ultimately "see."

Technology, for instance, for many of us is mysterious. The advent of the CT scanner revolutionized neurosurgery forever, and it has been a nonstop whirlwind of advancing technology, creativity, and innovation. We have anatomic and physiologic "glimpses" into the nervous system like we have never had before—and it seems to change every day. Surely, millions of lives have been impacted, and the future impact is beyond the dreams of even the most visionary.

The use of computers in the operating room has ushered in the era of image-guided surgery. Intraoperative imaging is an emerging field, sure to evolve into the mainstream. Robotics already has entered the operating rooms of our colleagues and clearly will hold an important future in neurosurgery.

We must always continue on the road of lifelong education.

Joe Maroon, in his 1986 CNS Presidential Address (1), spoke about the importance of spiritual balance in a neurosurgeon's life. He recounts a book entitled *I Dare You,* by William Danforth, which implores the reader to create a square diagram, with each arm of the square proportional to one's personal commitment in four major areas: professional, family/social, spiritual, and physical. Dr. Maroon further describes the typical neurosurgeon's square, with an imbalanced emphasis on the professional arm of the square and a resulting shortening of the other three. Through an eloquent dialog, Dr. Maroon concludes that a triangle may best depict a physician's approach to equilibrium—with spirituality permeating all aspects of our professional, family, and physical lives (*Fig. 1.4*).

We must keep our mind and hearts spiritually receptive.

In closing, I would like to read to you a passage from the book entitled *Mortal Lessons: Notes on the Art of Surgery* (2), by Dr. Richard Selzer, a retired surgeon from Yale School of Medicine in New Haven, Connecticut.

> I stand by the bed where a young woman lies, her face postoperative, her mouth twisted in palsy, clownish. A tiny twig of the facial nerve, the one to the muscles of her mouth, has been severed. She will be thus from now on. The surgeon had followed with religious fervor the curve of her flesh; I promise you that. Nevertheless, to remove the tumor in her cheek, I had cut the little nerve.
>
> Her young husband is in the room. He stands on the opposite side of the bed, and together they seem to dwell in the evening lamplight, isolated from me, private. Who are they, I ask myself, he and this wry-mouth I have made, who gaze at and touch each other so generously, greedily? The young woman speaks.
>
> "Will my mouth always be like this?" she asks.

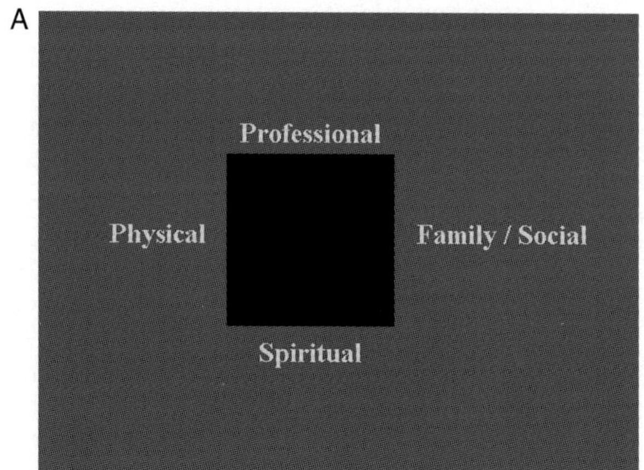

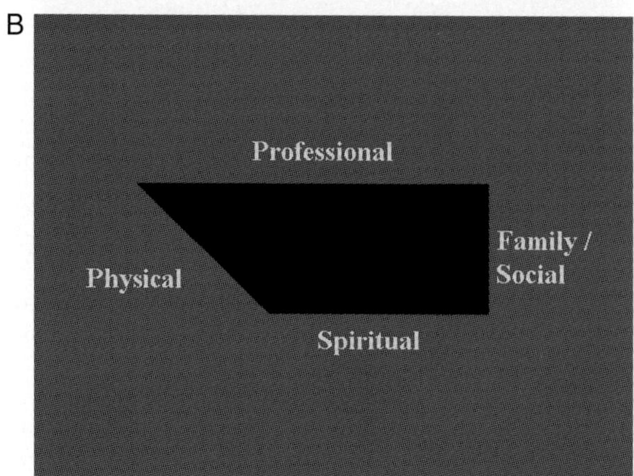

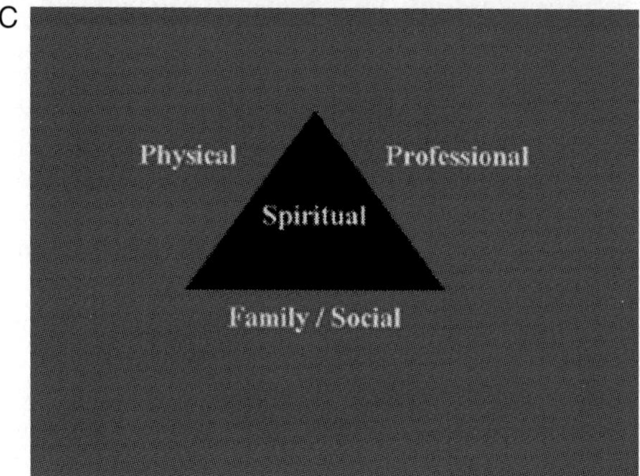

FIG. 1.4 (*A*) Commitment square. (*B*) Typical neurosurgeon's square. (*C*) Equilibrium.

"Yes," I say, "it will. It is because the nerve was cut."

She nods, and is silent. But the young man smiles.

"I like it," he says. "It is kind of cute."

All at once I know who he is. I understand, and I lower my gaze. One is not bold in an encounter with a god. Unmindful, he bends to kiss her crooked mouth, and I so close I can see how he twists his own lips to accommodate to hers, to show her that their kiss still works. I remember that the gods appeared in ancient Greece as mortals, and I hold my breath and let the wonder in.

Hold your breath and let the wonder in.
Thank you.

REFERENCES

1. Maroon JC: Presidential address: From Aequanimitas to Icarus. **Clin Neurosurg** 34:3–15, 1986.
2. Selzer R: *Mortal Lessons: Notes on the Art of Surgery.* Fort Washington, PA: Harvest Books, 1996, pp 45–46.

I

General Scientific Session I Discovery

CHAPTER

2

From Discovery to Design: Image-Guided Surgery

RICHARD D. BUCHOLZ, M.D., AND LEE McDURMONT

Each of us defines ourself in unique ways. For many of us, we define ourselves within our role in a family, such as father, mother, husband, or wife. Many of us define ourselves within a business venture, such as a chair, professor, manager, or assistant. But for the vast majority of us, especially those of us within the field of neurological surgery, we define ourselves by what we do. Each of us within our specialty has experienced a particular acknowledgement when we indicate to others that neurosurgery is our profession. The mention of neurosurgery evokes many reactions in almost everyone, a testimony to the remarkable history of achievements and of audacity within the field. The specialty is typified by an extreme confidence in one's capability to enter, navigate through, and repair the most complex structure known to mankind. Furthermore, it is marked by a group of professionals who are united in their desire to learn and to grow over the course of their professional lives. Finally, these individuals are known as having a compassion and a compulsion for meticulous detail, bordering on the obsessive. Indeed, it could be stated that a slavish devotion to accuracy and precision are true hallmarks of the neurosurgical specialty above and beyond any other distinctions between our field of specialization and the remainder of medicine.

If one looks at the definition of *accurate*, the first entry is "conforming exactly to fact, errorless." The second entry is "deviating only slightly or within acceptable limits from a standard." An accurate procedure, then, embodies the concept of a successful neurosurgical procedure in that little deviation occurs from a narrowly defined path to a specific target. Obviously, an accurate procedure is not only desirable but is mandatory in pursuing a target through the most important and intricate structure within the human body.

Individuals who embraced the concept of accuracy created neurosurgery. Cushing's meticulous technique defined neurosurgery at the onset of its creation and has stood as a model for all subsequent neurosurgeons to reduce and minimize injury to the tissue surrounding an intracerebral target. Walter Dandy was the first to employ localization of pathology using imaging to improve the ability to diagnose and reach neurological pathology. Our specialty was the first to embrace microscopic magnification to allow precise movements through delicate and complex tissues. The history of neurosurgery is a history marked by the pursuit of accuracy and precision.

Neurosurgeons have pursued diverse alternatives for improving the accuracy of their surgical technique. Cushing's contributions include detailed pathological review of brain tumor tissue removed operatively to better define prognosis. Dandy introduced new radiographic techniques to improve his ability to localize abnormal tissue. Egas Moniz was the first to employ contrast-enhanced radiography in the localization of cerebrovascular disease. Finally, Sir Victor Horsley was the first to design and implement a stereotactic instrument to guide a surgeon with extreme precision to a preselected surgical target.

For many of us, neurosurgery was the only logical choice as we entered medical school and considered our lives' options. Meticulous attention to detail suits the personality of a prospective neurosurgeon, and the complexity of the brain itself promises to many of us a life full of research and learning. Finally, for me personally, the structure of the brain paralleled my pre-existing interest in computers and electronics.

Doctor Dennis Spencer introduced me to stereotactic surgery shortly after I entered the neurosurgical residency program at Yale. He employed the Todd Wells frame for implantation of depth electrodes in the evaluation of patients with epilepsy intractable to medical intervention. Hours were spent with Dr. Spencer pouring over Vernier scales and waiting for radiographs to be developed at the West Haven Veterans Administration Hospital. I was struck by the dramatic results experienced by these patients who had been devastated by their chronic epilepsy. At the same time, I was also frustrated over the limitations imposed by a mechanical device that seemed to have its roots more in the nineteenth rather than the twentieth century. My frustration with the stereotactic frame led to a conviction that I could improve or replace it.

My first task was to learn the history of stereotactic instrumentation, which in itself is a fascinating topic. The efforts by Wycis and others to improve the accuracy of surgery should be a source of inspiration to all of us in neurosurgery. Although stereotactic surgery had reached an advanced state of development when I entered neurosurgical training in 1977, it was obvious that stereotactic surgeons constituted a minority—and a breed apart—from the mainstream of neurosurgery. Stereotactic surgeons were, in general, individuals who enjoyed mechanical instrumentation, engineering, and physics and who had the skills needed to use the simple computers that enabled the process of stereotactic registration. Clearly, the majority of neurological surgeons did not manifest or embrace these skills and, therefore, avoided any employment of stereotactic technique.

Rather than embracing stereotaxis, during my residency neurosurgery was focusing on improving the vision of the surgeon through the use of operative magnification. Many individuals within the field of neurological surgery, such as Prof. Yasargil of Zurich, were instrumental in adapting and using microscopes for surgical interventions. Through their efforts, a variety of approaches to specific intracranial lesions were devised that minimized damage to the surrounding tissue. These approaches have now become the standard of care in the routine approach to difficult vascular lesions. Shortly after the advent of the use of surgical microscopes, Dr. Patrick Kelly, currently of New York University, coupled a computer to the surgical microscope to assist in the navigation to deep-brain structures. Dr. Kelly saw the logical connection in using preoperative images to guide a microscope-equipped surgeon through the small recesses of the brain. His resultant device tracked the eye of the surgeon, consisting of the microscope, and aligned it with a surgical plan selected before the procedure. Although his solution was elegant, it still relied upon the concept of framed stereotaxy and, therefore, would not appeal to the vast majority of neurological surgeons, who avoided the frame. The optimal solution did not yet exist.

As Dr. Kelly was making his pioneering achievements in the field of stereotactic surgery, I graduated from the Yale program and became an Assistant Professor at Saint Louis University, recruited by the chair of the division, Dr. Kenneth Smith. Shortly after arriving at Saint Louis University, he was able to arrange the purchase of the first stereotactic device at the medical center through the benevolence of a donor. Doctor Smith also gave me protected time to follow my interests in the development of a stereotactic device, even during times when failure seemed to be imminent.

A few years after my arrival at Saint Louis University, Dr. David Roberts, currently the chair at Dartmouth University, produced a sonically guided microscope that could be registered to preoperative images without the use of a stereotactic frame. Dr. Roberts took advantage of improvements in digital scanners that, for the first time, produced image data sets with uniform intersection thickness and orientation. Previous scanners had produced data sets comprised of scans and images at random orientation and spacing to each other. By utilizing data sets with regular orientation, Dr. Roberts was able to forego the requirement of having numerous markers appear on every scanned image and use only a few point markers, or fiducials, attached to the patient. By identifying these fiducials within the operating room using a sonic, three-dimensional digitizer and equipping microscope with sound emitters, he was able to achieve guidance to deep-seated targets in a manner similar to that achieved by Kelly with a mechanical device and framed patient.

Both systems, however, guided the virtual eye of the surgeon and not his hand, which seemed to be ergonomically more attractive. This goal was achieved shortly after Dr. Roberts' publication by Dr. Watanabe of Tokyo University, who employed a mechanical arm, linked by several joints, to track the surgeon's hand. By determining the position of each joint, he was able to determine the position of the point at the end of the jointed arm within the patient's body. As with the Roberts device, Dr. Watanabe's instrument employed frameless registration using 4 to 5 fiducials on the patient's body. Although the instrument was an elegant solution and a major advance, its ergonomics were less than optimal given the frustrations associated with using a mechanical arm having multiple joints and limited range of rotation.

I became committed to a goal of building upon these advances by coupling preoperative imaging directly to surgical instrumentation through tracking the tip of surgical instruments held by the surgeon free of any connection between the instrument, the patient, or the operating table. This implied that the localization technology employed by the system would have to be built into the instruments, as opposed to adding dedicated stereotactic instrumentation to the surgical field. In the simplest possible terms, the goal was to build an instrument that was already used by surgeons but that knew where it was. It was apparent that the instrument would have to broadcast its position by the emission or reflection of energy to some form of receptive array. It also became clear that the position of the instrument had to be related to the patient's anatomy. Because the position of the instrument within the patient's body was the critical item of interest to a surgeon, it was not sufficient simply to know where the tip of the instrument was in three-dimensional space. The patient's anatomy had to be tracked as well. Therefore, the system would require that a similar form of tracking technology be attached or coupled to the patient's head and that patient's head be registered to the preoperative images using fiducials in a fashion similar to that suggested by Kelly or Roberts.

Rather than developing a frameless technique for our initial prototype, we decided to simplify the computational demands required of the system by the use of a stereotactic frame, thereby limiting the utility of the initial prototype to cranial interventions. The design of the initial prototype was then drawn up using a stereotactic frame with a reference system for the localization technology mounted in the plane of origin of the stereotactic co-ordinate system. Because our stereotactic frame was a CRW system, we developed and fabricated a reference system in the form of a ring that had sound emitters used by our sonic digitizer located within the plane origin of the BRW co-ordinate system. By making the localization technique have a plane of reference coaxial with the reference system of the stereotactic frame, the calculations necessary to determine the position of the instrument would be minimized (*Fig. 2.1*).

The next important consideration, once the technique of localization was finalized, was how to display a digital diagnostic image within the operating room. Given the limited amount of computer power that could be purchased with the funding available for our project, it was difficult to find a low-cost system that was capable of displaying images from a CT scanner. This problem was solved through a collaboration wit Dr. Peter Heilbrun, currently at Stanford University, who was then the chair at the University of Utah. Doctor Heilbrun had developed a stereotactic display system based upon an IBM 80286 computer that, through the use of a separate graphics card, was able to depict a CT section and display it at high resolution on a dedicated

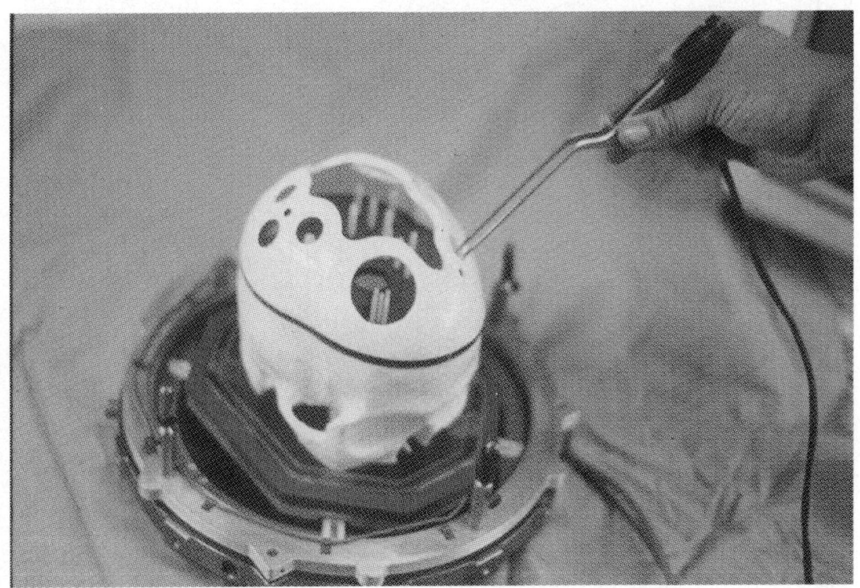

FIG. 2.1 "Herbie" in the CRW frame with sonic ring and sonic forceps.

monitor in the operating room. This was the first PC-based system that was portable and capable of handling large image data sets. This system came with a magnetic tape drive capable of reading the tapes produced by common CT scanners. Finally, Dr. Heilbrun offered support to generate a software algorithm that would take a BRW co-ordinate and depict the position on a section of the CT data set with a set of crosshairs superimposed on the CT scan through the position of interest. This, then, left the issue of programming the digitizer unit to generate this co-ordinate system and transfer it into the software display routines offered by the stereotactic computer to our group, greatly simplifying our programming effort.

With the advent of Dr. Heilbrun's computer system, all elements were present for the fabrication of a clinical prototype. Of paramount importance was insuring the accuracy of the system, which required days of work determining those factors associated with error. Our team was made complete by the addition of Lee McDurmont, who was brought on to support the information technology backbone of the surgery department. Lee quickly went from support of office personnel to finding himself within the operating room supporting our efforts to develop image-guided surgery (*Fig. 2.2*).

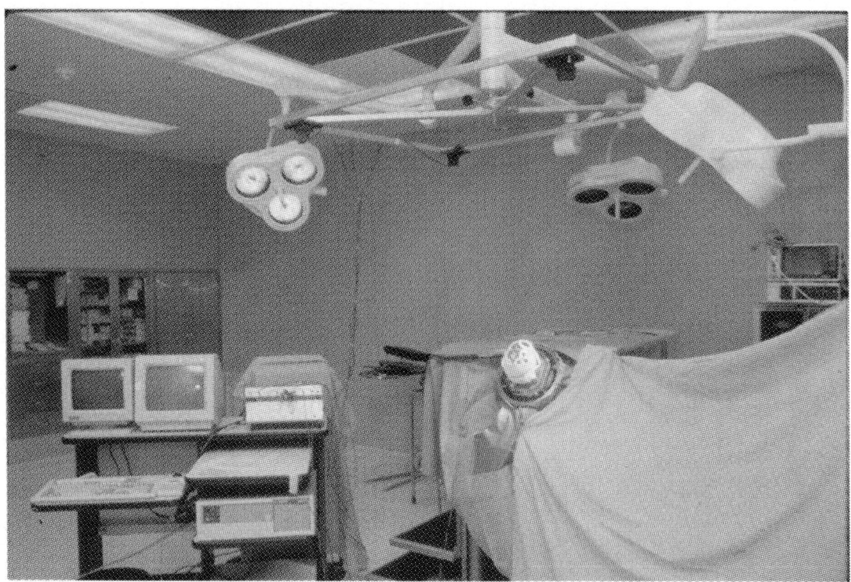

FIG. 2.2 Operation room setup with a stereotactic display system (based upon an IBM 80286 PC) and microphone array suspended over the operating table.

Accuracy was then determined by using the sonic digitizer with its microphone array fabricated in a basement suspended over a desk listening to a forceps held within a BRW phantom base that also held the reference arc. The position of the tip of the instrument was determined through the range of a typical surgical field, and the accuracy of the device depicting the location of the tip was carefully determined. Studies were also performed on a phantom ("Herbie") produced by Dr. Heilbrun that was scanned literally hundreds of times in an attempt to improve and insure the accuracy of the system. When MR imaging became routinely available, the phantom was suspended in water and accuracy testing performed using that imaging modality as well (*Fig. 2.3*).

Once the accuracy of the device was sufficient to warrant use in a clinical situation, approval for use of the device in surgery was ob-

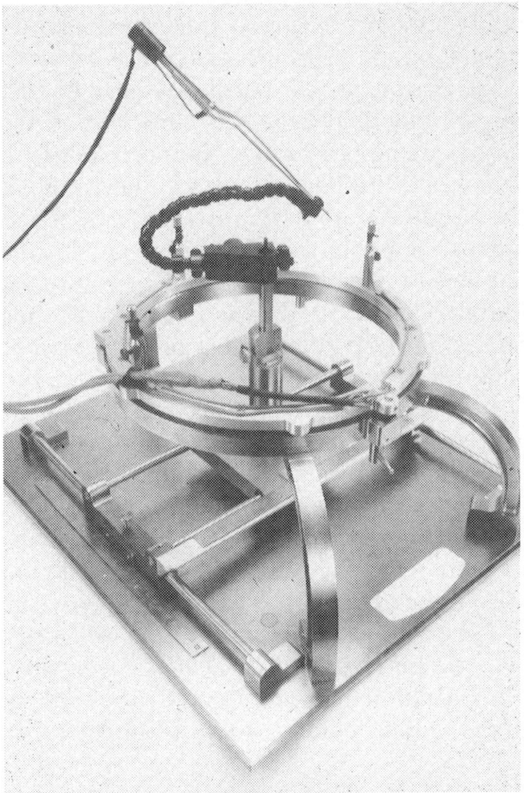

FIG. 2.3 BRW phantom base with sonic ring and sonic forceps.

tained from our Institutional Review Board. Critical to this acceptance was that conventional stereotactic surgery involving use of the BRW arc system was always available as a backup to the investigational sonic device. Using a forceps altered by the Storz Company (St. Louis, MO), eight operations were performed. Almost immediately, a problem with echoes was encountered. The sonic digitizer determined the time of flight of sound emitted by spark-gap emitters to each of the four microphones in the array. By comparing the time of flight to each microphone, the position of the emitter could be triangulated from the microphone array. It became apparent that sound could travel not only directly from the emitters on the instruments to the microphone array but also could echo off the tiled wall of the operating room and then to the microphone array with an appreciable delay. This would cause erratic localization with occasionally gross error in localization of the tip of the forceps. This problem was so intractable that the viability of the project came into question.

At that time, two events occurred that reversed our negative fortunes and were pivotal to our eventual success. I had the opportunity to meet Dr. Kurt Smith, an electrical engineer at Southern Illinois University at Edwardsville, who at the time was developing a digital audio tape recorder using Silicon Graphics computers. Doctor Smith's research interest was to build a device that allowed musicians to record separate tracks of music onto different segments of a hard drive and then mix the tracks down to a stereophonic pair. Although this concept is routinely used today, in 1989 it was revolutionary and a topic of intense research. Doctor Smith was introduced to me by his uncle, Dr. Ken Smith, as an individual with expertise in programming the high-power computers that would be necessary for the next generation of display consisting of three orthogonal images (*Fig. 2.4*). A second development was the advent of optical digitizers that, for the first time, could match the accuracy previously seen only with sonic digitizers. These optical devices relied upon either reflected or emitted light focused upon charged coupled devices (CCDs) that had a fixed relationship to each other. By comparing the location of focused light on either two two-dimensional CCD cameras or three one-dimensional CCD cameras, the position of the emitted or reflected light could be determined with a high degree of precision. Given the difficulty with echoes in the operating room encountered by the sonic digitizer, it was decided to switch the development work to employ an optical digitizer (*Fig. 2.5*).

A whole new set of problems, however, was then encountered with the use of light-emitting diodes (LEDs), which served as our emitted points of light. The available LEDs were highly directional and re-

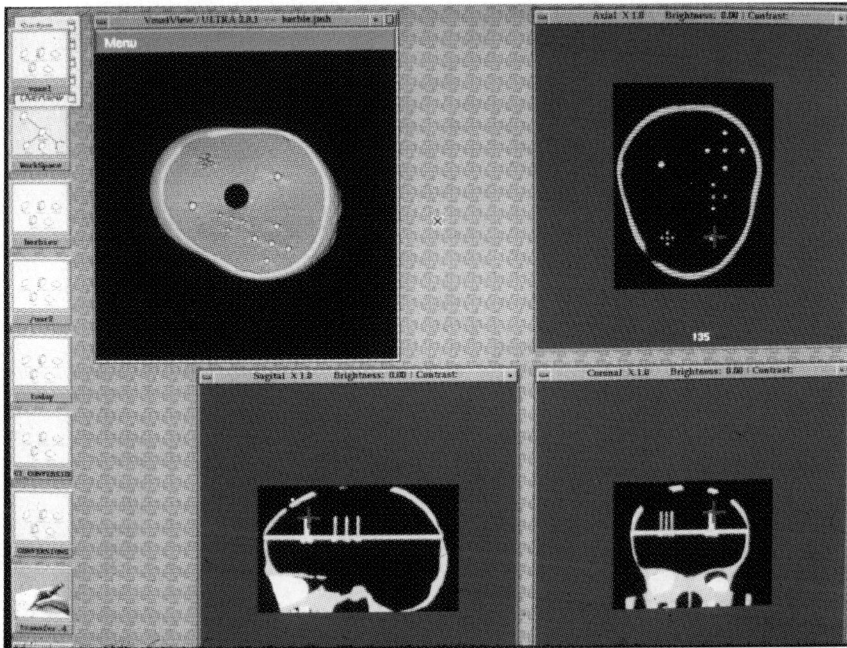

FIG. 2.4 Early orthogonal display of "Herbie" showing tip co-ordinates of forceps with red cross.

quired a gimbaled system to direct their output to the camera array. As the exact point of emission was critical to the accuracy of the system, great attention had to be focused on ensuring that the gimbal pivoted around the point of origin of light from the LED. In addition, the camera array had to be positioned carefully at a specified distance and orientation to the surgical field to guarantee accuracy. This led to a series of prototypes for the reference arc to address the limitations of the LED arrays. At the same time, stereotactic localization was replaced by the use of paired-point registration using the technique developed by Roberts. With this programming effort, the goal of eliminating the stereotactic was realized, and the problems of the sonic digitizer were eliminated. The accuracy of the optical system had to be proven in a fashion reminiscent of the sonic digitizer (*Fig. 2.6*). A whole new set of experiments was devised to test the accuracy of the system, and these were carried out by a computer-orientated resident, Dr. Jaimie Henderson. Now at the Cleveland Clinic, Dr. Henderson also pioneered a whole new set of applications based upon his work with the initial accuracy of the device as well as subsequent work in the area of functional neurosurgery.

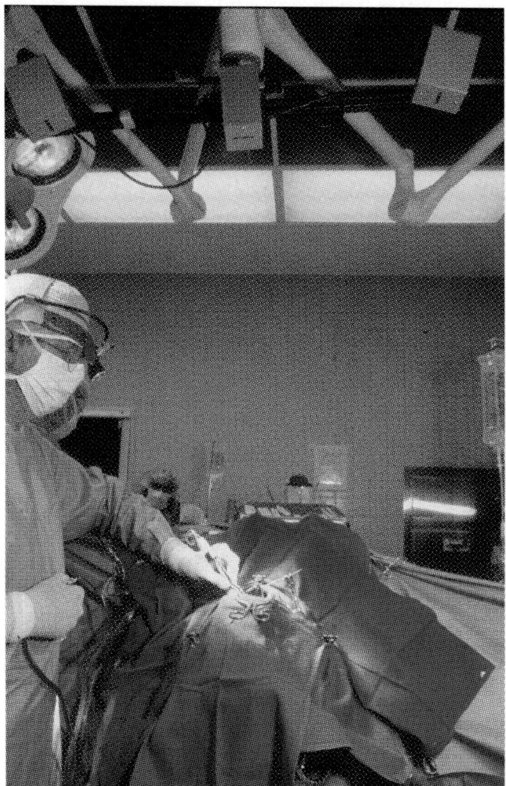

FIG. 2.5 The author with a three-camera array over the operating table and infrared LED forceps and infrared ring on the patient.

With the advent of the frameless registration techniques, new phantom studies were also required. Doctor Smith's group developed a new user interface and registration technique based upon paired-point matching. These had to be tested through the use of a modified phantom, which had skin similar to that of a human subject. The image presentation software was also changed to allow depiction of the position of three images positioned at right angles to each other. This, then, gave an appreciation of the three-dimensional position of the tip of the instrument as opposed to relying upon a single image, as used in the initial prototype.

With the advent of an alternative registration technique, Dr. Kevin Foley of the University of Tennessee at Memphis appreciated the utility of the device for surgery outside of the cranium. Doctor Foley employed anatomical landmarks, such as bony protrusions on the posterior aspect of the spine, to allow registration of images to the system. By adapting our reference arc to a device that would attach to the

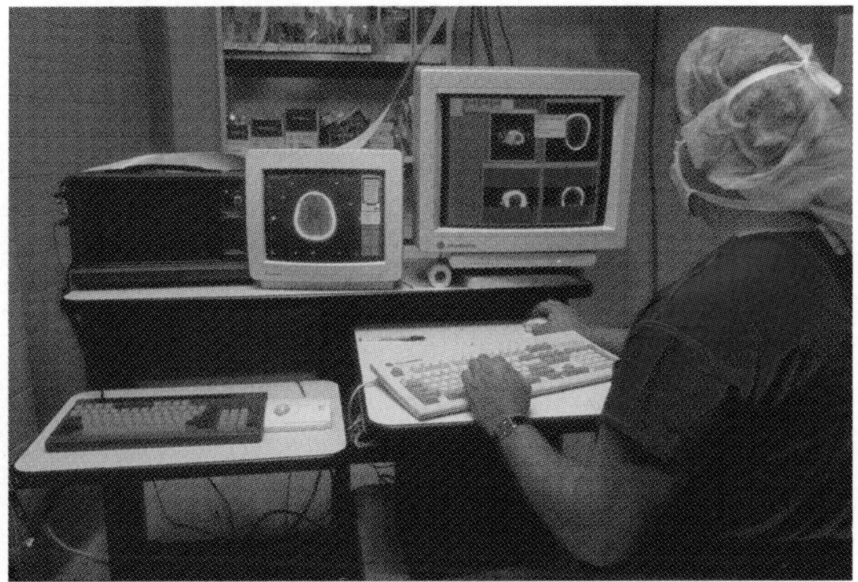

FIG. 2.6 Lee McDurmont at a hybrid workstation. The original two-dimensional CT display is on the left, and the upgraded, three-dimensional display is on the right.

spinous process and by registering the vertebral body using bony anatomical landmarks, Dr. Foley was able to develop a stereotactic application for the insertion of pedicle screws into the spine. This application was critical for increasing the overall interest in the device, especially within the commercial field.

The addition of Dr. Foley at the University of Tennessee completed the membership of our development team. Stealth Technologies, a company set up by Dr. Kurt Smith with programmers from the original digital recorder team, produced software and prototypes employed by both clinical centers. Cranial applications and accuracy testing were performed and revised at Saint Louis University. Prototypes were rapidly developed and used operatively, only to be critiqued and replaced to maximize the ergonomics and ease of use of the device. Spinal applications were similarly developed and refined at the University of Tennessee at Memphis by Dr. Foley. By 1995, the development work was sufficiently advanced to warrant the production of 16 units, which were purchased by a beta test group.

After a year of intensive work by the beta test group at the test sites, an application to the U.S. Food and Drug Administration (FDA) was submitted and approved in 1996. This approval came at a time when the finances of Stealth Technologies were extremely tenuous. With

U.S. FDA approval and transfer of the firm to a larger corporate entity, however, frameless stereotaxis was rapidly accepted by mainstream neurosurgeons and was translated into its own field of image guidance, or neuronavigation (*Fig. 2.7*). Use of navigational systems then became an accepted part of residency training, and the StealthStation name, which was selected to be attractive to musicians and potential rock stars, was now synonymous with surgical accuracy.

It is my firm conviction that image guidance supplies the platform for development of the vast majority of new surgical procedures within cranial neurosurgery. By employing such a system, any information that can be obtained about the organization of a particular patient's brain can be related to that patient's anatomy during the course of surgical intervention. This information can be culled from a variety of sources, and it allows the accurate positioning of any therapeutic intervention (*Fig. 2.8*). As miniature therapeutic devices, such as those for deep-brain stimulation, are developed, image guidance will insure their placement within a precisely defined area of maximal. Further-

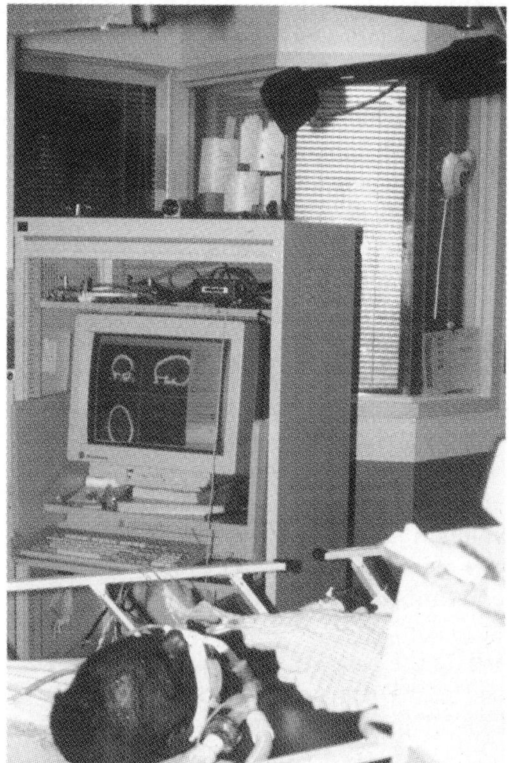

FIG. 2.7 The system became portable enough to use in the intensive care unit circa 1994.

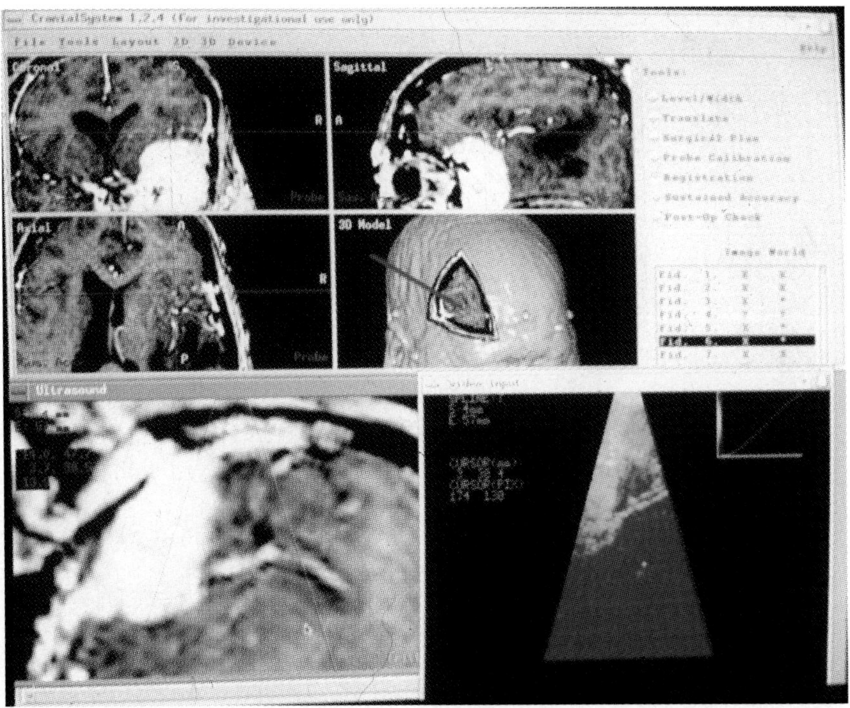

FIG. 2.8 Early, coregistered MR and ultrasound images.

more, the acceptance of image guidance by neurosurgeons will ensure that the association of neurosurgery with the pursuit of accuracy will continue for our surgical specialty. Image guidance, like the majority of major developments within surgery, will be developed by neurosurgeons who are committed to improving the state of the surgical art. Only by encountering a problem will individuals be motivated to answering that problem by diligent work, and surgeons are the only individuals who will face these problems within the operative environment. Through the formation of alliances with talented individuals within the field of engineering, surgical problems will be resolved, and the outcome of our patients will be improved. Thus, we will be true to the legacy left by our neurosurgical predecessors, a legacy of accuracy and precision.

CHAPTER

3

Endovascular Neurosurgery: An Evolution in Process

JAY U. HOWINGTON, M.D., LEE R. GUTERMAN, Ph.D., M.D., AND L. NELSON HOPKINS, M.D.

> Humanity does not pass through phases as a train passes through stations: being alive, it has the privilege of always moving yet never leaving anything behind. Whatever we have been, in some sort we are still.
>
> C.S. Lewis (18)

INTRODUCTION

With the recent publication of the results of the International Subarachnoid Aneurysm Trial (ISAT) (22), Mr. Lewis' words could not be more apropos. The 1990s saw the emergence of interventional neuroradiology as a catheter-based treatment modality that was performed, in large part, by radiologists. Many neurosurgeons saw this new technology as nonneurosurgical and a "phase" that would have a minimal impact on their specialty, if it had any staying power at all. The ISAT results summon the neurosurgeon of today to embrace endovascular therapies and include them in the management strategy of cerebrovascular diseases or else remain on the station's platform, watching the train of progress pass. Historically, neurosurgeons have been the health care provider of choice with regard to cerebrovascular disease, and this should not change. What should change is the way in which neurosurgeons care for patients with vascular lesions. Instead of resisting the inevitable shifts in treatment that endovascular innovations will bring, the vascular neurosurgeon should strive to understand these new techniques and tools, if not to master them altogether. Vascular neurosurgery will evolve into a specialty that incorporates both the knife and the catheter and, in so doing, will move forward without "leaving anything behind." Our objective with this manuscript is to describe the current state of endovascular therapy in an effort to increase the neurosurgeon's awareness of and participation in these treatment modalities.

INTRACRANIAL ANEURYSMS

The ISAT results have already generated considerable discussion in the neurosurgery community, much of which revolves around the accuracy and validity of the study. The Section on Cerebrovascular Surgery of the American Association of Neurological Surgeons and the Congress of Neurological Surgeons (AANS/CNS) has published a position statement in which the authors seek to educate fellow neurosurgeons with regard to the trial's conclusions (9). The authors of this statement claim that the results of the trial have been inaccurately reported by the media. An article in the *New York Times* shortly after the study was published in *The Lancet* focused on the *relative* rather than the *absolute* risk reduction rate of endovascular therapy compared with surgical therapy (21). The difference between the absolute risk reduction rate of 6.9% and the relative risk reduction rate of 22.6% is dramatic, and the authors of the AANS/CNS position statement have a valid argument in their complaint against the media's representation of this study's results. These authors also argue that the results of the trial may not apply to patients in the United States because of differences in practice patterns that exist between the European and American neurosurgical communities. A question not answered by the study was the level of experience of each practitioner. Specifically, the number of craniotomies for aneurysm that each surgeon had performed or the number of coiling procedures that each interventionist had performed, and how that number correlated with outcome, was not analyzed as a part of the ISAT. Finally, the long-term results of the study are a few years away from publication, and already the questions of recurrent hemorrhage and recanalization rates are evident. In the short-term, 2.6% of the patients who underwent coil embolization experienced a posttreatment hemorrhage, compared with 0.9% of those who were treated surgically. The authors of the position statement claim that this increased hemorrhage rate, combined with the increased need for additional treatments in the endovascular group, might act to nullify the 6.9% absolute risk reduction rate conferred by coil embolization in the short term. Long-term results are definitely needed, but which treatment modality will prove to be the preferred option for ruptured intracranial aneurysms is a question that, although extremely important, the neurosurgeon of the twenty-first century needs to look beyond to see a bigger picture.

Endurance of the short-term results in the ISAT is important, but of far greater importance is that a prospective, randomized trial was conducted and the results demonstrated that coil embolization of ruptured intracranial aneurysms exists as a viable (and safer) option compared to traditional surgical therapy. Publication of the ISAT results coincides with an ever-increasing number of coil manufacturers and endovascular innovations. The growing coil marketplace signifies a rise in the number of coil embolizations being done globally as well as in the United States. Neurosurgeons are quickly finding that they no longer are "taking the point" with regard to treatment of these lesions and that craniotomy for aneurysm will soon be relegated to the status of "another option." The care of intracranial aneurysms is already a big business, and the Internet-versed patient no longer seeks care as the "patient" but as the "health care consumer." Whether good or bad, when given a choice between a craniotomy and a needle stick in the groin, most consumers will seek the latter. As this happens, the natural reaction of the neurosurgery community will be anger and opposition, but such a response is shortsighted. The shift toward endovascular therapy is inevitable, and neurosurgeons would do well to embrace the change and modify their own practice patterns in the process. Embracing the changes produced by endovascular therapy, however, does not mean leaving old practices behind. Neurosurgeons need to proceed with caution, because the growing bias toward embolization sets up a troubling treatment paradigm.

The vast majority of coil embolizations for intracranial aneurysms are currently being performed by interventional neuroradiologists, whereas the pre- and postprocedural management is left to the neurosurgeon. These two groups, neurosurgeons and neuroradiologists, possess a limited knowledge, at best, of what goes on in the realm of the other, and in no other area of medicine does such a schism exist between treatment and management. Interventional neuroradiologists should coil aneurysms, and neurosurgeons should care for patients with subarachnoid hemorrhage. Neuroradiologists, however, must understand and participate in the care of patients with subarachnoid hemorrhage outside of the angiography suite, and neurosurgeons must acquire a working knowledge of endovascular procedures. For the neurosurgeon, this means more than being well versed on the ISAT results, and for the neuroradiologist, it means more than recognizing the presence of hydrocephalus. At our institution, we feel that, at the very least, the neurosurgeon caring for patients with aneurysms should be able to perform an angiogram and understand the tools and strategies that might be applied in the embolization process. In the optimal setting, such a neurosurgeon should possess the knowledge and requisite skills to perform the actual embolization itself. The care provided in that type of situation benefits the patient immensely and lacks the discontinuity that is so readily apparent when one physician treats the aneurysm and another manages the intensive care. Ideally, neurosurgeons, with their strong clinical and intensive care skills, should merge with interventional neuroradiologists, with their strong imaging and image anatomy skills. In the future, it is quite possible that the labels *interventional neuroradiologist* and *vascular neurosurgeon* will cease to exist, that the physicians who care for patients with aneurysms will be known as *endovascular neurosurgeons*. This new breed of physician will retain the best of both worlds and have the knowledge and skill to provide the patient with complete care. The question is how we, as neurosurgeons, plan to continue in our role as aneurysm caretakers while at the same time modifying our skill set to meet the demands of an evolving discipline.

The areas of spinal surgery and stereotactic radiosurgery demonstrate two different ways in which neurosurgery has adapted to changes in the health care environment and how neurosurgeons have remained at the forefront as both care providers and researchers. As the advances in spinal instrumentation came about, neurosurgeons chose not to stand back and watch. Spinal instrumentation was incorporated into the neurosurgery curriculum so that every graduating neurosurgery resident today is well qualified to perform standard instrumentation procedures. Historically, spinal instrumentation fell within the sphere of orthopedics, whereas neural decompression was left to neurosurgery. Neurosurgeons, however, have long played a significant role in the advancement of techniques and the understanding spinal fusion. In 1958, Cloward (2) published his modification of the technique described by Robinson and Smith (24) and spent the remainder of his career studying spinal biomechanics in an effort to improve fusion techniques. The emphasis on spinal fusion was slow to take hold in the neurosurgical community. Today, however, some of the major figures in spinal surgery are neurosurgeons, and the neurosurgical residency curriculum reflects this shift. Neurosurgeons often work in tandem with orthopedists to provide optimal care for patients, and many neurosurgical and orthopedic departments collaborate with each other to offer their residents as complete an education as possible. Each discipline brings a unique perspective to the practice of spinal surgery, and there is no reason why both cannot—and should not—continue to advance the field both clinically and scientifically.

In 1951, Leksell (15) described the concept of focusing many beams of radiation on a stereotactically defined target and coined the term *radiosurgery*. The result of this concept was the Gamma knife. Neurosurgeons created this new technique and have expanded the indications for its use through meticulous research. Neurosurgeons work in conjunction with radiation oncologists in the clinical setting to create an ideal treatment plan for each patient and in the research setting to further our understanding of stereotactic radiosurgery as a treatment modality. Every neurosurgical residency in the United States now has access to a Gamma knife, and every resident now completing a residency has knowledge of the technology behind its use as well as of the lesions for which radiosurgery is most suitable. Both spinal instrumentation and stereotactic radiosurgery have changed the neurosurgical landscape immensely, and neurosurgeons have responded to this change by modifying practice patterns and ensuring that the neurosurgical curriculum provides an adequate education in both areas. And in both areas, neurosurgeons work with physicians from other disciplines in a relationship that enjoys the benefit of multiple perspectives. In so doing, neurosurgeons have done much more than simply step off the platform and onto the train of progress. They have taken control of the train and now guide its future. The management of aneurysmal subarachnoid hemorrhage should be no different.

ARTERIOVENOUS MALFORMATIONS

The morbidity associated with the surgical treatment of intracranial arteriovenous malformations (AVMs) has decreased over the past two decades, mainly because of advances in endovascular therapy. The aim of endovascular therapy is to alter the hemodynamics of the malformation and thereby reduce its size and enhance the patient's outcome. The rationale behind such an aim stems from the results of several studies that have demonstrated the direct relationship between AVM size and both surgical difficulty and operative morbidity (10, 19, 26, 27). Polyvinyl alcohol particles were once the mainstay of AVM embolization, but in recent years, they have been replaced by cyanoacrylates and a nonadhesive agent known as Onyx (Micro Therapeutics, Inc., Irvine, CA). *N*-butyl-cyanoacrylate (NBCA) and Onyx are thought of as liquid agents, because they are injected through a microcatheter that has been positioned as close to the nidus of the AVM as possible (23). The U.S. Food and Drug Administration has given its approval for NBCA (Trufill; Cordis Neurovascular, Inc., Miami Lakes, FL) to be used as an embolic agent for AVMs and is evaluating clinical trial results in consideration of the approval of Onyx.

Small AVMs with a single feeding pedicle can often be obliterated with endovascular therapy, and when complete casting of the nidus has been achieved, the AVM is usually cured (6, 12, 20, 28–30). With larger AVMs, such a cure is difficult to achieve, because the complexity of the nidus and the multiplicity of arterial feeders preclude a complete filling of the nidus (5, 8). Embolization serves as an adjunct to surgical or radiosurgical therapy by decreasing the size of the nidus. The reduction in the size of the nidus achieved by embolization transforms an AVM that was previously too large for either surgery or radiosurgery into a manageable lesion (3, 4, 6, 7, 13, 23, 28, 29).

Angiography has long been the imaging modality of choice in evaluating AVMs, but this could change with recent advances in both MR imaging and CT. These relatively noninvasive techniques provide relatively accurate images without exposing the patient to the risks of cerebral angiography; however, one often has trouble discerning the edge of the nidus from the draining veins. The authors feel that high-speed angiography (15–30 frames/sec) provides the physician with a more complete understanding of the AVM. When compared with CT, MR imaging, and even conventional angiography, high-speed angiography enables the treating physician to define the boundaries of the malformation more effectively and to estimate the transit time of blood through the lesion. Such knowledge enhances the treatment plan.

So what does all of this have to do with the neurosurgeon? *Everything.* With the standard of care for the treatment of cerebral AVMs rapidly moving toward an "embolize first" protocol, the neurosurgeon treating patients with AVMs must understand all that takes place in the angiography suite. As with the management of intracranial aneurysms, the best way for the neurosurgeon to do this is to have a place at the angiography table. At the very least, neurosurgeons should have a collaborative relationship with their neuroradiology colleagues, and ideally, they should participate in the endovascular procedures that are required in the evaluation and management of these lesions. Neurosurgeons need to fully understand current endovascular techniques and materials as well as keep abreast of future directions in the field if they are to continue playing a significant role in the treatment of AVMs. The authors feel that for this understanding to take place, a change must be made in the neurosurgery curriculum. Basic endovascular training deserves a place in neurosurgery resident education.

CEREBROVASCULAR OCCLUSIVE DISEASE

Since the 1990s, the disciplines of cardiology and interventional neuroradiology have focused much effort on the development and refinement of carotid artery angioplasty and stenting as an alternative to carotid endarterectomy (CEA). The results of the first randomized study comparing carotid angioplasty with CEA were published in 2001 (1). This study showed equivalency of the two procedures with regard to major outcome events during the first 30 days as well as the rate of ipsilateral stroke, with survival analysis extending to 3 years after randomization. This study did show that severe (70–99%) ipsilateral stenosis was more common in the endovascular group, however, and only 26% of the endovascular group underwent stenting in conjunction with angioplasty. This study also did not evaluate the use of a device that protects the brain from the embolic shower associated with angioplasty. For these reasons, another study was designed that focused on those patients deemed to be at high risk and randomized them to either CEA or angioplasty and stenting with a distal protection device. This second study is known as the Stenting and Angioplasty with Protection in Patients at High Risk for Endarterectomy (SAPPHIRE) study (14).

In the SAPPHIRE study, 409 patients were enrolled at 30 centers in the United States, and they had to meet the following criteria: either asymptomatic with at least 80% stenosis or symptomatic with at least 50% stenosis and at least onc feature that would put them at high risk for either endoluminal or surgical revascularization. The high-risk factors included age older than 80 years, congestive heart failure, severe chronic obstructive pulmonary disease, restenosis after CEA, previous radiation therapy or radical neck surgery, and lesions that were deemed either too distal or proximal for adequate surgical exposure. Patients had to be considered good candidates for either method of revascularization to be randomized, which resulted in a total of 307 patients in the randomization (151 to CEA and 156 to stenting). The primary end point was the incidence of major adverse cardiac or neurologic events. At 30 days, the incidence of a major event was reduced by more than 50% in the stenting group compared to the CEA group. Although the SAPPHIRE trial focused on those patients who are at higher risk for CEA than for stenting, the National Institutes of Health is currently sponsoring another trial that compares stenting with surgery in lower-risk patients; this study is known as the Carotid Revascularization versus Stenting Trial (CREST) (11).

With advances in endovascular technology, physicians are now able to treat symptomatic stenosis of the intracranial vessels. At our institution, we have published our results with staged stent-assisted angioplasty (angioplasty followed by repeated angioplasty and stent placement ≥1 mo later) for symptomatic vertebrobasilar artery stenosis (17). With this technique, we have been able to reduce the mean stenosis from 78% to 30% in these vessels. Technologic advances in the arena of coronary angioplasty and stenting have also led to the evaluation of drug-eluting stents in the intracranial circulation. We have assessed these stents using a canine model, with results that suggest a lower percentage of occlusion occurs after implantation of heparin-coated versus uncoated stents, and have begun testing these devices in humans (16).

Cerebrovascular occlusive disease, once considered to be a surgical disease, is now being treated more often by endovascular means, and if they do not adapt, neurosurgeons will soon find themselves no longer in a position to care for these patients. The neurosurgeon is uniquely qualified to manage cerebrovascular occlusive disease, but there must be more to the armamentarium than the 10 blade. To optimally care for these patients, the neurosurgeon must know which therapeutic modality would benefit the patient most and why. The best way to gain this knowledge is for the neurosurgeon to be present during—and to participate in—endovascular procedures and for neurosurgery residents to participate in them as well. Otherwise, neurosurgeons run the risk of being poorly informed, which translates into suboptimal patient care.

CONCLUSIONS

Throughout its history, neurosurgery has been a specialty defined by constant innovation. In most areas of neurosurgery, these innovations have led to changes in methods for the treatment of neurological diseases. In the area of cerebrovascular disease, however, much progress is being made, but the changes are not coming from neurosurgeons. If neurosurgeons are to remain in the forefront of this field, they must recall their history as innovators and adapt to these new changes.

> Progress, far from consisting in change, depends on retentiveness. When change is absolute there remains no being to improve and no direction is set for possible improvement: and when experience is not retained, as among savages, infancy is perpetual.
>
> George Santayana (25)

REFERENCES

1. Endovascular versus surgical treatment in patients with carotid stenosis in the Carotid and Vertebral Artery Transluminal Angioplasty Study (CAVATAS): A randomised trial. **Lancet** 357:1729–1737, 2001.
2. Cloward RB: The anterior approach for removal of ruptured cervical disks. **J Neurosurg** 15:602–617, 1958.
3. Debrun GM, Aletich V, Ausman JI, Charbel F, Dujovny M: Embolization of the nidus of brain arteriovenous malformations with *N*-butyl cyanoacrylate. **Neurosurgery** 40:112–121, 1997.

4. DeMeritt JS, Pile-Spellman J, Mast H, et al.: Outcome analysis of preoperative embolization with *N*-butyl cyanoacrylate in cerebral arteriovenous malformations. **AJNR Am J Neuroradiol** 16:1801–1807, 1995.
5. Fournier D, Terbrugge K, Rodesch G, Lasjaunias P: Revascularization of brain arteriovenous malformations after embolization with bucrylate. **Neuroradiology** 32:497–501, 1990.
6. Fournier D, TerBrugge KG, Willinsky R, Lasjaunias P, Montanera W: Endovascular treatment of intracerebral arteriovenous malformations: Experience in 49 cases. **J Neurosurg** 75:228–233, 1991.
7. Frizzel RT, Fisher WS III: Cure, morbidity, and mortality associated with embolization of brain arteriovenous malformations: A review of 1246 patients in 32 series over a 35-year period. **Neurosurgery** 37:1031–1040, 1995.
8. Gobin YP, Laurent A, Merienne L, et al.: Treatment of brain arteriovenous malformations by embolization and radiosurgery. **J Neurosurg** 85:19–28, 1996.
9. Harbaugh RE, Heros RC, Hadley MN: AANS/CNS Section on Cerebrovascular Surgery: position statement on the International Subarachnoid Aneurysm Trial (ISAT). **Neurosurgery News** 3(18):4–5, 2002.
10. Heros RC, Tu YK: Unruptured arteriovenous malformations: A dilemma in surgical decision making. **Clin Neurosurg** 33:187–236, 1986.
11. Hobson RW II: Update on the Carotid Revascularization Endarterectomy versus Stent Trial (CREST) protocol. **J Am Coll Surg** Suppl 1, 194:S9–S14, 2002.
12. Hurst RW, Berenstein A, Kupersmith MJ, Madrid M, Flamm ES: Deep central arteriovenous malformations of the brain: The role of endovascular treatment. **J Neurosurg** 82:190–195, 1995.
13. Jafar JJ, Davis AJ, Berenstein A, Choi IS, Kupersmith MJ: The effect of embolization with *N*-butyl cyanoacrylate prior to surgical resection of cerebral arteriovenous malformations. **J Neurosurg** 78:60–69, 1993.
14. Jeffrey S: SAPPHIRE: Carotid stenting superior to endarterectomy in high-risk patients. In: *Heartwire, 2002*. Available at http://www.theheart.org/index.cfm?doc_id=33213 [Accessed 01/20/03].
15. Leksell L: The sterotaxic method and radiosurgery of the brain. **Acta Chir Scand** 102:316–319, 1951.
16. Levy EI, Boulos AS, Hanel RA, et al.: In vivo model of intracranial stent implantation: A pilot study examining the histological response of cerebral vessels after randomized implantation of heparin-coated and uncoated endoluminal stents in a blinded fashion. **J Neurosurg** 98:532–541, 2003.
17. Levy EI, Hanel RA, Bendok BR, et al.: Staged stent-assisted angioplasty for symptomatic intracranial vertebrobasilar artery stenosis. **J Neurosurg** 97:1294–1301, 2002.
18. Lewis CS: *The Allegory of Love: A Study in Medieval Tradition.* Oxford: Clarendon Press, 1936.
19. Luessenhop AJ, Gennarelli TA: Anatomical grading of supratentorial arteriovenous malformations for determining operability. **Neurosurgery** 1:30–35, 1977.
20. Mansmann U, Lasjaunias P, Meisel HJ: Treatment of patients with cerebral arteriovenous malformations. **Radiology** 223:879–881, 2002.
21. McNeil DG: Fixing aneurysms without surgery. In: *New York Times.* New York, 2002, p 5.
22. Molyneux A, Kerr R, Stratton I, et al.: International Subarachnoid Aneurysm Trial (ISAT) of neurosurgical clipping versus endovascular coiling in 2143 patients with ruptured intracranial aneurysms: A randomised trial. **Lancet** 360:1267–1274, 2002.

23. Pasqualin A, Scienza R, Cioffi F, et al.: Treatment of cerebral arteriovenous malformations with a combination of preoperative embolization and surgery. **Neurosurgery** 29:358–368, 1991.
24. Robinson RA, Smith G: Anterolateral cervical disc removal and interbody fusion for cervical disc syndrome. **Bull Johns Hopkins Hosp** 96:223–224, 1955.
25. Santayana G: *Life of Reason,* vol. 1. New York: Scribner, 1905.
26. Spetzler RF, Martin NA: A proposed grading system for arteriovenous malformations. **J Neurosurg** 65:476–483, 1986.
27. Tamaki N, Ehara K, Lin TK, et al.: Cerebral arteriovenous malformations: Factors influencing the surgical difficulty and outcome. **Neurosurgery** 29:856–863, 1991.
28. Vinuela F, Dion JE, Duckwiler G, et al.: Combined endovascular embolization and surgery in the management of cerebral arteriovenous malformations: Experience with 101 cases. **J Neurosurg** 75:856–864, 1991.
29. Wikholm G: Occlusion of cerebral arteriovenous malformations with *N*-butyl cyanoacrylate is permanent. **AJNR Am J Neuroradiol** 16:479–482, 1995.
30. Wikholm G, Lundqvist C, Svendsen P: Embolization of cerebral arteriovenous malformations: Part I—Technique, morphology, and complications. **Neurosurgery** 39:448–459, 1996.

CHAPTER

4

Discovering the Novel Surgical Approach

RICHARD E. CLATTERBUCK, M.D., Ph.D., ANTONIO BERNARDO, M.D., AND ROBERT F. SPETZLER, M.D.

Historically, voyages of discovery were launched on the courage to ignore conventional wisdom and explore uncharted territory to identify something that existed but was previously unrecognized. Dispelling the myths of centuries required a leap of faith, tempered by knowledge and rational thought. The historian Daniel J. Boorstin (1) said this of discovery:

> The obstacles to discovery—the illusions of knowledge—are also part of our story. Only against the forgotten backdrop of the received common sense and myths of their time can we begin to sense the courage, the rashness, the heroic and imaginative thrusts of the great discoverers. They had to battle against the current "facts" and dogmas of the learned.

The same could be said, to some extent, of discovering the novel surgical approach. Requiring a commanding knowledge of anatomy and the ability to look beyond conventional neurosurgical wisdom, the novel surgical approach allows surgeons greater access to areas of the neuraxis, such as the brain stem, once considered either hard to reach or inaccessible.

Lesions in and around the brain stem are perhaps the best examples of difficult surgical targets for which novel surgical approaches are still forging new frontiers. Regardless of whether aneurysms along the basilar trunk and apex or intrinsic mesencephalic vascular and neoplastic lesions are the concern, surgery in and around the brain stem may be the most challenging and treacherous activity confronting neurosurgeons. By discovering novel surgical approaches that decrease the working depth, increase the working area, and increase the angle of attack, access to deep-seated, confined lesions is improved. In turn, these improvements decrease retraction, thereby decreasing patient morbidity and improving patient outcomes.

This article discusses the two-point method for determining the best corridor of approach to any brain stem lesion as well as the principles of working depth, working area, and angle of attack. Two examples of novel approaches to the upper and mid brain stem, the extreme lateral supracerebellar infratentorial and the extended orbitozygomatic, are used as paradigms for discovering the novel surgical approach to highlight the application of these ideas.

THE TWO-POINT METHOD

The two-point method (2, 5) is not a novel surgical approach. Rather, it is a logical method for determining the best corridor of approach to a given brain stem lesion. In this simple method, a point is placed in the center of the lesion. A second point is placed on the perimeter of the lesion, where it comes nearest to the surface of the brain stem. A line extending from the first point through the second point and out through the skull is then drawn. This line indicates the best angle for approaching the lesion (*Fig. 4.1*). A craniotomy along this line of at-

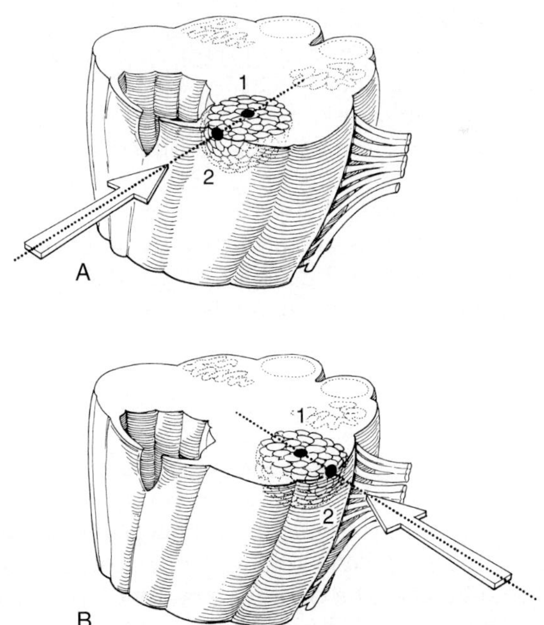

FIG. 4.1 The two-point method for determining the best approach to brain stem lesions. The first point is placed at the center of the lesion, and the second point is placed where the lesion comes closest to the surface of the brain stem. A line is then drawn from the first point through the second point and out through the skull. The trajectory of this line dictates the corridor of approach to the lesion. Examples are shown for suboccipital (*A*) and far-lateral (*B*) approaches. [Reprinted with permission from Barrow Neurological Institute.]

tack is planned, and the principles of working depth, working area, and angle of attack are applied to optimize the surgical approach.

FIRST PRINCIPLES IN DEVELOPING A NOVEL SURGICAL APPROACH

The need to discover the novel surgical approach is driven by the necessity to access a region of the neuraxis that is difficult to reach with conventional approaches. Conventional approaches are inadequate when they require excessive retraction or excessive bone removal, either of which may increase patient morbidity. Conventional approaches are often modified to develop an alternative, superior approach. The three most important principles used to modify existing approaches or to design novel ones are working depth, working area, and angle of attack (3).

Working depth refers to the distance between the surgeon's hands when held in the working position and the surgical target. Minimizing working depth can be as simple as minimizing the profile of the retraction system being used. High-profile retractors for holding the scalp flap should be replaced by fish hooks or similar low-profile means. Higher-profile, articulated retractors could add several millimeters to more than a centimeter to the working depth. In designing a novel approach, extending the amount of bone that is removed can bring the surgeon closer to the target, thereby decreasing the working depth.

Working area refers to the sum of the contiguous polygonal surfaces viewed by the surgeon at working depth by tilting the microscope. This working area is maximized by thorough dissection of the arachnoid and by optimizing the exposure of a given craniotomy by removing enough bone. This optimization means extending the craniotomy to maximize the working area without incurring additional morbidity and mortality.

Angle of attack is the angle measured between the relaxed brain and the surface of the skull or regional dural reflection (*Fig. 4.2*). Again, this angle is maximized by thorough arachnoid dissection and by optimizing the extension of bone removed during the craniotomy. Removing additional bone at the edges of a craniotomy increases the angle over which structures at the working depth can be viewed.

Extreme Lateral Supracerebellar Infratentorial Approach

The extreme lateral supracerebellar infratentorial (ELSI) approach provides access to the posterolateral mesencephalon (6) (*Fig. 4.3*). Standard approaches to this region either fail to provide adequate exposure or are associated with unacceptable risks. The mid-

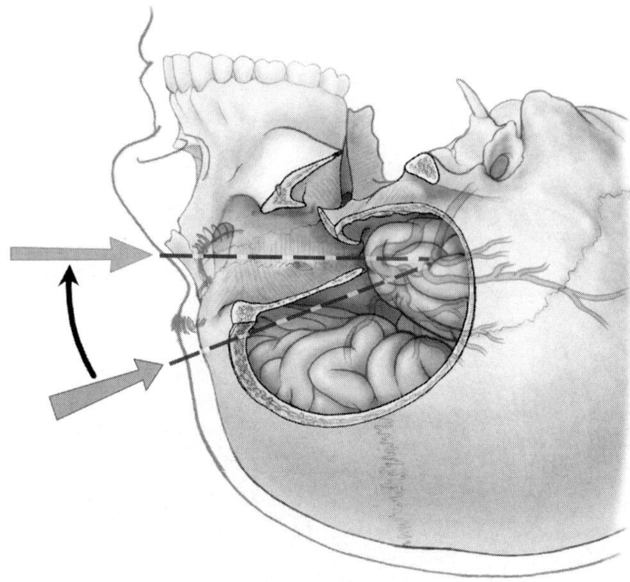

FIG. 4.2 Angle of attack. The line drawing depicts the increase in the working angle between the surface of the brain and skull base when a pterional craniotomy is modified to an orbitozygomatic craniotomy. [Reprinted with permission from Barrow Neurological Institute.]

line and paramedian supracerebellar infratentorial approaches provide inadequate exposure. The transpetrosal approaches that provide adequate exposure involve drilling through the bony labyrinth and cochlea and manipulating the facial nerve. Hearing loss and transient facial weakness result, and the risk of cerebrospinal fluid (CSF) leak is increased. The subtemporal approach risks injury to the vein of Labbé and an associated venous infarction. The ELSI approach to the posterolateral mesencephalon maximizes working area and angle of attack. Concomitantly, working depth is minimized, and the unnecessary morbidities associated with the transpetrosal approaches are avoided.

Patients can be positioned either prone or in the park bench position with the lesion-side up or supine with the ipsilateral shoulder elevated and the head turned away from the side of the lesion if their habitus is favorable. The Mayfield headholder is used for rigid fixation. The mastoid should be at the highest point of the surgical field. Image-guided, frameless stereotaxy can be used to optimize head positioning for any given lesion and to appreciate the course of the sigmoid and transverse sinuses. Preoperatively, a lumbar drain can be

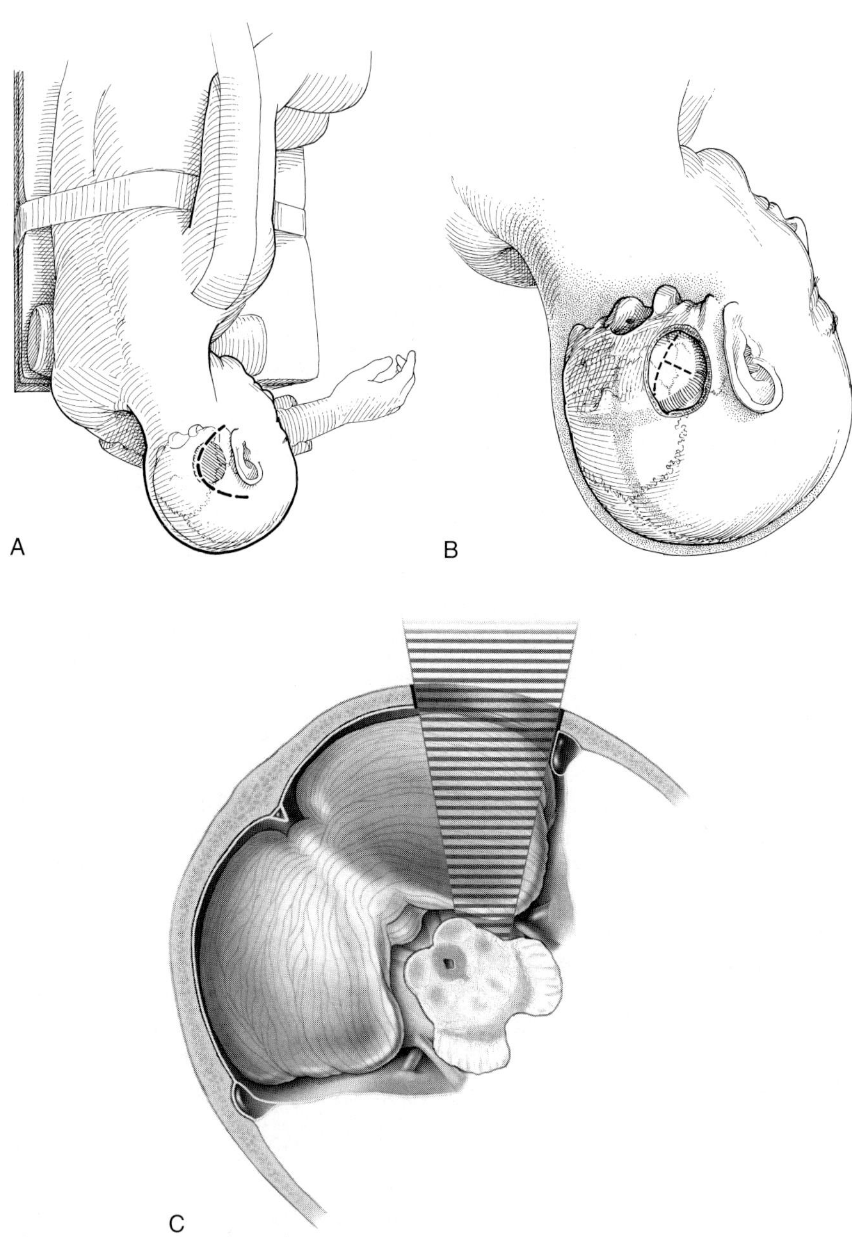

FIG. 4.3 The extreme lateral supracerebellar infratentorial approach. (*A*) The patient is placed in the park bench position. The extent of the craniotomy is shown. (*B*) The corridor of approach to the posterolateral mesencephalon. (*C*) The subsequent exposure of this region. [Reprinted with permission from Barrow Neurological Institute.]

placed to remove CSF to maximize brain relaxation. The incision is C-shaped and based laterally. The mastoid tip and the posterior temporal region lie at its extremes.

A high-speed drill is used to create a burr hole that exposes the edge of the sigmoid sinus. The dura is cleared from the underside of the skull, and a craniotomy is completed using a side-cutting bit with a guard and footplate. The craniotomy extends several centimeters above the transverse sinus but is predominantly suboccipital. The dura is opened based on the sinuses. The transverse sinus is uncovered so that it can be retracted with tack-up sutures placed through oblique holes drilled into the occipital edge of the craniotomy to maximize the working area and angle of attack.

CSF is removed from the lumbar drain or cisterna magna to optimize cerebellar relaxation. Dissection of the arachnoid between the tentorium and the cerebellum increases the working area by allowing further cerebellar relaxation. A retractor is used on the surface of the cerebellum if needed. Bridging veins are coagulated and cut only as necessary to supply the needed exposure. Section of the proximal tentorium also can be used to increase the exposure and working area at the working depth. Once the exposure is completed, the specifics of lesion resection are dictated by the pathology.

Extended Orbitozygomatic Approach

The extended orbitozygomatic (EOZ) approach is used to access the midbasilar region (4) (*Fig. 4.4*). Before this novel surgical approach was developed, lesions in this region were treated through transpetrosal approaches. Like the ELSI approach, radical transpetrosal approaches afford adequate working depth, working area, and angle of attack, but the costs are hearing loss and the risk of damage to facial nerve function. The EOZ approach is based on the standard orbitozygomatic craniotomy (7), which already optimizes working depth, working area, and angle of attack for surgery in the region of the basilar apex. With the addition of resection of the anterior clinoid process and the upper clivus, working area and angle of attack are optimized for an anterior approach to the midbasilar region.

The patient is positioned supine with the head turned away from the lesion in the Mayfield fixation system. The malar eminence should be at the highest point in the field. The incision extends from a point 1 cm in front of the tragus near the zygomatic root to near the hairline over the contralateral midpupillary line in a gentle arc. The skin flap is elevated in continuity with the superficial temporalis fascia to protect the frontalis branch of the facial nerve. Subperiosteal dissec-

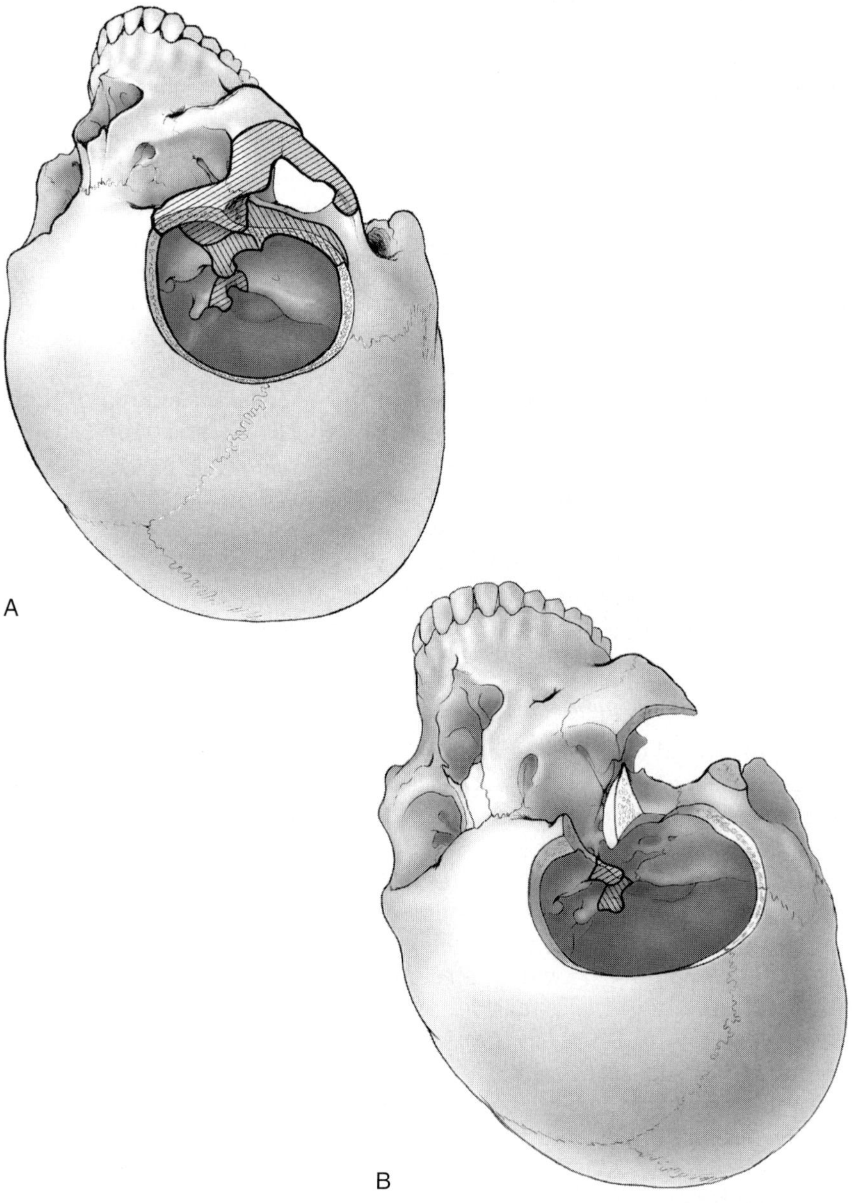

FIG. 4.4 The extended orbitozygomatic approach showing the view of the midbasilar region obtained through a pterional approach (*A*) and through a standard orbitozygomatic approach (*B*). Cross-hatching indicates the bone impeding the view of the midbasilar artery.

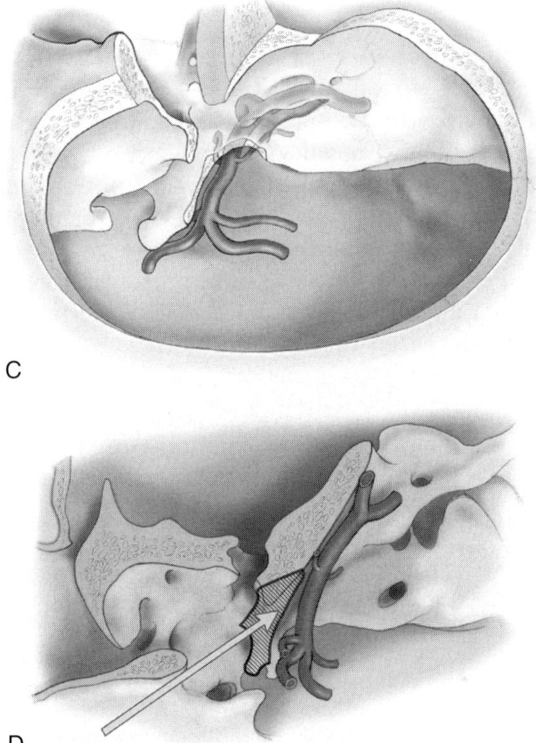

FIG. 4.4 *Continued.* The view achieved with additional removal of the anterior clinoid process (*C*) and upper clivus (*D*) is also shown. [Reprinted with permission from Barrow Neurological Institute.]

tion is used to expose the frontal bone, orbital rim, malar eminence, and zygomatic arch. The temporalis muscle is mobilized from the underlying skull. The periorbita is then freed from the superior and lateral orbital walls medial to the supraorbital nerve.

A burr hole is created in the temporal bone, and a standard pterional craniotomy flap with an attached myofascial temporalis cuff is created using a side-cutting burr with guard and footplate. The orbitozygomatic bar is removed using a reciprocating saw as described previously (7). The dura is incised in a semilunar fashion based anteriorly and is then tacked down over the periorbita. The anterior clinoid and the upper portion of the clivus on the ipsilateral side are removed intradurally using a high-speed drill to complete the exposure of the midbasilar region.

SUMMARY

Discovering the novel surgical approach requires surgeons to look beyond the dogma of current practices. By applying simple principles and concepts, such as the two-point method, working depth, working area, and angle of attack, novel approaches can evolve from existing approaches to improve exposure and decrease patient morbidity. The EOZ and ELSI are two examples in which these principles have been applied to generate novel surgical approaches by modifying existing ones. Compared to the previously used approaches, both of these novel approaches afford superior access to their respective regions of the brain stem with decreased rates of morbidity.

REFERENCES

1. Boorstin DJ: *The Discovers. A History of Man's Search to Know His World and Himself,* 1st ed. New York, Vintage Books (Random House), 1985.
2. Brown AP, Thompson BG, Spetzler RF: The two-point method: Evaluating brain stem lesions. **BNI Quarterly** 12:20–27, 1996.
3. Gonzalez LF, Crawford NR, Horgan MA, et al.: Working area and angle of attack in three cranial base approaches: Pterional, orbitozygomatic, and maxillary extension of the orbitozygomatic approach. **Neurosurgery** 50:550–557, 2002.
4. Lawton MT, Daspit CP, Spetzler RF: Technical aspects and recent trends in the management of large and giant midbasilar artery aneurysms. **Neurosurgery** 41: 513–521, 1997.
5. Porter RW, Detwiler PW, Spetzler RF: Surgical approaches to the brain stem. **Operative Techniques in Neurosurgery** 3:114–123, 2000.
6. Vishteh AG, David CA, Marciano FF, et al.: Extreme lateral supracerebellar infratentorial approach to the posterolateral mesencephalon: Technique and clinical experience. **Neurosurgery** 46:384–389, 2000.
7. Zabramski JM, Kiris T, Sankhla SK, et al.: Orbitozygomatic craniotomy. Technical note. **J Neurosurg** 89:336–341, 1998.

CHAPTER

5

Honored Guest Presentation: Discovery of the Spine Specialist: Instrumentation of the Cervical Spine

ERIC W. NOTTMEIER, M.D., AND VOLKER K.H. SONNTAG, M.D.

For several decades, spinal instrumentation has been used to augment spinal fusions and to correct deformities as well as an alternative or supplement to external orthosis. Only recently, however, has instrumentation become an almost routine technique in the treatment of cervical spine disorders. This explosion of cervical instrumentation in the last 10 to 15 years has paralleled the development of the spine specialist in the fields of neurosurgery and orthopedics. The following discussion describes and documents the development of cervical instrumentation.

POSTERIOR WIRING TECHNIQUES

The first spinal fusion using instrumentation was described by B.E. Hadra in 1891 (30). He used wire to hold together adjacent spinous processes in a patient with a fracture-dislocation of the cervical spine. Hadra's description of spinous process wiring was the beginning of an evolution in spinal surgery instrumentation that still continues. In 1942, W.A. Rogers (55) described the principles of posterior cervical fusion for trauma, which included using intraoperative traction, fracture reduction, wire fixation around the spinous processes, and bone grafting. This technique involved stabilizing adjacent vertebrae by passing a cerclage wire or cable through a hole made in the spinous process of each vertebrae and then tightening it accordingly (*Fig. 5.1*). Autogenous bone graft was then placed over the decorticated spinous processes and laminae or packed within the joint space (55). This technique proved to be efficient and reliable. All 11 patients in Rogers' series achieved sound fusion. Subsequent modifications of the Rogers interspinous wiring technique include the Whitehill modification (69) (*Fig. 5.2*), the Bohlman triple-wire technique (41) (*Fig. 5.3*), the Benzel-Kesterson modification (6) (*Fig. 5.4*), the Murphy-Southwick

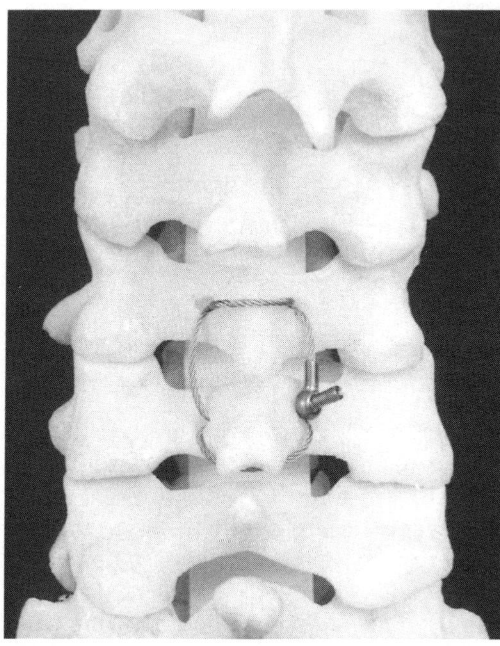

FIG. 5.1 The Rogers interspinous wiring technique. [From Sawin P, Sonntag VKH: Techniques of posterior subaxial cervical fusion. **Operative Techniques in Neurosurgery** 1(2): 72–83, 1998; reprinted with permission from WB Saunders.]

modification (49) (*Fig. 5.5*), and the Cahill oblique facet wiring technique (13) (*Fig. 5.6*).

In 1977, Callahan et al. (14) described a technique of cervical fusion using facet wiring. The technique was used in postlaminectomy patients

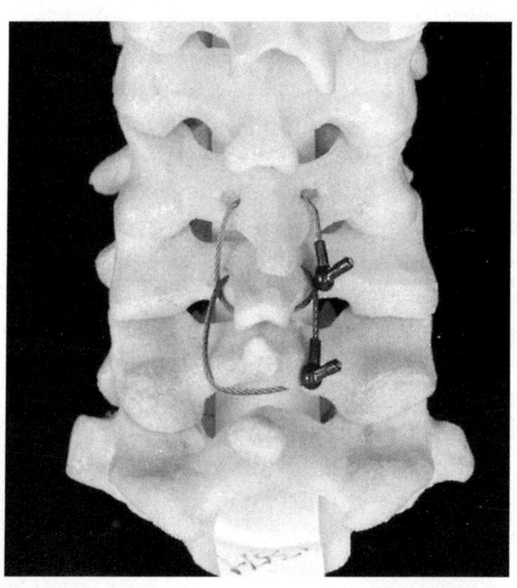

FIG. 5.2 The Whitehill modified wiring technique. [From Sawin P, Sonntag VKH: Techniques of posterior subaxial cervical fusion. **Operative Techniques in Neurosurgery** 1(2):72–83, 1998; reprinted with permission from WB Saunders.]

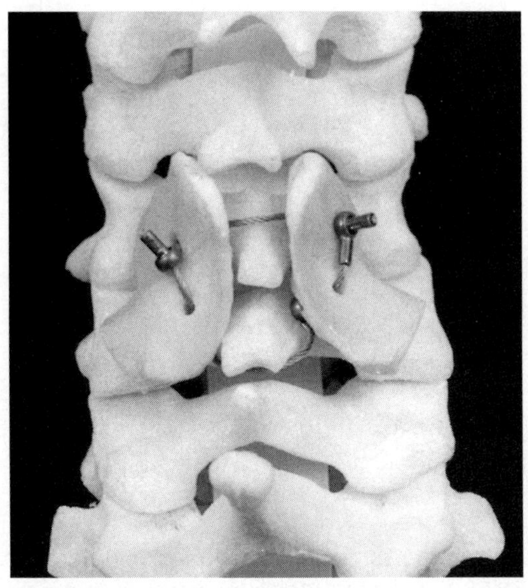

FIG. 5.3 The Bohlman triple-wire technique. [From Sawin P, Sonntag VKH: Techniques of posterior subaxial cervical fusion. **Operative Techniques in Neurosurgery** 1(2):72–83, 1998; reprinted with permission from WB Saunders.]

to prevent postlaminectomy kyphosis. This procedure involved drilling holes perpendicularly through the inferior articular processes of the facet joints to be fused, disrupting these facet joints by removing the articular cartilage, and then fastening a corticocancellous graft over these facets using a wire or cable passed through the drilled hole (*Fig. 5.7*). The posterior surface of the facet was decorticated before the graft was

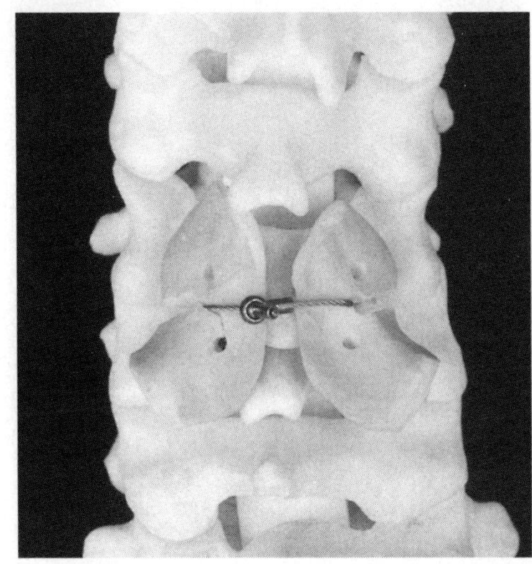

FIG. 5.4 The Benzel-Kesterson wiring technique. [From Sawin P, Sonntag VKH: Techniques of posterior subaxial cervical fusion. **Operative Techniques in Neurosurgery** 1(2):72–83, 1998; reprinted with permission from WB Saunders.]

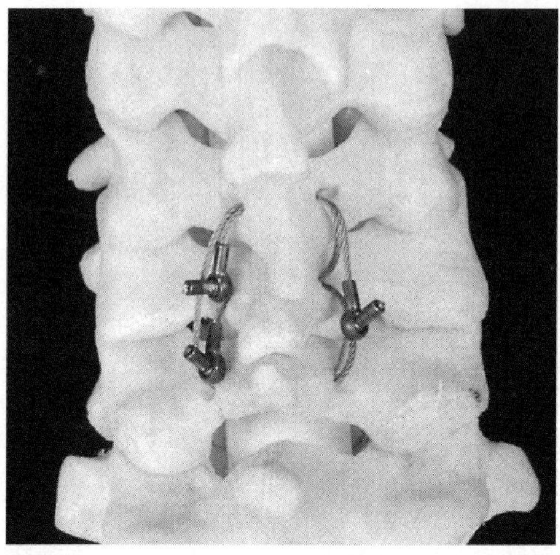

FIG. 5.5 The Murphy-Southwick wiring technique. [From Sawin P, Sonntag VKH: Techniques of posterior subaxial cervical fusion. **Operative Techniques in Neurosurgery** 1(2):72–83, 1998; reprinted with permission from WB Saunders.]

placed to promote bony fusion. A significant advantage of this technique is that it did not require intact spinous processes or laminae.

HALIFAX INTERLAMINAR CLAMP

Despite the multiple modifications of the Rogers' interspinous wiring technique, wire breakage and pullout from bone remained potential problems. Consequently, alternatives to wire fixation were developed. In 1975, Tucker (68) first described the use of an interlaminar clamp-

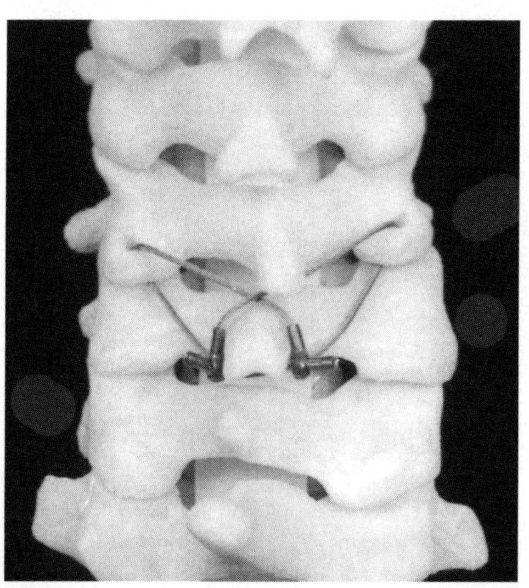

FIG. 5.6 The Cahill oblique facet wiring technique. [From Sawin P, Sonntag VKH: Techniques of posterior subaxial cervical fusion. **Operative Techniques in Neurosurgery** 1(2):72–83, 1998; reprinted with permission from WB Saunders.]

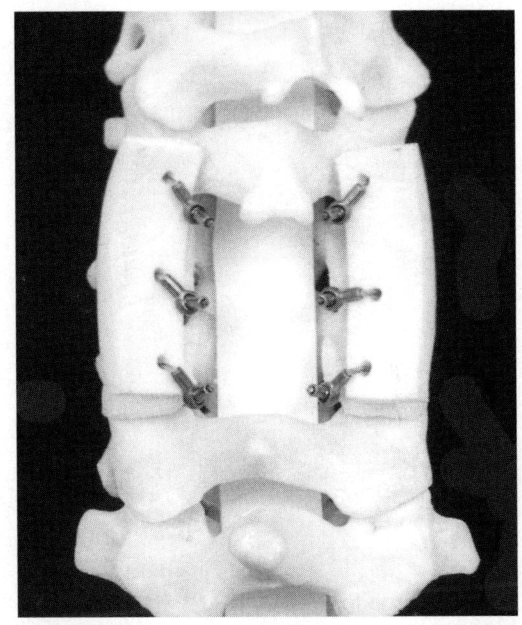

FIG. 5.7 Callahan facet fusion technique. [From Sawin P, Sonntag VKH: Techniques of posterior subaxial cervical fusion. **Operative Techniques in Neurosurgery** 1(2):72–83, 1998; reprinted with permission from WB Saunders.]

and-screw system to treat cervical subluxation inferior to C1-C2. After Holness et al. (34) published their experience with 51 patients having cervical injuries treated with the system in 1984, the popularity of the cervical interlaminar clamp increased. Two patients needed a reoperation and replacement of the clamps for recurrent subluxation, but all 51 patients eventually achieved solid fusion. Holness et al. practiced in Halifax (Nova Scotia, Canada), and the system was referred to and marketed as the Halifax clamp (American Medical Electronics, Inc., Richardson, TX), as mentioned in an article by Schulder in 1996 (61). Composed of titanium, the Halifax clamp system consisted of clamps and screws of various sizes. Bilateral application of the clamps (*Fig. 5.8*), supplemented with autogenous bone graft, was recommended. Halifax clamps proved to be useful in the treatment of subaxial incompetence of the posterior cervical ligament with traumatic or nontraumatic origins (2, 66). The use of Halifax clamps for atlantoaxial arthrodesis was associated with less favorable outcomes (2, 48, 62, 66).

POSTERIOR ATLANTOAXIAL ARTHRODESIS

In 1910, Mixter and Osgood (44) performed the first posterior atlantoaxial arthrodesis. They used a silk thread to fixate the posterior arch of C1 to the spinous process of C2. Approximately 30 years later,

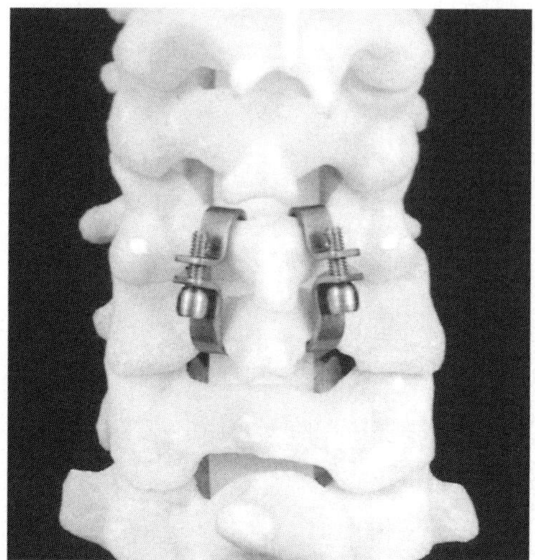

FIG. 5.8 The Halifax interlaminar clamp. [From Sawin P, Sonntag VKH: Techniques of posterior subaxial cervical fusion. **Operative Techniques in Neurosurgery** 1(2): 72–83, 1998; reprinted with permission from WB Saunders.]

Gallie used steel wire and bone grafting to perform posterior atlantoaxial arthrodesis. Although Gallie did not publish the specific technique, McGraw and Rusch (42) and Fielding et al. (21) later provided detailed descriptions. The technique involved passing steel wire under the arch of C1 and then around or through the spinous process of C2. An iliac crest graft was placed over the posterior aspects of C1 and C2. The graft was notched inferiorly to fit around the spinous process of C2. The ends of the wire were fastened on top of the graft to hold it in place (*Fig. 5.9*). This construct, however, allowed persistent rotation and translation at the C1-C2 level (26). The potential also existed for a posteriorly displaced, type II odontoid fracture to be further displaced when the posterior elements of C1 and C2 were forced together by tightening the wire over the graft (65).

In 1978, Brooks and Jenkins (9) described their method of posterior atlantoaxial arthrodesis, which involved wedging two tricortical iliac crest grafts between the posterior elements of C1 and C2. The grafts were placed laterally, one on each side, and held in place by wire passed through the sublaminar space of C1 and C2. The wire was then fastened over the graft (*Fig. 5.10*). This construct provided greater biomechanical stability than the Gallie technique (26), but the disadvantage of sublaminar wire passage at two adjacent cervical levels increased the risk of neurologic injury (65).

In 1989 Sonntag and Dickman (63) described a technique for posterior atlantoaxial arthrodesis that combined the principles of both the Gallie and Brooks technique. In this technique, a bicortical graft was

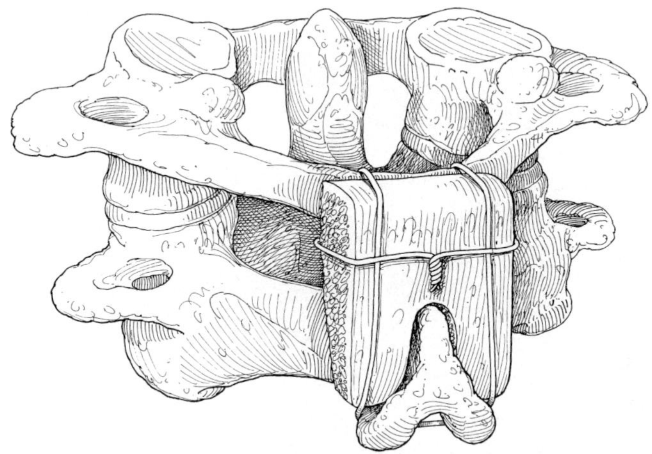

FIG. 5.9 The Gallie technique of posterior atlantoaxial arthrodesis. [Reprinted with permission from Barrow Neurological Institute.]

notched inferiorly to accommodate the C2 spinous process. The graft was held into place by a wire or cable passed in the sublaminar plane at C1 and then around the spinous process of C2. The wire or cable was tightened, compressing the graft between the posterior elements of C1 and C2 (*Fig. 5.11*). This technique avoided sublaminar passage of wire or cable at C2 while providing superb translational and rota-

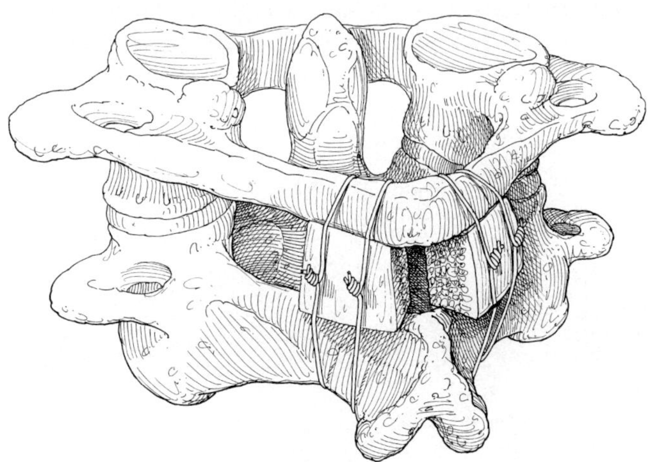

FIG. 5.10 The Brooks technique of posterior atlantoaxial arthrodesis. [Reprinted with permission from Barrow Neurological Institute.]

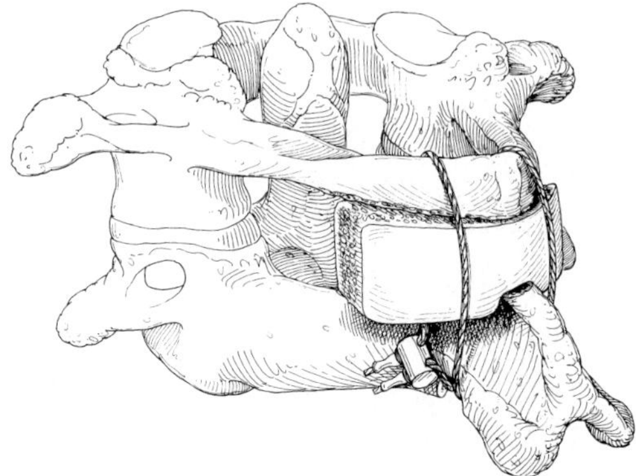

FIG. 5.11 The Sonntag method of posterior atlantoaxial arthrodesis. [Reprinted with permission from Barrow Neurological Institute.]

tional stability. When supplemented with external immobilization with a Halo brace, the fusion rate was 86% (63).

In 1987, Magerl and Seemann (40) first described posterior C1-C2 transarticular screw fixation. The advantages of this technique included greater stability in atlantoaxial rotation and translation compared to wiring techniques (46). When combined with interspinous wiring, posterior C1-C2 transarticular screw fixation provided excellent fusion rates without the need for the patient to wear a Halo orthosis after surgery (64) (*Fig. 5.12*). The technique, however, is technically challenging, with the potential for catastrophic injury even in experienced hands. Careful preoperative planning is essential. The anatomy of C1 and C2 must be studied carefully, with particular attention given to the course of the vertebral artery. An anomalous course of the vertebral artery can be a contraindication to using this

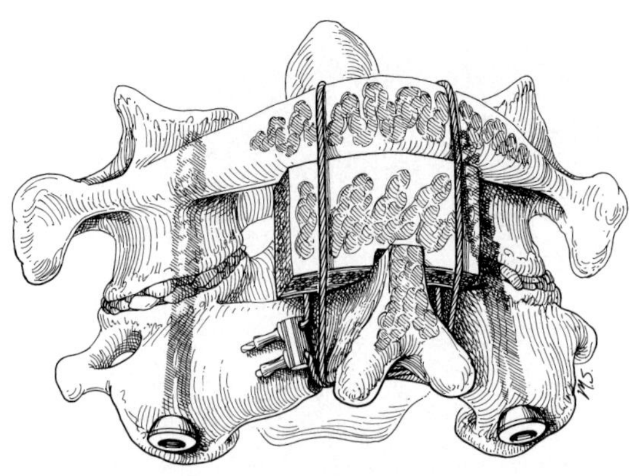

FIG. 5.12 Bilateral transarticular screws combined with posterior C1-C2 interspinous wiring. [With permission from Barrow Neurological Institute.]

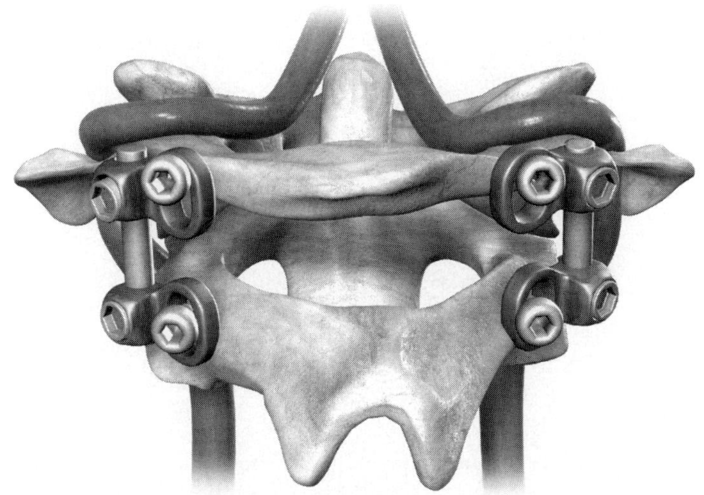

FIG. 5.13 C1 lateral mass–C2 pedicle screw construct. [Reprinted with permission from Barrow Neurological Institute.]

technique. If the anomalous vertebral artery course is unilateral, however, then a single, contralateral transarticular screw can be placed with acceptable clinical stability (50).

Recently, a new method of posterior atlantoaxial arthrodesis has been introduced. This technique consists of a connecting C1 lateral mass screw to a C2 pedicle screw or C2 pars interarticularis screw via a rod (22, 32, 67) (*Fig. 5.13*). Compared to C1-C2 transarticular screw fixation, this technique is associated with less risk of injuring the vertebral artery because of the differences in trajectory and locations of the C2 screws. An anomalous course of the vertebral artery is not necessarily a contraindication to using this technique, as it is with the placement of C1-C2 transarticular screws. Furthermore, this technique requires no preliminary reduction of C1 and C2 before the instrumentation is placed. The instrumentation can be placed and then subsequently used to reduce C1 and C2 by manipulating the screw-rod construct (32). A recent biomechanical study (39) demonstrated that the C1 lateral mass–C2 pedicle screw construct, although not as strong as transarticular screws, was stable enough to be used for posterior atlantoaxial arthrodesis. The authors have successfully combined C1 lateral mass screws with C3 lateral mass screws when instrumentation of C2 was impossible (Sonntag VKH, unpublished data, 2001) (*Fig. 5.14*).

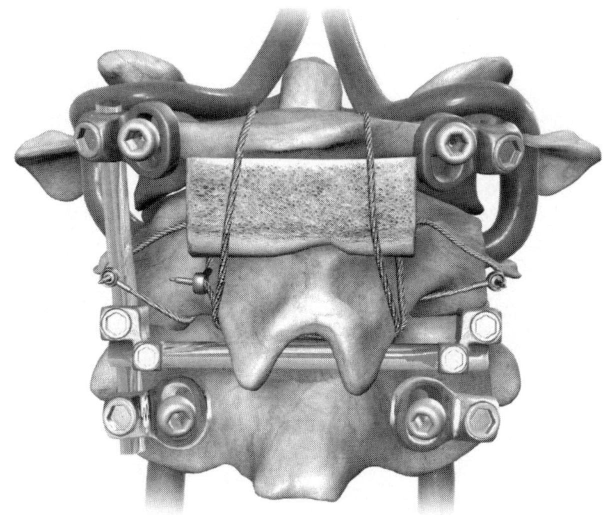

FIG. 5.14 C1-C3 lateral mass construct. [Reprinted with permission from Barrow Neurological Institute.]

ANTERIOR ODONTOID SCREW FIXATION

Traditionally, type II odontoid fractures have been treated with Halo immobilization, but high nonunion rates were associated with significantly displaced fractures (29). Furthermore, type IIA odontoid fractures with comminuted fragments at the base of the dens could not be aligned adequately with Halo immobilization (28). The overall nonunion rate of type II odontoid fractures varied from 15% to 85% (45). Traditionally, surgical treatment of these fractures consisted of posterior C1-C2 arthrodesis, with the resultant disadvantage of significantly limited atlantoaxial rotation. As discussed by Montesano et al. (45), Nakanishi et al., Magerl, and Bohler (8) first reported anterior odontoid screw fixation for the treatment of type II odontoid fractures (*Fig. 5.15*). Anterior odontoid screw fixation provides immediate fixation and is associated with high fusion rates while still maintaining normal atlantoaxial rotation. Whether one or two screws should be used when treating type II odontoid fractures was debated. The two-screw technique was thought to have provided greater rotational stability (19); however, subsequent studies demonstrated no significant biomechanical or clinical advantage to using two-screws compared with one in the treatment of type II odontoid fractures (23, 25, 59).

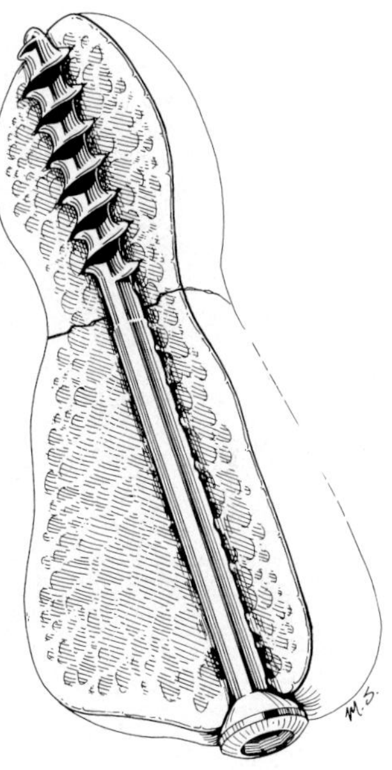

FIG. 5.15 Anterior odontoid screw fixation. [Reprinted with permission from Barrow Neurological Institute.]

OCCIPITOCERVICAL FUSION

In 1927, Foerster (23) described the first occipitocervical fusion. A decade later, Cone and Turner (15) described a method of occipitocervical fusion using iliac crest strut grafts fixated by wire. This technique (as well as other occipitocervical fusion techniques using only bone grafts) was used by surgeons for decades thereafter (24, 38, 43, 51, 52). These techniques, however, were associated with a high rate of pseudarthrosis. The lack of internal rigid stabilization also required postoperative Halo immobilization (20, 24, 38). To circumvent these disadvantages, some surgeons supplemented the wire with methylmethacrylate (10, 36, 70); however, excessive wound breakdown and wire breakage were reported as complications (10, 70).

Described in the late 1980s, the use of contoured rods with segmental wire fixation proved to be a reliable method of achieving internal rigid fixation (3, 20, 36, 52, 58, 65). Wire fixation was achieved via burr holes at the occiput and via interspinous or sublaminar wiring methods at the cervical spine level (*Fig. 5.16*). In addition to providing rigid internal fixation, the contoured rod technique was simple to perform. Using devices such as the BendMeister (Sofamor Danek, Memphis, TN) (*Fig. 5.17*), the rod also could be shaped to accommodate a wide variety of anatomic angles at the occipitocervical junction (4). A dis-

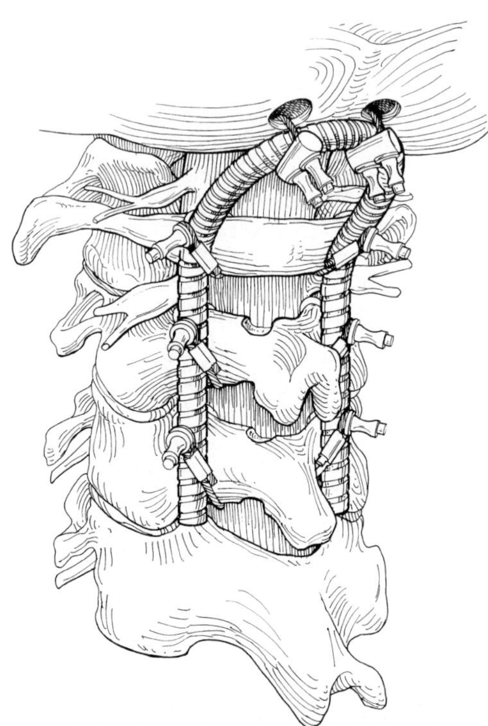

FIG. 5.16 Occipitocervical fusion with contoured rods. [Reprinted with permission from Barrow Neurological Institute.]

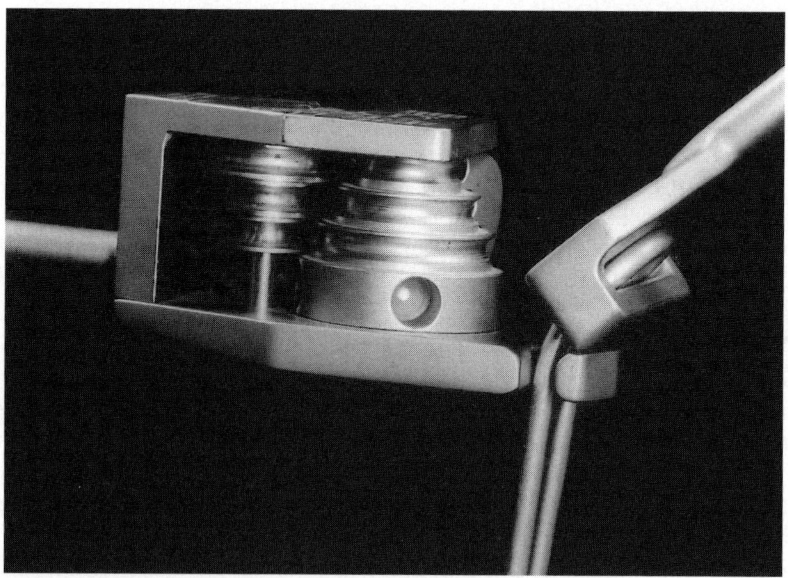

FIG. 5.17 The BendMeister allows the surgeon to place smooth primary and secondary curvatures in the rod for precise fitting to the patient's anatomy. [From (4); reprinted with permission from Lippincott Williams & Wilkins.]

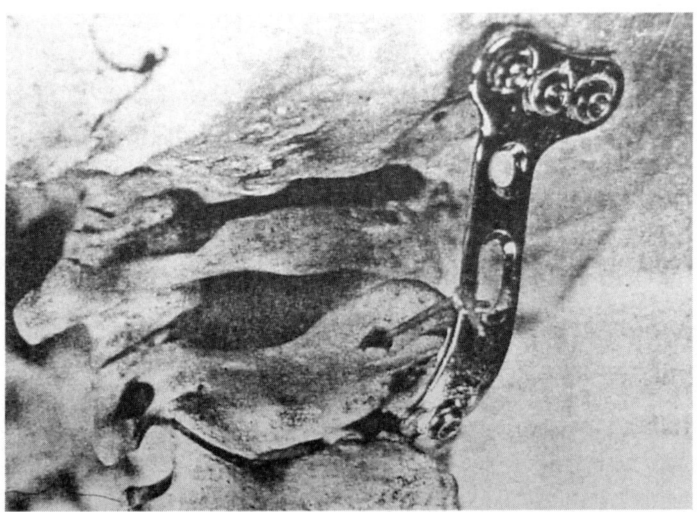

FIG. 5.18 Heywood T-plate. [From (33); reprinted with permission.]

advantage of the technique is that the posterior elements must be intact. Furthermore, biomechanical data have demonstrated that contoured rods are less resistant to cranial settling and rotation compared with plate and screw devices (35).

In 1966, Cregan (17) first described the use of plates and screws for occipitocervical fusion. In 1986, Roy-Camille (56) developed an occipitocervical plate, which was secured to the occiput by cancellous screws. Cervical fixation was obtained by placing C2 pedicle screws and subaxial lateral mass screws (20). In 1988, Heywood et al. (33) described the use of a T-plate for occipitocervical fusion. The plate was designed to be fixated to the midline, where the occiput is thickest (11–17 mm) (*Fig. 5.18*). In 1991, Grob et al. (27) described the use of an inverted Y-plate, which also was fixated to the midline occiput with screws; however, C1-C2 transarticular screws were used for spinal fixation (*Fig. 5.19*). In recent years, numerous instrumentation systems have been developed for occipitocervical fixation. The devices are fixed either to the midline or lateral occiput and linked to any of a variety of lateral mass fixation systems described below.

LATERAL MASS CONSTRUCTS

The use of lateral mass plates and screws for posterior stabilization of the cervical spine began in Europe in the 1970s. The earliest systems included the Louis system (Cremascoli, Milano, Italy), the Roy-

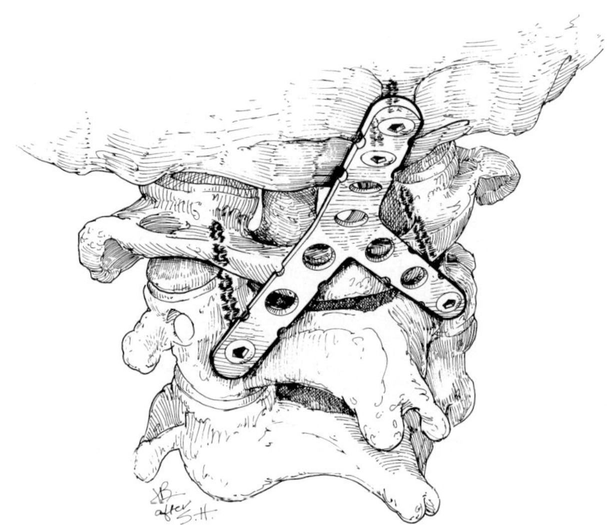

FIG. 5.19 The Y-plate for occipitocervical fusion. [Reprinted with permission from Barrow Neurological Institute.]

Camille system (Francobal, Bagneux, France), and the Magerl AO/ASIF system (Stratek Medical Waldenburg, Switzerland) (37).

The Louis system contained contoured, 6-mm thick, stainless-steel plates with depressed screw holes (*Fig. 5.20*). The self-tapping screws

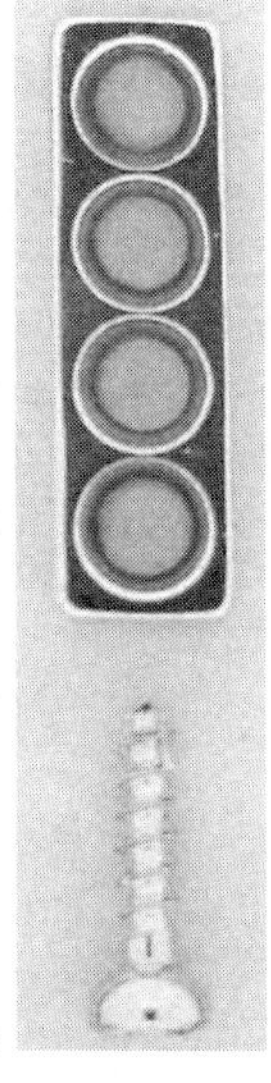

A

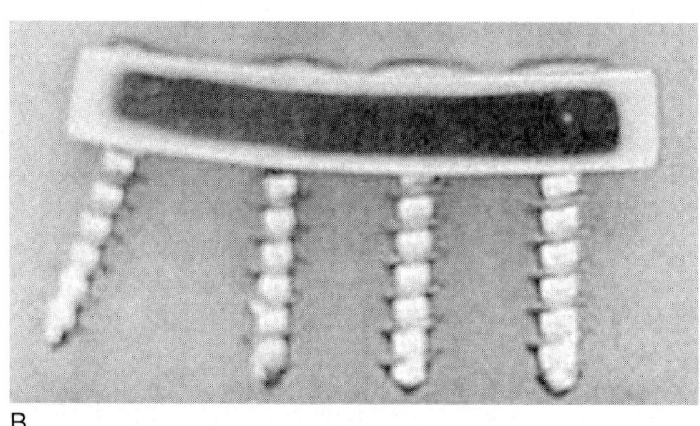

B

FIG. 5.20 Anteroposterior (*A*) and lateral (*B*) views of the Louis lateral mass system. [From (37); reprinted with permission from Lippincott Williams and Wilkins.]

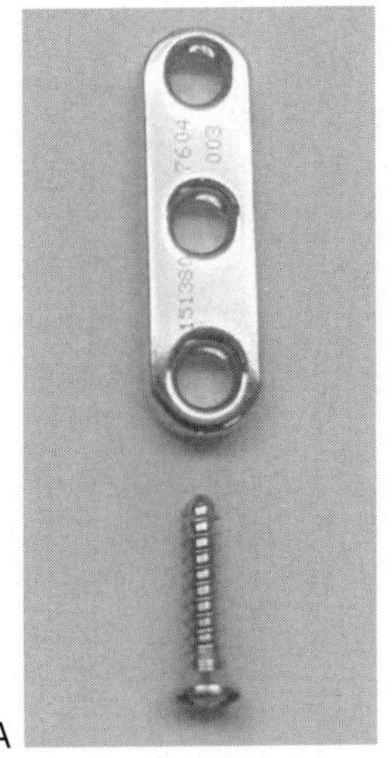

A

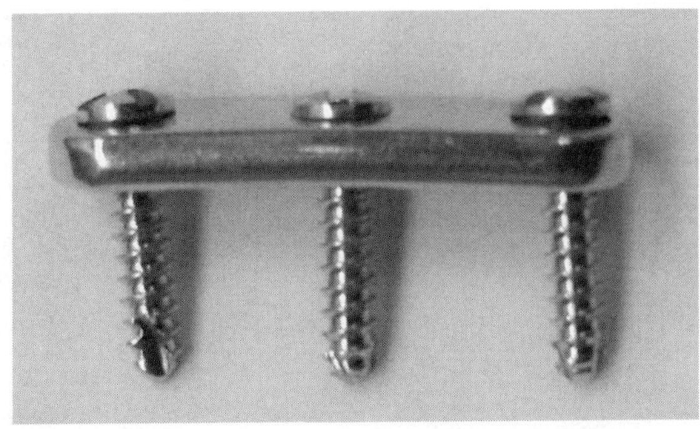

B

FIG. 5.21 Anteroposterior (*A*) and lateral (*B*) views of the Roy-Camille lateral mass system. [Reprinted with permission from Barrow Neurological Institute.]

were 4.5 mm in diameter and inserted perpendicular to the plate. The disadvantages of the Louis system included angulation of the screws toward the nerves as well as encroachment of the suprajacent facet joint by the thickened plate (37).

The Roy-Camille system used plates composed of chrome-cobalt and anchored with 3.5-mm diameter, self-tapping screws (37) (*Fig. 5.21*). The screws were placed in the center of the lateral mass and angled laterally 10° (57). Because the screws were not angled superiorly with the facet, the screw tip would penetrate the inferior facet joint. This configuration led to potential erosion of the facet joint inferior to the proposed levels to be fused.

The Magerl AO/ASIF system contained a thin, 1-mm hook plate with one to two holes (*Fig. 5.22*). The design of this system allowed a variable trajectory for the 4-mm diameter screws. Typically, screws were inserted at a point 2 to 3 mm superior and medial to the center of the facet joint, with a trajectory 20° to 30° superiorly and laterally. The oblique trajectory of the screws minimized injury to the nerve root and vertebral artery and provided significant resistance to the screw pulling out (37).

Lateral mass plating was used for almost two decades in Europe before it was introduced in the United States during the late 1980s. In 1988, Cooper et al. (16) were among the first groups to describe the use of lateral mass plating in the United States. Their series consisted of 20 patients with cervical instability who underwent posterior stabilization using the Roy-Camille plating system. Complications were

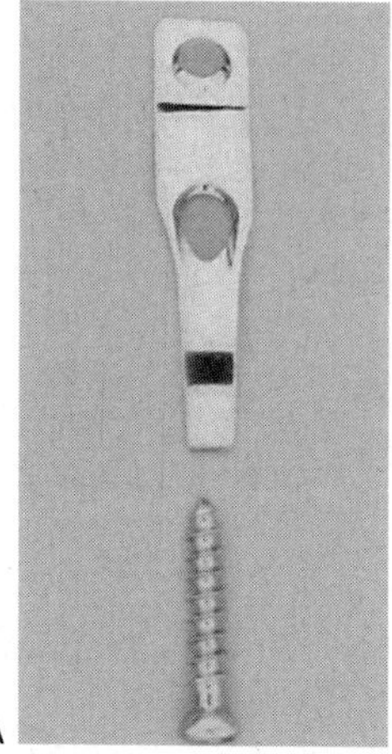

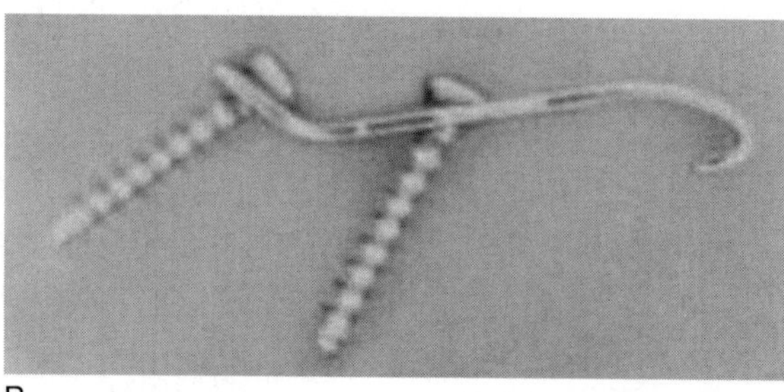

A B

FIG. 5.22 Anteroposterior (*A*) and lateral (*B*) views of the Magerl AO/ASIF lateral mass system. [From (37); reprinted with permission from Lippincott Williams and Wilkins.]

few, and adequate stabilization was achieved in 19 of 20 patients. As lateral mass plating became more popular in the United States, improved lateral mass plating systems were developed.

In 1989, the Haid Universal Bone Plate system was introduced. This system consisted of thick titanium plates containing two, three, or four

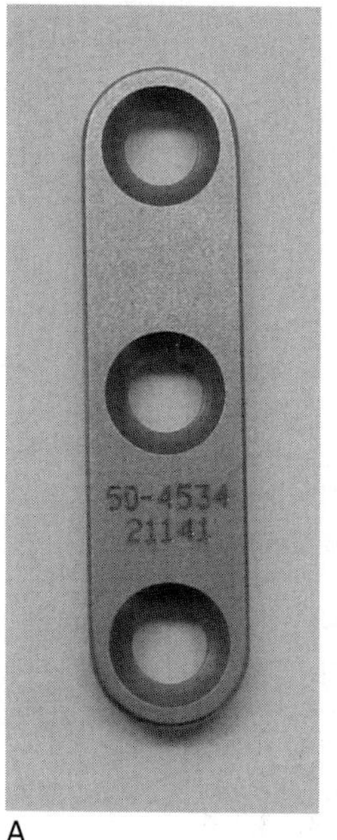

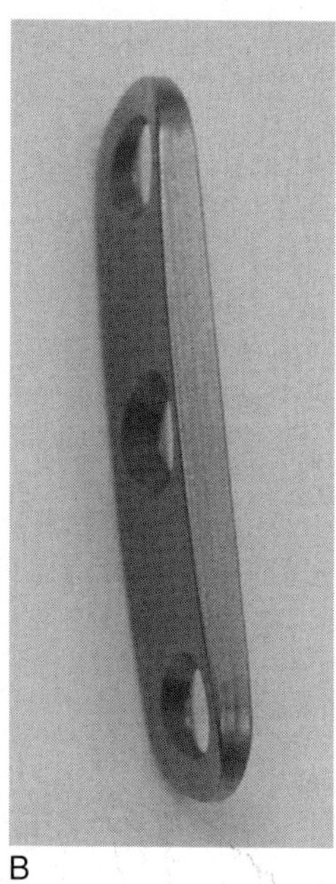

A B

FIG. 5.23 Anteroposterior (*A*) and lateral (*B*) views of the Haid Universal Bone Plate lateral mass system. [Reprinted with permission from Barrow Neurological Institute.]

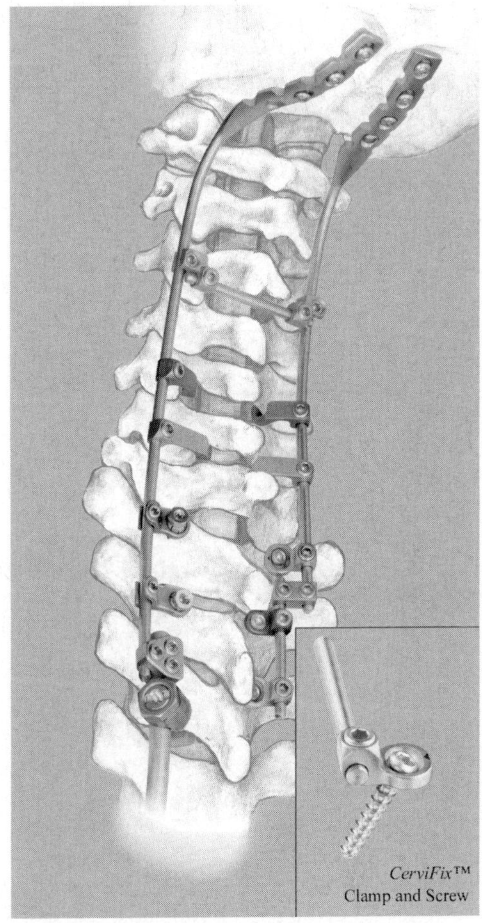

FIG. 5.24 The Cervifix system. [Reprinted with permission from Synthes Spine, Paoli, PA.]

holes (*Fig. 5.23*). The contoured undersurface of the plate allowed lordosis without having to bend the plate. The 15.5-mm long, self-tapping screws allowed bicortical purchase in most individuals (60).

The concept of a universal system for instrumentation of the thoracic and lumbar spine was then applied to the posterior cervical spine. Various elegant systems, which included lateral mass screws, interconnecting rods, and laminar hooks as integral components, were developed. These components enabled intraoperative compression or distraction as well as extension of instrumentation to involve the occiput superiorly or the upper thoracic spine inferiorly. Some examples of these systems include Cervifix (*Fig. 5.24*), Starlock (*Fig. 5.25*), and Vertex (*Fig. 5.26*).

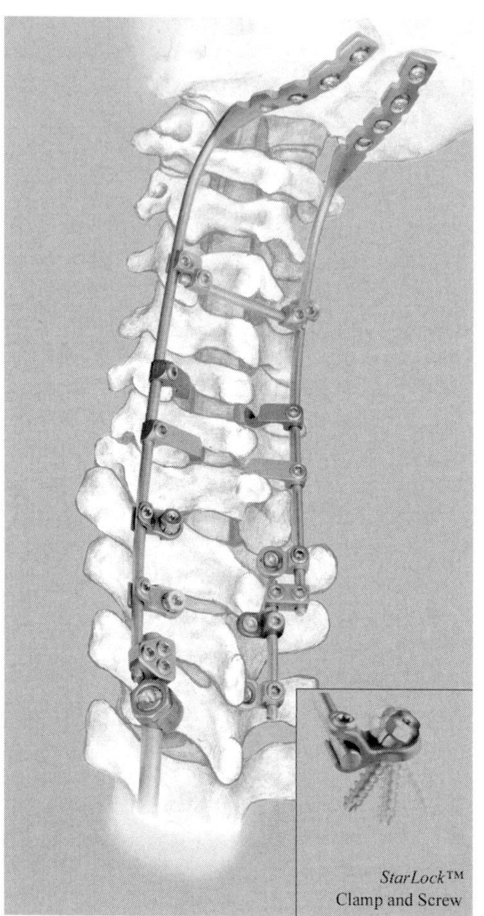

FIG. 5.25 The Starlock system. [Reprinted with permission from Synthes Spine, Paoli, PA.]

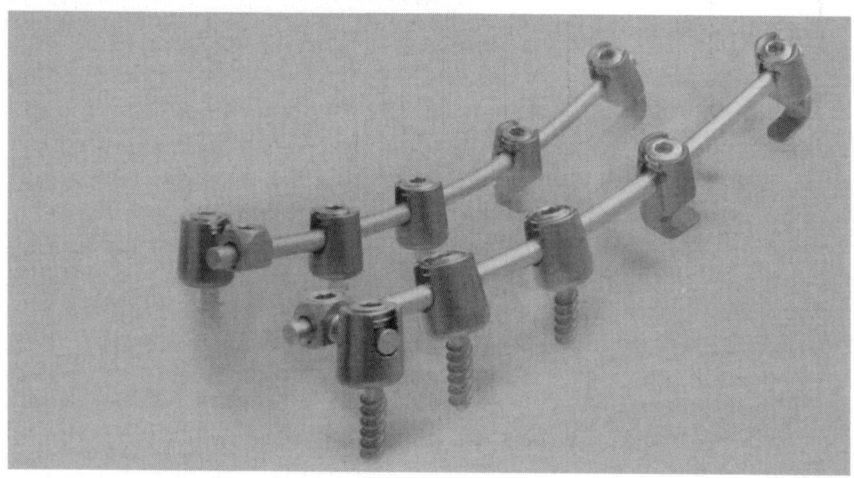

FIG. 5.26 The Vertex system. [Reprinted with permission from Medtronic, Sofamor Danek, Memphis, TN.]

ANTERIOR CERVICAL INSTRUMENTATION

The evolution of anterior cervical plating spans more than four decades and includes a wide variety of designs and concepts. Recently, Haid et al. (31) proposed a classification system that uses biomechanical properties to categorize anterior cervical plating *systems* (*Fig. 5.27*). This classification system clarifies the evolution of anterior cervical plating systems and categorizes the multiple cervical plates currently on the market.

Cervical plating dates to the early 1960s. According to most accounts (12), the earliest application of an anterior cervical plate appears to have occurred in Germany in 1964 by Bohler (7). In 1970, Orozco Delclos and Llovet Tapies reported the use of AO/ASIF small fragment plates and screws (18). Over the next decade, metal plates with bicortical or unicortical screw fixation in the cervical spine continued to be used in European countries.

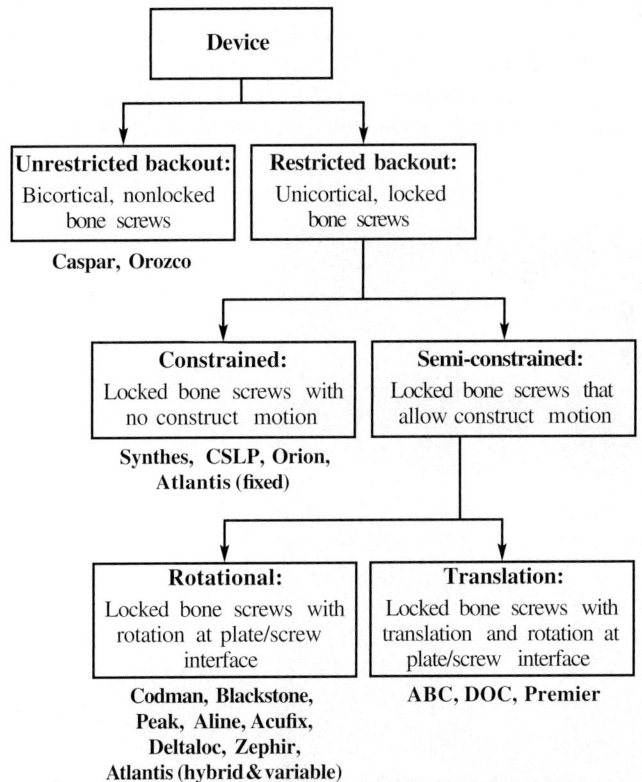

FIG. 5.27 Classification system for anterior cervical plates proposed by the Cervical Spine Study Group. [From (31); reprinted with permission from *Journal of Neurosurgery*.]

One year after Orozco Delclos and Llovet Tapies described the use of small fragment AO/ASIF plates for anterior cervical stabilization, they reported a modification of their technique, which consisted of an "H-" shaped plate (18a). By 1975, they were using double "H" plates to stabilize the cervical spine (54). These "H" plates were termed the *Orozco AO/ASIF cervical plate* and represented the first plate to be used routinely in stabilization of the cervical spine (*Fig. 5.28*). The plates were designed to be used with either one or two levels and contained holes both peripherally and centrally. Bicortical (3.5-mm) screws were used to anchor the plate to the vertebrae (1, 11). No locking mechanism was present on the plate.

The Caspar osteosynthetic plate (Aesculap, San Francisco, CA) was introduced in Europe in 1982 and in the United States in 1986 (*Fig. 5.29*). It was a nonconstrained system with no locking mechanism securing the screw head to the plate, but it required bicortical screw purchase with variable screw trajectory. The noncontoured plate was composed of stainless steel, which produced significant artifact on CT scans and MR images. The device was later manufactured from titanium, which had 90% of the strength of steel but markedly reduced artifact during CT scanning and MR imaging (5). Obtaining bicortical screw purchase was technically demanding even with the use of intraoper-

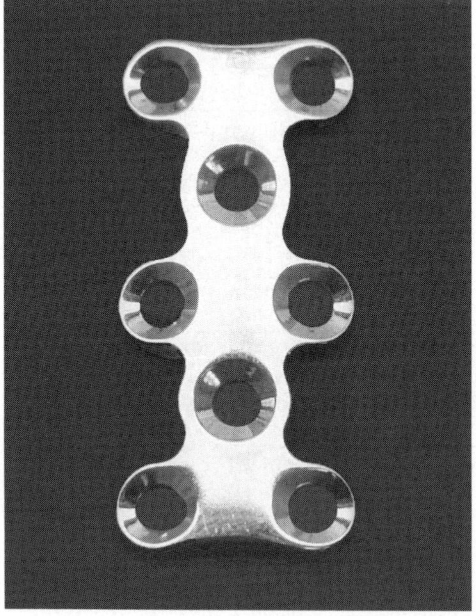

FIG. 5.28 The Orozco AO/ASIF plate. [Reprinted with permission from Barrow Neurological Institute.]

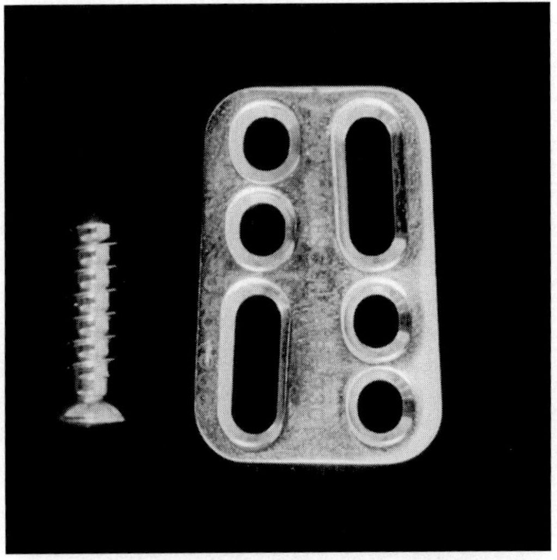

FIG. 5.29 The Caspar plate. [From (31); reprinted with permission from *Journal of Neurosurgery*.]

ative fluoroscopy (12). Although the Caspar plate was popular in its time, the potential risk of injury to the spinal cord and associated structures was a deterrent to some surgeons, and a different device was sought (5).

The Synthes (Synthes Spine; Paoli, PA) unicortical plate was introduced in Europe in 1986 and in the United States in 1991 (*Fig. 5.30*).

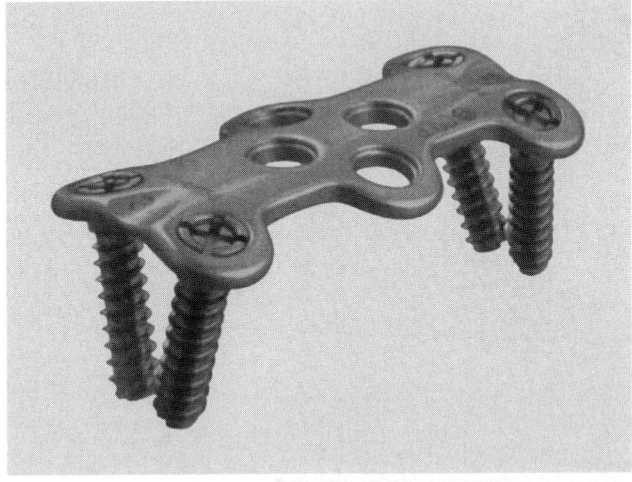

FIG. 5.30 The Synthes CSLP. [Reprinted with permission from Synthes Spine, Paoli, PA.]

It was developed in Switzerland by Morscher et al. (47) and represented a modification of the Orozco plate. Composed of titanium, the Synthes plate had unicortical screws with a locking mechanism consisting of an inner expansion screw. The original screw design was derived from a system designed by Raveh et al. (53) that was used to repair mandibular fractures. The screw in Raveh's system was perforated, hollow, and titanium-sprayed with an inner expansion bolt. This type of screw was originally used in the Synthes. After reports of the screw fracturing, however, it was later discontinued and replaced with a nonperforated screw (12). The screws for the Synthes plate were inserted in a rigidly fixed, convergent manner, making it a constrained

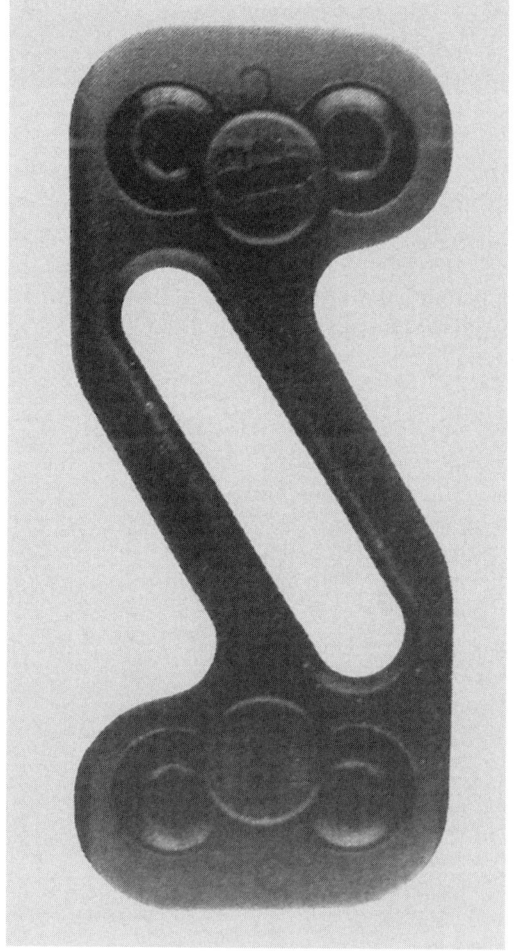

FIG. 5.31 The Orion plate. [From (31); reprinted with permission from *Journal of Neurosurgery*.]

system. The screws were available in 12-, 14-, and 16-mm lengths as well as in 4.0- and 4.35-mm diameters. The plate was manufactured with a preformed lordotic curvature (5).

Another constrained system, the Orion plate (Sofamor Danek, Memphis, TN), was introduced in 1993. It also consisted of a unicortical, rigidly fixed trajectory screw system with a preformed lordotic curve. The locking mechanism differed from that of the Synthes plate in that it involved a separate midline screw that fit over the two bone screws on each end of the plate instead of an inserted expansion screw (*Fig. 5.31*). In the central portion of the Orion plate, a diagonal slot extends superiorly to inferiorly to permit the placement of additional screws. Only one of these additional screws could be inserted per level, and no locking mechanism existed for these screws (5). Screw diameters were the same as those for the Synthes system, and the screws were 11-, 13-, or 15-mm long.

In 1996, the Codman contoured titanium plate (Codman Anterior Cervical Plating System; Johnson & Johnson Professional, Inc., Raynham, MA) was launched (*Fig. 5.32*). This plate was lordotically curved

FIG. 5.32 The Codman plate. [From (31); reprinted with permission from *Journal of Neurosurgery*.]

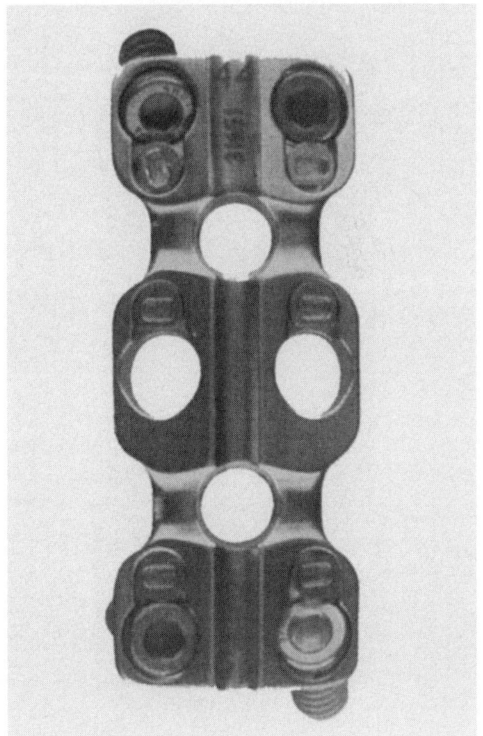

and used an integrated cam as a locking device for its unicortical screws. The screws could be placed at various angles. Additionally, the design of the plate-screw interface allowed a pivoting motion, making the plate the first semiconstrained, rotational device to be produced.

Introduced in March 1998, the DOC anterior cervical stabilization system represented the first semiconstrained, translational device to be produced. It allowed graft subsidence via a sliding mechanism at the plate-screw interface (*Fig. 5.33*). An adjustable, locking cross-connector determined how much translation and, therefore, subsidence the construct would allow. An inner expansion screw was used as a locking mechanism for the unicortical screws. The open design of the construct made it one of the first to allow adequate visualization of the bone graft during application.

The Atlantis plate (Sofamor Danek, Memphis, TN) was introduced in June 1998 and represented the first multiconstruct system ever produced (*Fig. 5.34*). The device used two types of screws: variable angle

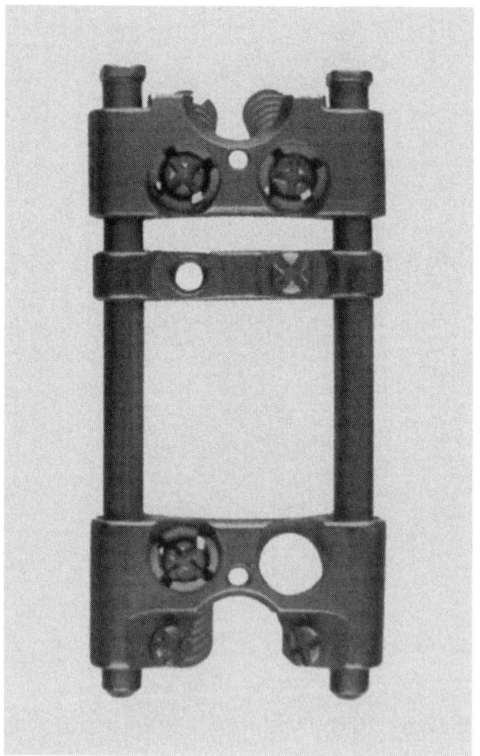

FIG. 5.33 The DOC anterior cervical stabilization system. [From (31); reprinted permission from *Journal of Neurosurgery*.]

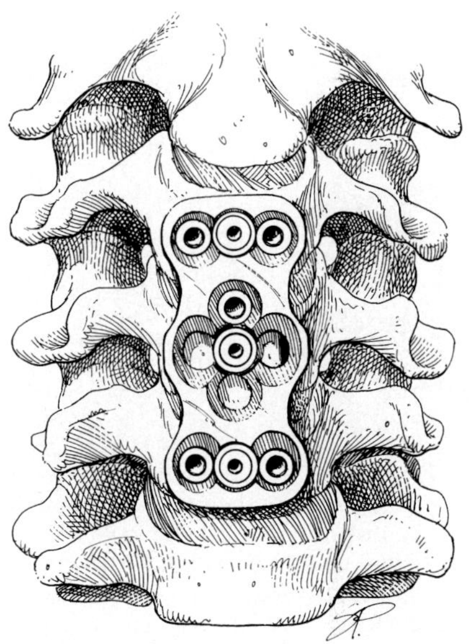

FIG. 5.34 The Atlantis plate. [Reprinted with permission from Barrow Neurological Institute.]

and fixed angle (*Fig. 5.35*). Placement of variable-angle screws resulted in a semiconstrained, rotational device, because the round screw head allowed pivoting at the plate-screw interface (*Fig. 5.36*). Accordingly, placement of fixed-angle screws resulted in a constrained device. A hybrid device was also possible by placing variable-angle screws at the cephalad end and fixed-angle screws at the caudal end. The locking mechanism on the Atlantis plate consisted of an integrated floating washer design. The recently introduced Atlantis "Vision" plate combines all of the features of the original Atlantis plate, but the design

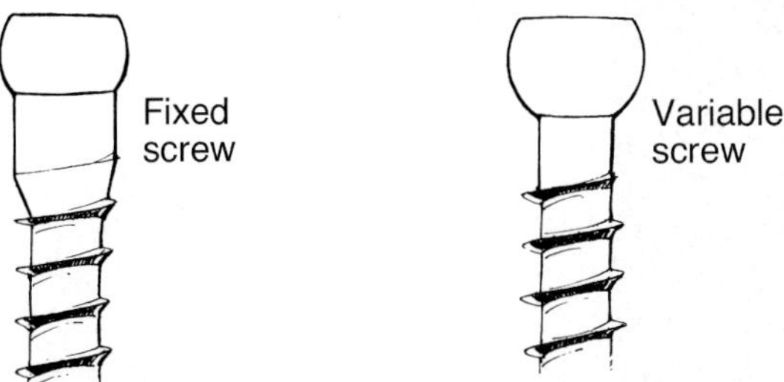

FIG. 5.35 Illustration showing the fixed and variable trajectory screws (Atlantis system). The configuration of the head and proximal shaft of the fixed screw results in a rigid or constrained interface with the Atlantis plate. [Reprinted with permission from Barrow Neurological Institute.]

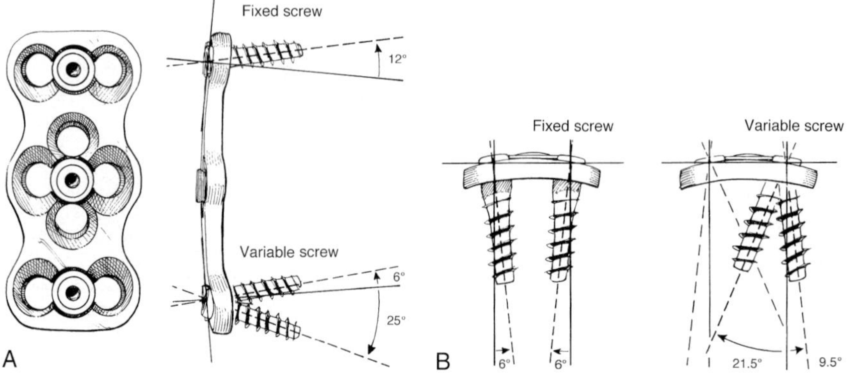

FIG. 5.36 (*A*) Anterior and lateral views of the Atlantis plate demonstrating the screw trajectories in the sagittal plane for fixed and variable screws. Fixed screws are used at the rostral screw site and are angled 12° rostral to a line perpendicular to the plate. Variable screws are used at the caudal screw site. For a 4-mm diameter screw, the arc of rotation possible in the sagittal plane is 6° rostrally or 25° caudally from the perpendicular. (*B*) Axial views of the Atlantis plate demonstrating the degree of angulation in the axial plane for fixed and variable screws. Fixed screws are angled 6° medially from the perpendicular. Variable screws can rotate 9.5° laterally or 21.5° medially from the perpendicular. The degree of angulation possible in the axial and sagittal planes is less with the larger, 4.5-mm diameter screw. [Reprinted with permission from Barrow Neurological Institute.]

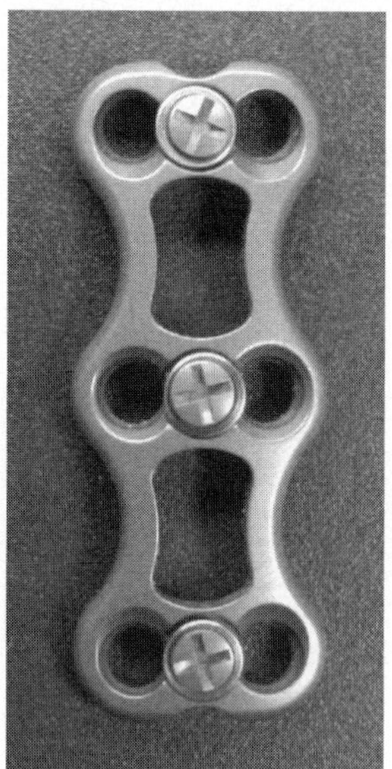

FIG. 5.37 The Atlantis "Vision." [Reprinted with permission from Barrow Neurological Institute.]

of the plate has been modified to allow direct visualization of the bone graft during application of the plate (*Fig. 5.37*).

In the past few years, numerous anterior cervical plating devices have been introduced, with a variety of characteristics demonstrated in the plates above.

CONCLUSIONS

Although the evolution of cervical instrumentation spans more than a century, the most numerous and significant advances have occurred during the past two decades. Rudimentary wiring techniques have been replaced by cervical instrumentation that allows not only rigid internal fixation but also graft subsidence, compression, and distraction and extension of instrumentation to the occiput superiorly and to the thoracic spine inferiorly. On the horizon are bone morphogenic protein and other bone growth stimulators, artificial discs, resorbable implants, genetically driven fusion, and other advances, all of which will play a role in the continuing evolution of cervical instrumentation. In turn, these developments will fuel the continued discovery and development of the spine specialist.

REFERENCES

1. Aebi M, Zuber K, Marchesis D: Treatment of cervical spine injuries with anterior plating. Indications, techniques, and results. **Spine** Suppl 3, 16:S38–S45, 1991.
2. Aldrich FE, Weber PB, Crow WN: Halifax interlaminar clamp for posterior cervical fusion: A long-term follow-up review. **J Neurosurg** 78:702–708, 1993.
3. Apostolides PJ, Dickman CA, Golfinos JG, et al.: Threaded Steinmann pin fusion of the craniovertebral junction. **Spine** 21:1630–1637, 1996.
4. Apostolides PJ, Karahalios DG, Yapp RA, et al.: Use of the BendMeister rod bender for occipitocervical fusion. Technical note. **Neurosurgery** 43:389–391, 1998.
5. Baskin JJ, Vishteh AG, Dickman CA, et al.: Techniques of anterior cervical plating. **Operative Techniques in Neurosurgery** 1:90–102, 1998.
6. Benzel EC, Kesterson I: Posterior cervical interspinous compression wiring and fusion for mid to low cervical spine injuries. **J Neurosurg** 70:893–899, 1989.
7. Bohler J: Immediate and early treatment of traumatic paraplegias [in German]. **Z Orthop Ihre Grenzgab** 103:512–529, 1967.
8. Bohler J: Anterior stabilization for acute fractures and non-unions of the dens. **J Bone Joint Surg Am** 64:18–27, 1982.
9. Brooks AL, Jenkins EB: Atlanto-axial arthrodesis by the wedge compression method. **J Bone Joint Surg Am** 60:279–284, 1978.
10. Bryan WJ, Inglis AE, Sculpo TP, et al.: Methylmethacrylate stabilization for enhancement of posterior cervical arthrodesis in rheumatoid arthritis. **J Bone Joint Surg Am** 64:1045–1050, 1982.
11. Cabanela ME, Ebersold MJ: Anterior stabilization for bursting teardrop fractures of the cervical spine. **Spine** 13:888–891, 1988.

12. Cahill DW: Anterior cervical instrumentation. In: Menezes AH, Sonntag VKH. (eds.), *Principles of Spinal Surgery*. New York: McGraw-Hill, 1996, pp 1105–1120.
13. Cahill DW, Bellegarrigue R, Ducker TB: Bilateral facet to spinous process fusion: A new technique for posterior fusion after trauma. **Neurosurgery** 13:1–4, 1983.
14. Callahan RA, Johnson RM, Margolis RM, et al.: Cervical facet fusion for control of instability following laminectomy. **J Bone Joint Surg Am** 59:991–1002, 1977.
15. Cone W, Turner WG: The treatment of fracture-dislocations of the cervical vertebrae by skeletal traction and fusion. **J Bone Joint Surg** 19:583–602, 1937.
16. Cooper PR, Cohen A, Rosiello A, et al.: Posterior stabilization of cervical spine fractures and subluxations using plates and screws. **Neurosurgery** 23:300–306, 1988.
17. Cregan JC: Internal fixation of the unstable rheumatoid cervical spine. **Ann Rheum Dis** 25:242–252, 1966.
18. Orozco Delclos R, Llovet Tapies J: Osteosintesis en las fracturas de raquis cervical. Nota de Tecnica. **Revista de Orthopedia y Traumatologia** 14:285–288, 1970.
18a. Orozco Delclos R, Llovet Tapies J: Osteosintesis en las lesiones traumaticas y degenerativas de la columna cervical. **Revista Traumatol Cirurg Rehabil** 1:45–52, 1971.
19. Etter C, Coscia M, Jaberg H, et al.: Direct anterior fixation of dens fractures with a cannulated screw system. **Spine** Suppl 3, 16:S25–S32, 1991.
20. Fehlings MG, Errico T, Cooper PR, et al.: Occipitocervical fusion with a five-millimeter malleable rod and segmental fixation. **Neurosurgery** 32:198–207, 1993.
21. Fielding JW, Hawkins RJ, Ratzan SA: Spine fusion for atlanto-axial instability. **J Bone Joint Surg Am** 58:400–407, 1976.
22. Fiore AJ, Haid RW, Rodts GE, et al.: Atlantal lateral mass screws for posterior spinal reconstruction. Technical note. **Neurosurgical Focus** 12:Article 5, 2002.
23. Foerster O: *Die Leitungsbahnen des Schmerzgefühls Und Die Chirurgische Behadlung der Schmerzzustaüde.* Berlin: Urban und Schwarzenberg, 1927.
24. Grantham SA, Dick HM, Thompson RC, Jr., et al.: Occipitocervical arthrodesis. Indications, technique and results. **Clin Orthop** 65:118–129, 1969.
25. Graziano G, Jaggers C, Lee M, et al.: A comparative study of fixation techniques for type II fractures of the odontoid process. **Spine** 18:2383–2387, 1993.
26. Grob D, Crisco JJI, Panjabi MM, et al.: Biomechanical evaluation of four different posterior atlantoaxial fixation techniques. **Spine** 17:480–490, 1992.
27. Grob D, Dvorak J, Panjabi MM, et al.: Posterior occipitocervical fusion. A preliminary report of a new technique. **Spine** Suppl 3, 16:S17–S23, 1991.
28. Hadley MN, Browner C, Liu SS, et al.: New subtype of acute odontoid fractures (type IIA). **Neurosurgery** 22:67–71, 1988.
29. Hadley MN, Browner C, Sonntag VK: Axis fractures: A comprehensive review of management and treatment in 107 cases. **Neurosurgery** 17:281–290, 1985.
30. Hadra BE: Wiring the spinous processes in Pott's disease. **Trans Am Orthop Assoc** 4:206–210, 1891.
31. Haid RW, Foley KT, Rodts GE, et al.: The Cervical Spine Study Group anterior cervical plate nomenclature. **Neurosurgical Focus** 12:Article 15, 2002.
32. Harms J, Melcher RP: Posterior C1-C2 fusion with polyaxial screw and rod fixation. **Spine** 26:2467–2471, 2001.
33. Heywood AW, Learmonth ID, Thomas M: Internal fixation for occipito-cervical fusion. **J Bone Joint Surg Br** 70:708–711, 1988.
34. Holness RO, Huestis WS, Howes WJ, et al.: Posterior stabilization with an interlaminar clamp in cervical injuries: Technical note and review of the long term experience with the method. **Neurosurgery** 14:318–322, 1984.

35. Hurlbert RJ, Crawford NR, Choi WG, et al.: A biomechanical evaluation of occipitocervical instrumentation: Screw compared to wire fixation. **J Neurosurg** 90:84–90, 1999.
36. Itoh T, Tsuji H, Katoh Y, et al.: Occipito-cervical fusion reinforced by Luque's segmental spinal instrumentation for rheumatoid diseases. **Spine** 13:1234–1238, 1988.
37. Jonsson H, Jr., Rauschning W: Anatomical and morphometric studies in posterior cervical spinal screw-plate systems. **J Spinal Disord** 7:429–438, 1994.
38. Lipscomb PR: Cervico-occipital fusion for congenital and post-traumatic anomalies of the atlas and axis. **J Bone Joint Surg Am** 39:1289–1301, 1957.
39. Lynch JJ, Crawford NR, Chamberlain RH, et al.: Biomechanics of lateral mass/pedicle screw fixation at C1-2 (abstract). **18th Annual Meeting AANS/CNS Section on Disorders of the Spine and Peripheral Nerves, February, Lake Buena Vista, FL,** 2002.
40. Magerl F, Seemann PS: Stable posterior fusion of the atlas and axis by transarticular screw fixation. In: Kehr P, Weidner A. (eds.), *Cervical Spine I.* Vienna: Springer-Verlag, 1987, pp 322–327.
41. McAfee PC, Bohlmann HH, Wilson WL: The triple wire fixation technique for stabilization of acute cervical fracture-dislocations. A biomechanical analysis (abstract). **Orthop Trans** 9:142, 1985.
42. McGraw RW, Rusch RM: Atlanto-axial arthrodesis. **J Bone Joint Surg Br** 55:482–489, 1973.
43. Menezes AH, VanGilder JC, Clark CR, et al.: Odontoid upward migration in rheumatoid arthritis. An analysis of 45 patients with "cranial settling." **J Neurosurg** 63:500–509, 1985.
44. Mixter SJ, Osgood RB: Traumatic lesions of the atlas and axis. **Ann Surg** 51: 193–207, 1910.
45. Montesano PX, Anderson PA, Schlehr F, et al.: Odontoid fractures treated by anterior screw fixation. **Spine** Suppl 3, 16:S33–S37, 1991.
46. Montesano PX, Juach EC, Anderson PA, et al.: Biomechanics of cervical spine. **Spine** Suppl 3, 16:S10–S16, 1991.
47. Morscher E, Sutter F, Jenny H, et al.: Anterior plating of the cervical spine with the hollow screw-plate system of titanium [in German]. **Chirurg** 57:702–707, 1986.
48. Moskovich R, Crockard HA: Atlantoaxial arthrodesis using interlaminar clamps: An improved technique. **Spine** 17:261–267, 1992.
49. Murphy MJ, Southwick WO: Posterior approaches and fusions. In: Cervical Spine Research Society Editorial Committee (ed.), *The Cervical Spine.* Philadelphia: Lippincott Williams and Wilkins, 1989, pp 775–791.
50. Naderi S, Crawford NR, Song GS, et al.: Biomechanical comparison of C1-C2 posterior fixations. Cable, graft, and screw combinations. **Spine** 23:1946–1955, 1998.
51. Newman P, Sweetnam R: Occipito-cervical fusion. An operative technique and its indications. **J Bone Joint Surg Br** 51:423–431, 1969.
52. Ransford AO, Crockard HA, Pozo JL, et al.: Craniocervical instability treated by contoured loop fixation. **J Bone Joint Surg Br** 68:173–177, 1986.
53. Raveh J, Sutter F, Hellem S: Surgical procedures for reconstruction of the lower jaw using the titanium-coated hollow screw reconstruction plate system: Bridging of defects. **Otolaryngol Clin North Am** 20:535–558, 1987.
54. Ripa DR, Kowall MG, Meyer PR, Jr., et al.: Series of ninety-two traumatic cervical spine injuries stabilized with anterior ASIF plate fusion technique. **Spine** Suppl 3, 16:S45–S46, 1991.

55. Rogers WA: Treatment of fracture-dislocation of the cervical spine. **J Bone Joint Surg Am** 24:245–258, 1942.
56. Roy-Camille R, Gagna G, Lazennec JY: L'arthrodäse occipitcervicale. In: Roy-Camille R (ed.), *Cinqièes Journées d'Orthopédie de la Pitié. Rachis Cervical Supérieur*. Paris: Masson, 1986, pp 49–51.
57. Roy-Camille R, Saillant G, Mazel C: Internal fixation of the unstable cervical spine by posterior osteosynthesis with plates and screws. In: Cervical Spine Research Society Editorial Committee (ed.), *The Cervical Spine*. Philadelphia: Lippincott Williams and Wilkins, 1989, pp 390–404.
58. Sakou T, Kawaida H, Morizono Y, et al.: Occipitoatlantoaxial fusion using a rectangular rod. **Clin Orthop** 239:136–144, 1989.
59. Sasso R, Doherty BJ, Crawford MJ, et al.: Biomechanics of odontoid fracture fixation. Comparison of the one- and two-screw technique. **Spine** 18:1950–1953, 1993.
60. Sawin PD, Traynelis VC: Posterior articular mass plate fixation of the subaxial cervical spine. In: Menezes AH, Sonntag VKH (eds.), *Principles of Spinal Surgery*. New York: McGraw-Hill, 1996, pp 1081–1104.
61. Schulder M: Interlaminar clamps: Indications, techniques, and results. In: Menezes AH, Sonntag VKH (eds.), *Principles of Spinal Surgery*. New York: McGraw-Hill, 1996, pp 1121–1132.
62. Seex K, Johnston RA: Interlaminar clap for posterior fusions (letter). **J Neurosurg** 75:495, 1991.
63. Sonntag VKH, Dickman CA: Occipitocervical and high cervical stabilization. In: Rengachary SS, Wilkins RH (eds.), *Neurosurgical Operative Atlas*. Baltimore: Williams and Wilkins, 1991, pp 327–339.
64. Sonntag VKH, Dickman CA: Posterior occipital C1-C2 instrumentation. In: Menezes AH, Sonntag VKH (eds.), *Principles of Spinal Surgery*. New York: McGraw-Hill, 1996, pp 1067–1079.
65. Sonntag VKH, Kalfas I: Innovative cervical fusion and instrumentation techniques. **Clin Neurosurg** 37:636–660, 1991.
66. Statham P, O'Sullivan M, Russel T: The Halifax Interlaminar Clamp for posterior cervical fusion: Initial experience in the United Kingdom. **Neurosurgery** 32: 396–398, 1993.
67. Stokes JK, Villavicencio AT, Liu PC, et al.: Posterior atlantoaxial stabilization: New alternative to C1-2 transarticular screws. **Neurosurgical Focus** 12:Article 6, 2002.
68. Tucker HH: Technical report: Method of fixation of subluxed or dislocated cervical spine below C1-C2. **Can J Neurol Sci** 2:381–382, 1975.
69. Whitehill R, Reger SI, Fox E, et al.: The use of methylmethacrylate cement as an instantaneous fusion mass in posterior cervical fusions: A canine in vivo experimental model. **Spine** 9:246–252, 1984.
70. Zygmunt SC, Ljunggren B, Alund M, et al.: Realignment and surgical fixation of atlanto-axial and subaxial dislocations in rheumatoid arthritis (RA) patients. **Acta Neurochir (Wien)** 43:79–84, 1988.

II

General Scientific Session II Leadership

CHAPTER

6

The Neurosurgeon as a Spine Surgeon: An Historical Perspective

FREDERICK A. SIMEONE, M.D.

I have been asked to review the role of the neurosurgeon in the development of spine surgery.

Actually, it is far more difficult to define *neurosurgeon* than it is to define *spine surgery*. When does one actually become a neurosurgeon? Is it when a full specialty with associated boards is created, or is it when an individual devotes the majority of his or her surgical practice to neurosurgery?

Obviously, there were individuals who focused their surgical efforts on the brain and spine before there were accrediting agencies. These individuals, rightfully, should be called neurosurgeons. I will resist the temptation to compare the role of neurosurgeons versus orthopedic surgeons in the development of spine surgery in order to focus the limited space available on the subject at hand. Nevertheless, orthopedists have made significant contributions, notably in the area of spine stabilization, which is currently a subject of dominant interest (perhaps overemphasized) amongst spine surgeons of all disciplines.

To best define *neurosurgeon*, one should refer to the father of American neurosurgery, William Williams Keen, who while a Professor of Surgery at the Women's Medical College, now the Medical College of Pennsylvania, performed the first successful brain operation in America in 1887 (*Fig. 6.1*). His own curriculum vitae indicates that in 1889, while at the same institution, he wrote both on surgery of the spine as well as on surgery of the brain (7). Later, he became editor of *Keen's Surgery,* which was popular from 1908 to 1913 and which helped to advance the field of spine surgery (6). From 1886 onward, he was the editor of *Gray's Anatomy.*

Other American neurosurgeons who were prolific in the study of spine surgery include Charles Harrison Frazier, Professor of Clinical Surgery and Surgeon to the Hospital of the University of Pennsylvania in Philadelphia, who in 1918 published *Surgery of the Spine and Spinal Cord* (4). This 970-page text innovated surgical procedures for

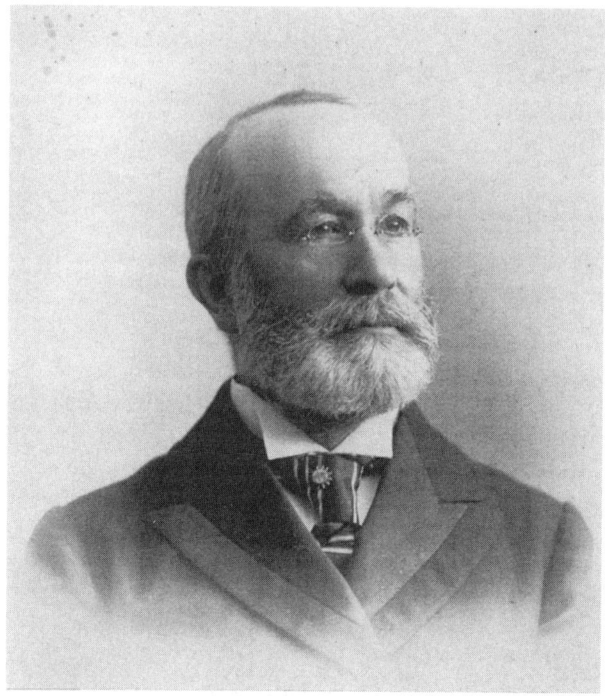

FIG. 6.1

infections and injuries and delineated rhizotomy for pain and spasticity (*Fig. 6.2*).

Charles A. Elsberg, who referred to himself as Professor of Clinical Surgery at the New York University and Bellevue Hospital Medical College and attending surgeon to the Mount Sinai Hospital and the New York Neurological Institute, wrote extensively on spinal cord diseases, both from their medical and their surgical aspects. His pivotal text, *Diagnosis and Treatment of Surgical Diseases of the Spinal Cord and Its Membranes* (2), was published in 1916 and generally referred to a broad range of spinal disorders with an emphasis on surgery (*Fig. 6.3*). Later, in 1925, he published a specific text, *Tumors of the Spinal Cord* (3), which was the first detailed American treatise on the surgical management of the broad range of spinal tumors. This exhaustive work of over 420 pages was the standard surgical text for spinal cord tumors for decades. *Figure 6.4* is his illustration of an anteriorly placed, intradural spinal cord tumor before removal (without the aid of microscope or fine microsurgical instrumentation).

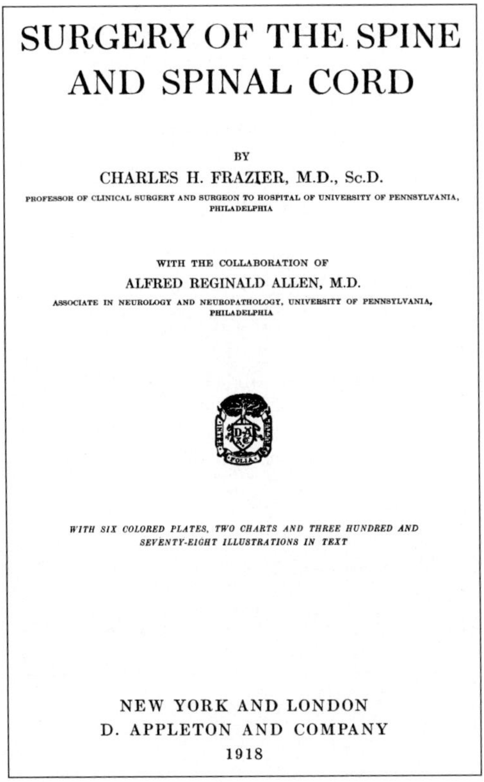

SURGERY OF THE SPINE AND SPINAL CORD

BY

CHARLES H. FRAZIER, M.D., Sc.D.

PROFESSOR OF CLINICAL SURGERY AND SURGEON TO HOSPITAL OF UNIVERSITY OF PENNSYLVANIA, PHILADELPHIA

WITH THE COLLABORATION OF

ALFRED REGINALD ALLEN, M.D.

ASSOCIATE IN NEUROLOGY AND NEUROPATHOLOGY, UNIVERSITY OF PENNSYLVANIA, PHILADELPHIA

WITH SIX COLORED PLATES, TWO CHARTS AND THREE HUNDRED AND SEVENTY-EIGHT ILLUSTRATIONS IN TEXT

NEW YORK AND LONDON
D. APPLETON AND COMPANY
1918

FIG. 6.2

In 1934, William Jason Mixter, who was referred to as visiting surgeon, Massachusetts General Hospital, but who restricted most of his activities to neurosurgery, published "Rupture of the intervertebral disc with involvement of the spinal canal" (8) along with orthopedist Joseph S. Barr. Although herniation of the intervertebral disc was recognized for some time as a source of symptoms, there was confusion as to the exact nature and pathological mechanisms. Indeed, Walter Dandy discovered "enchondromas," which were presumed to be tumors of the intervertebral disc cartilage compressing the spinal cord and spinal nerves. Mixter s paper received wide attention. It reviewed 19 cases, studied in detail, with disc herniations throughout the entire spine, and it delineated some of the symptoms of cervical, thoracic, and lumbar disc herniation. As such, it represented the most complete American work on the subject to that time, and it caused a height-

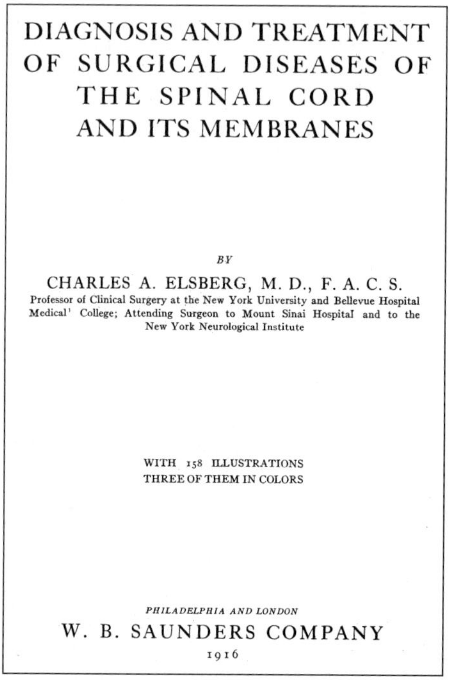

DIAGNOSIS AND TREATMENT OF SURGICAL DISEASES OF THE SPINAL CORD AND ITS MEMBRANES

BY

CHARLES A. ELSBERG, M. D., F. A. C. S.
Professor of Clinical Surgery at the New York University and Bellevue Hospital Medical College; Attending Surgeon to Mount Sinai Hospital and to the New York Neurological Institute

WITH 158 ILLUSTRATIONS
THREE OF THEM IN COLORS

PHILADELPHIA AND LONDON
W. B. SAUNDERS COMPANY
1916

FIG. 6.3

ened index of suspicion for what turned out to be the neurosurgeon's most common operative focus. (The authors did mention a paper published in 1893 by G. Mauric that was also apparently an extensive review of symptomatic disc herniations.) Other neurosurgeons completed exhaustive reviews of disc surgery in several texts, such as *The Intervertebral Disc* (1), published in 1941 by neurosurgeons F. Keith Bradford and R. Glenn Spurling.

EUROPEAN CONTRIBUTIONS

There will be no attempt in this discussion to summarize the history of spine surgery throughout Europe or even the role of the neurosurgeon. Among the many texts on surgery published from the beginning of medical writings to the late nineteenth century, there are few references to spine surgery, and dramatically few to *successful* spine surgery. These surgical texts, which often include operations on the skull and brain, notably trepanation for various presumed diseases, still did not include sections on spine surgery.

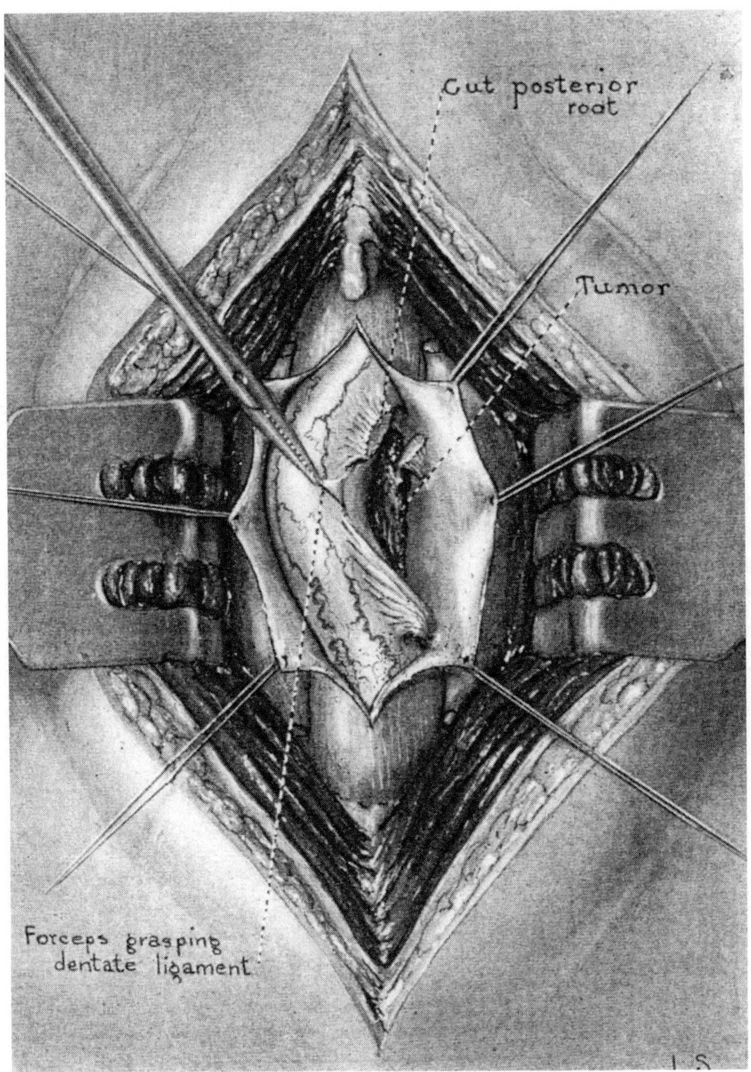

FIG. 6.4

Notable is the work of Percival Pott, who apparently successfully drained paraspinal tuberculous abscesses with improvement in some of his reports. These patients often presented with kyphosis and even draining abscesses, which led to the concept that surgical drainage might be effective. In his book, *The Chirurgical Works of Percival Pott*

(10), he illustrated the ravages of tuberculosis on the spine and reported symptomatic improvement following drainage (*Figs. 6.5 and 6.6*).

The remarkable case of Horsley (an individual specializing in neurosurgery) and Gowers perhaps could be recognized as the dawn of modern scientific spine surgery. In this remarkable instance, in 1887 neurologist Gowers diagnosed an intraspinal tumor and encouraged Horsley to successfully remove what was apparently a meningioma. The patient made a satisfactory recovery (5).

NINETEENTH CENTURY SPINE SURGERY TEXTS

Few texts in neurosurgery appeared before the turn of the twentieth century. Some referred specifically to trauma, such as *Injuries of the Spine and Spinal Cord* (9) by Herbert W. Page of St. Mary's Hospital and the Cumberland Infirmary in 1883 (*Fig. 6.7*). Little of surgery was discussed therein.

In 1889, William Thorburn of the Manchester Royal Infirmary made a significant analysis in his *A Contribution to the Surgery of the Spinal*

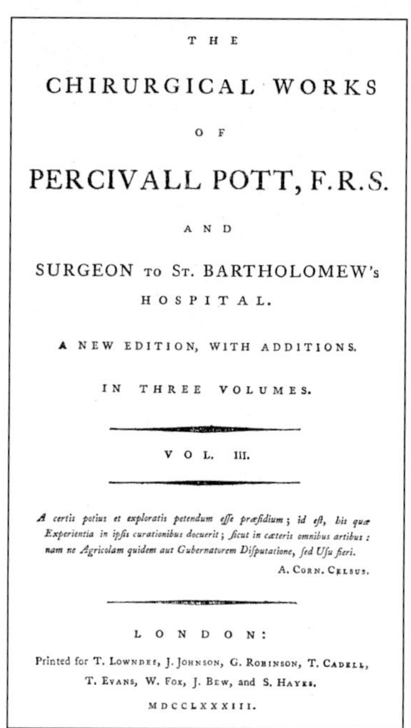

THE

CHIRURGICAL WORKS

OF

PERCIVALL POTT, F.R.S.

AND

SURGEON TO ST. BARTHOLOMEW'S HOSPITAL.

A NEW EDITION, WITH ADDITIONS.

IN THREE VOLUMES.

VOL. III.

A certis potius et exploratis petendum esse præsidium; id est, his quæ Experientia in ipsis curationibus docuerit; sicut in cæteris omnibus artibus: nam ne Agricolam quidem aut Gubernatorem Disputatione, sed Usu fieri.

A. CORN. CELSUS.

LONDON:

Printed for T. LOWNDES, J. JOHNSON, G. ROBINSON, T. CADELL, T. EVANS, W. FOX, J. BEW, and S. HAYES.

MDCCLXXXIII.

FIG. 6.5

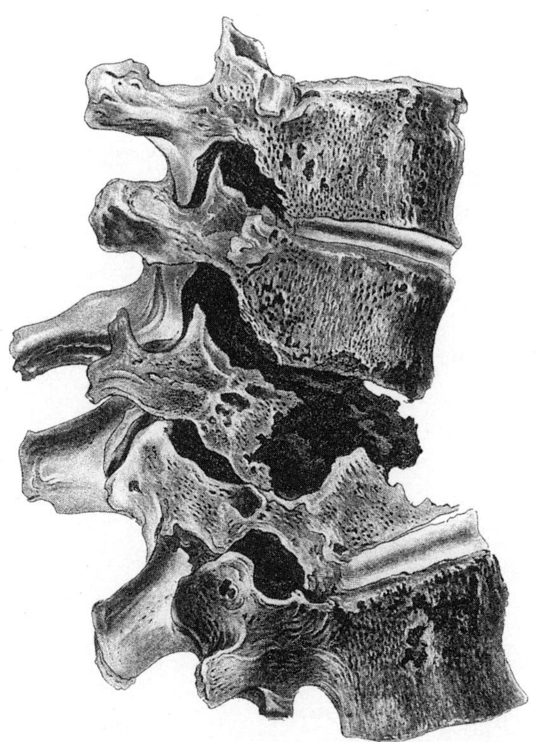

FIG. 6.6

Cord (11) (*Fig. 6.7*). This work is notable, because he reviewed in detail some 56 cases of spine surgery, all for trauma, published in the English literature from 1814 through 1889. This series is also remarkable not only for its high percentage of postoperative deaths but also for the occasional dramatic partial or complete recovery following such rudimentary surgery.

These few sentences highlight anecdotally some early observation on spine surgery before the specialty of neurosurgery was formalized.

THE NEUROSURGEON AND MODERN SPINE SURGERY

As spine surgery passed into the twentieth century, neurosurgeons contributed with the introduction of the operating microscope; specific microsurgical instruments; operations on the spinal cord for relief of pain and spasticity; improved methods for removing tumors in the intradural, intramedullary and extraspinal sites; and methods for reconstruction of the spine. In the latter instance, the orthopedist's

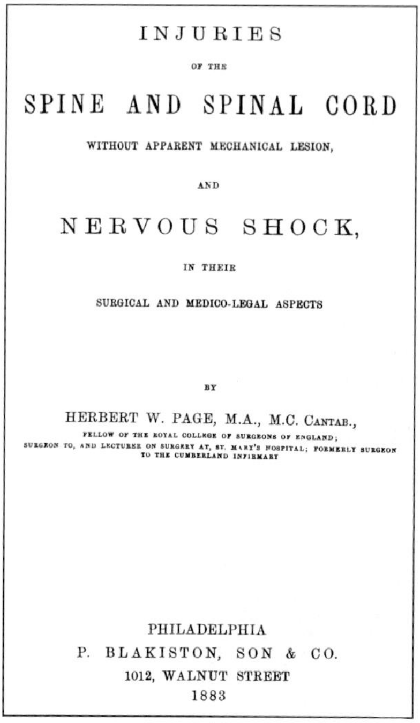

INJURIES

OF THE

SPINE AND SPINAL CORD

WITHOUT APPARENT MECHANICAL LESION,

AND

NERVOUS SHOCK,

IN THEIR

SURGICAL AND MEDICO-LEGAL ASPECTS

BY

HERBERT W. PAGE, M.A., M.C. CANTAB.,

FELLOW OF THE ROYAL COLLEGE OF SURGEONS OF ENGLAND;
SURGEON TO, AND LECTURER ON SURGERY AT, ST. MARY'S HOSPITAL; FORMERLY SURGEON TO THE CUMBERLAND INFIRMARY

PHILADELPHIA
P. BLAKISTON, SON & CO.
1012, WALNUT STREET
1883

FIG. 6.7

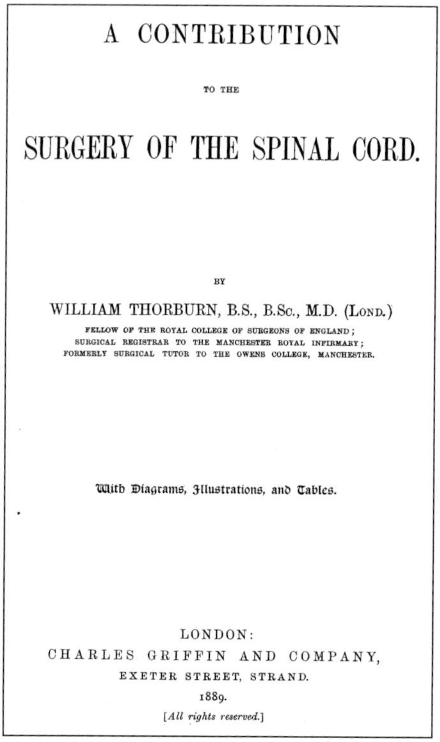

A CONTRIBUTION

TO THE

SURGERY OF THE SPINAL CORD.

BY

WILLIAM THORBURN, B.S., B.Sc., M.D. (LOND.)

FELLOW OF THE ROYAL COLLEGE OF SURGEONS OF ENGLAND;
SURGICAL REGISTRAR TO THE MANCHESTER ROYAL INFIRMARY;
FORMERLY SURGICAL TUTOR TO THE OWENS COLLEGE, MANCHESTER.

With Diagrams, Illustrations, and Tables.

LONDON:
CHARLES GRIFFIN AND COMPANY,
EXETER STREET, STRAND.
1889.
[*All rights reserved.*]

FIG. 6.8

interests in bone formation and healing has lead to a dominant contribution by that discipline to instrumentation and other methods to amplify bone fusion and deformity correction. From a practical viewpoint, spine surgery represents the majority of the average practicing neurosurgeon's operative activity. In some instances, neurosurgeons have elected to include nonoperative treatment of spinal disorders in their sphere of interests, though apparently not as commonly as orthopedic surgeons, who generally spend more time in the office. In the laboratory, neurosurgeons have been focused on methods of spinal cord regeneration, spinal cord circulation, and the function of the contents of the spine, whereas other disciplines have helped to understand the biology of the spine itself in co-operation with those neurosurgeons interested in the subject. The neurosurgeon s role in spine surgery tends to be both regional and, sometimes, traditional. In some instances, the lines are drawn sharply between neurosurgical and orthopedic activity, whereas in others, cases tend to gravitate to whatever discipline is most interested in pursuing comprehensive treatment of these patients.

As time progresses, interventional techniques will lead neurosurgical cerebrovascular surgeons into other methods of treatment. Similarly, focused-beam radiation will encourage neurosurgical tumor surgeons to expand their armamentarium. Spine surgery is evolving not only to include major reconstructions but also minimally invasive therapies that offer better or equal cure with less disability. In this regard, neurosurgeons have been particularly fruitful in opening new avenues of therapy in a field that promises to expand at least as rapidly as any other area in the surgery of the nervous system.

REFERENCES

1. Bradford KF, Spurling R: *The Intervertebral Disc.* Baltimore: Charles C. Thomas, 1941.
2. Elsberg CA: *Diagnosis and Treatment of Surgical Diseases of the Spinal Cord and Its Membranes.* Philadelphia: WB Saunders, 1916.
3. Elsberg CA: *Tumors of the Spinal Cord, the Symptoms of Irritation and Compression of the Spinal Cord and Nerve Roots.* New York: Paul B. Hoeber, 1925.
4. Frazier CH: *Surgery of the Spine and Spinal Cord.* New York and London: D. Appleton and Company, 1918.
5. Gowers WR, Horsley V: *A Case of Tumour of the Spinal Cord. Removal; Recovery.* **Medico-Chirurgical Transactions** 53:377–428, 1888.
6. Keen WWW: *Surgery, Its Principles and Practice.* Philadelphia and London: WB Saunders Company, 1921.
7. Keen-James WW: *The Memoirs of William Williams Keen, MD.* Doylestown, PA: Privately published as a Keen book, 1990, pp 321–322.
8. Mixter WJ, Barr JS: Rupture of the intervertebral disc with involvement of the spinal canal. **N Engl J Med** 211:210–214, 1984.
9. Page HW: *Injuries of the Spine and Spinal Cord.* Philadelphia: Blakiston and Son, 1883.
10. Pott P: *The Chirurgical Works of Percival Pott.* London: Lowndes etc., 1783.
11. Thorburn W: *A Contribution to the Surgery of the Spinal Cord.* London: Charles Griffin and Company, 1889.

CHAPTER

7

The Essentials of Spine Biomechanics for the General Neurosurgeon

EDWARD C. BENZEL, M.D.

> Give me a lever long enough and a fulcrum on which to place it, and I shall move the world.
>
> Archimedes

This chapter essentially is an abridged version of the book *The Biomechanics of Spine Stabilization* (1). Obligatorily, it is incomplete by virtue of the fact that it does not—and cannot—cover the entirety of spine biomechanics. It therefore is intended as an introductory review, not as a replacement for the original text regarding content, educational value, and reference value. The bibliography for this chapter is intentionally brief. The only references provided in this bibliography are two books. For additional references, both books included in the bibliography should be consulted, particularly the first. This chapter is intended to provide information in the form of the illustrations and written text. It is hoped that it will stimulate the reader to pursue the fundamentals of spine surgery to greater depths, perhaps by delving further into either of the reference texts. It is also hoped that each surgeon who considers himself or herself to be a spine surgeon will embrace the principles presented herein and in the two books included in the bibliography. After all, one cannot proceed to the complex without a firm grasp of the fundamentals.

BIOMECHANICALLY RELEVANT ANATOMY

The vertebral column complex consists of ventrally located vertebral bodies and intervening intervertebral discs that collectively assume most of the axial load-bearing responsibilities of the spine. The pedicles connect the ventral and the dorsal components of each spinal segment. The laminae provide a roof for the spinal canal, whereas the facet joints limit rotation, flexion, extension, lateral bending, and translation. The muscles and ligaments provide for and limit torso movement. They also provide for some axial load-bearing (1).

The Vertebral Body

Both the width and depth of the vertebral bodies increase as one descends the spine in a rostral-to-caudal direction (*Fig. 7.1*). The vertebral body height also increases in a rostral-to-caudal direction, with the exception of a slight reversal of this relationship at the C6 and lower lumbar levels (*Fig. 7.2*). The height of the C6 vertebral body is usually less than those of the C5 and C7 bodies, and the heights of the lower lumbar vertebral bodies are usually less than that of the L2 vertebral body. In the cervical spine, the uncinate process projects from the rostral-dorsal-lateral aspect of each vertebral body (C3 through C7). The uncovertebral joint provides an articulation of this process with the caudal-dorsal-lateral aspect of the vertebral body above. This is essentially an extension of the intervertebral disc that plays a role in the coupling phenomenon and in rotation (1).

The progressive increase in size of the vertebral bodies, observed as one descends the spine, correlates with strength or stress-resisting abilities. The decreased incidence of spine fractures observed in the lower lumbar spine is related, at least in part, to the increased strength of the vertebrae in this region. This correlates with the axial load-resisting ability of the spine (1) (*Fig. 7.3*).

The shape of the vertebral body varies from region to region. Al-

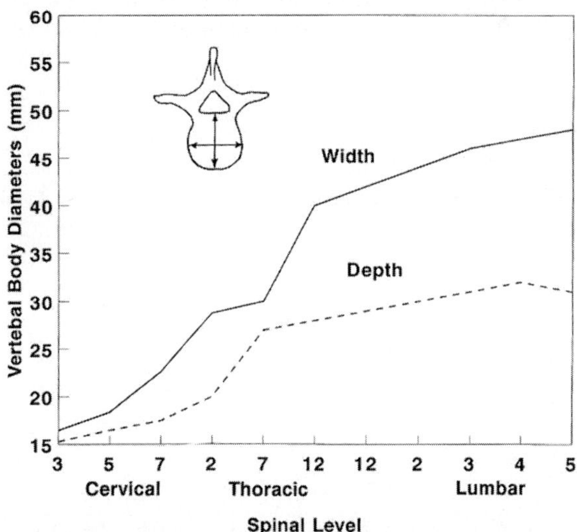

FIG. 7.1 Vertebral body diameter versus spinal level. The width (solid line) and depth (dashed line) of the vertebral bodies are depicted separately. [From (1); copyright © 2001 by the American Association of Neurological Surgeons.]

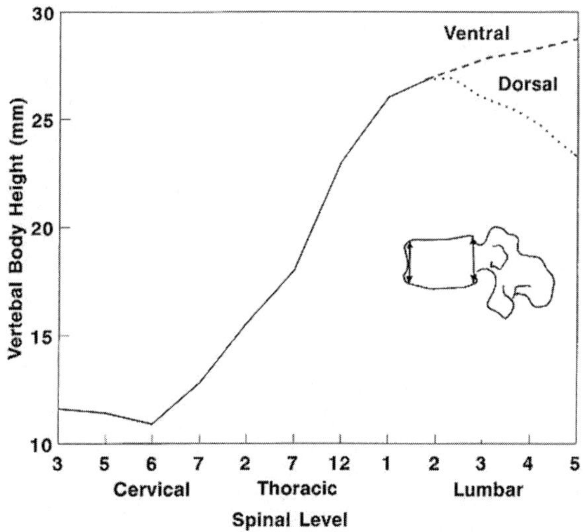

FIG. 7.2 Vertebral body height versus spinal level. The dorsal height (dotted line) and ventral height (dashed line) where significantly different, are depicted separately. [From (1); copyright © 2001 by the American Association of Neurological Surgeons.]

though its shape is generally that of a solid cylinder, the dorsal aspect of the vertebral body (surface facing the spinal canal) is concave dorsally. This is particularly significant in ventral spinal operations in which screw purchase of the dorsal vertebral body cortex is critical.

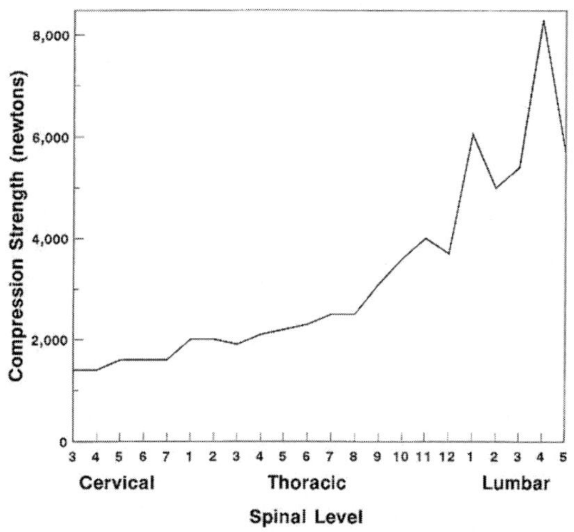

FIG. 7.3 Vertebral compression strength versus spinal level. [From (1); copyright © 2001 by the American Association of Neurological Surgeons.]

Misinterpretation of the lateral radiograph may lead to neural impingement by the screw.

The costovertebral joint contributes to spinal stability by providing an articulation to the rib. This is particularly true with respect to lateral bending and axial rotation (1).

The Facet Joints

The facet joints do not, in and of themselves, substantially support axial loads unless the spine is in an extension posture (lordosis). They are apophyseal joints that have a loose capsule and a synovial lining. In the cervical spine, the facet joints are primarily oriented in a coronal plane. The orientation of the facet joints changes significantly as one descends the thoracic and lumbar spine. The angle (from midline) increases from L1 to L5.

The facet joint surfaces of C3 through C7 face the instantaneous axis of rotation (IAR; the axis about which a vertebral segment rotates) and are not particularly restrictive of gliding movements. The abilities of the cervical spine facet joint to resist flexion-extension, lateral bending, and rotation are relatively diminished because of this coronal plane orientation. Thus, such movement is substantial in this region. Cervical facet joint anatomy should be carefully scrutinized before placement of a lateral cervical mass screw; otherwise, joint violation by the screw may be an undesirable result, particularly at the caudal joint.

In the lumbar region, the facet joints are oriented in a sagittal plane. Their ability to resist flexion or translational movement in this region is minimal, whereas their ability to resist rotation is substantial.

The nearly coronal facet orientation at L5/S1 is a factor in the relatively decreased incidence of subluxation, in the presence of intact facet joints, at the lumbosacral joint. That is, in degenerative spondylolisthesis, subluxation is more common at L4-L5 than at L5/S1, despite the relative vertical orientation of the L5/S1 disc interspace.

The aforementioned variations of facet joint orientation, as well as ligamentous strength and the moment arms through which they act (see below), affect spinal segmental motion. Such motion at each segmental level can be depicted in graphic form (1) (*Fig. 7.4*).

The facet joints absorb a greater fraction of the axial load-bearing if the spine is oriented in extension (see *Configuration of the Spine* before). This varies with the type of load.

The Pedicles

A knowledge of pedicle anatomy is relevant regarding appropriate surgical intervention. The pedicles of the cervical spine are shorter and proportionally of greater diameter than other regions of the spine.

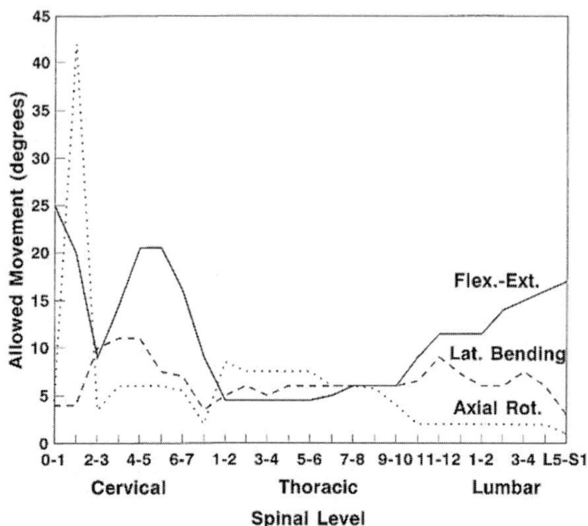

FIG. 7.4 Segmental motions allowed at the various spinal levels (combined flexion and extension, solid line; unilateral lateral bending, dashed line; and unilateral axial rotation, dotted line). [From (1); copyright © 2001 by the American Association of Neurological Surgeons.]

The transverse pedicle width gradually decreases from the cervical to the midthoracic region and then increases as one descends in the lumbar spine. The pedicle height (sagittal pedicle width) increases gradually (except at C2) from the cervical to the thoracolumbar region and then decreases as one descends in the lumbar spine. This relationship is favorable for transpedicular screw placement in the lumbar spine, because pedicle width is more important than height in this regard. A small variation in pedicle height (sagittal pedicle width) in the lumbar region is not clinically significant because of the already generous dimension.

The transverse pedicle angle decreases from the cervical spine to the thoracolumbar region and then increases as the lumbar spine is descended. This necessitates a wider angle of approach for the placement of pedicle screws in the low lumbar spine. An appreciation of vertebral anatomy is similarly important when pedicle screws are to be placed in the sacral region. Usually, however, there is a greater margin of safety with regard to screw placement.

Also important, particularly regarding pedicle screw placement in the upper lumbar and thoracic spine (where the margin of safety is less than that in the low lumbar region), is the sagittal pedicle angle and the relationship of adjacent neural structures. In the upper lumbar and thoracic spine, the sagittal pedical angle becomes relatively steep.

The unique relationship between the thoracic pedicle and adjacent transverse process has been described. This, in fact, can be objectively portrayed by the equation

$$D = 7.9 - (1.2 \cdot TL)$$

where D = rostral-caudal distance of the thoracic pedicle from the midpoint of the pedicle and TL = thoracic level. This may provide assistance to the surgeon during the placement of thoracic pedical screws. Of note is that pedicle morphology is relatively unaffected by race but is significantly affected by age (youth) (1).

The Intervertebral Disc

The annulus fibrosus is composed of several layers of radiating fibers attached to the cartilaginous end plates (inner fibers) and the cortical bone on the walls of the vertebral body (Sharpey's fibers). In the cervical region, the anulus is more like a crescent-shaped anterior interosseous ligament. These components incompletely resist deformation. Because of their angled orientation ($\approx 30°$ with respect to the end plate), the annulus fibrosis fibers resist rotation with relative effectiveness. They do not, however, resist compression as well. Note that disc bulging occurs on the concave side of a bending of the spine. This correlates with osteophyte formation. Disc bulging, however, should not be confused with disc herniation. The former is caused by distortion of the annulus fibrosus by compression; the latter is caused by migration of the nucleus pulposus from its normal anatomic location.

In contrast to the direction of disc (annulus) bulging (toward the concavity of a spinal bend), the nucleus pulposus moves in the opposite direction. Flexion therefore causes bulging of the annulus fibrosus ventrally. It also causes a tendency in the nucleus pulposus to migrate dorsally. Significant strains are placed on the annulus fibrosus by physiologic loads (1).

The Ligaments

A variety of well-studied spinal ligaments provide varying degrees of support for the spine. These include the interspinous ligament, the ligamentum flavum, the anterior and posterior longitudinal ligaments, the capsular ligaments, and the lateral ligaments of the spine. Their strength characteristics vary from ligament to ligament and from region to region. Other ligaments, such as the posterior epidural ligament and Hoffman's ligament, play roles in dural stabilization by anchoring the dorsal dura mater to adjacent structures.

The effectiveness of a ligament depends on its morphology and, particularly, on the moment arm through which it acts. To appreciate the contribution of an individual spinal ligament to the integrity of the spine, the length of the lever arm, as well as the strength of the ligament (*Figs. 7.5* and *7.6*), must be considered. The length of the lever arm (moment arm) is the perpendicular distance between the force vector (the force and its direction, as applied by the ligament) to the IAR. A very strong ligament that functions through a relatively short moment arm may contribute less to stability than a weaker ligament working a longer moment arm because of the latter's mechanical advantage (1).

CONFIGURATION OF THE SPINE

Under normal conditions, the cervical and lumbar regions of the spine assume a lordotic posture. A kyphosis, as exists in the thoracic and thoracolumbar regions, predisposes the spine to exaggerated

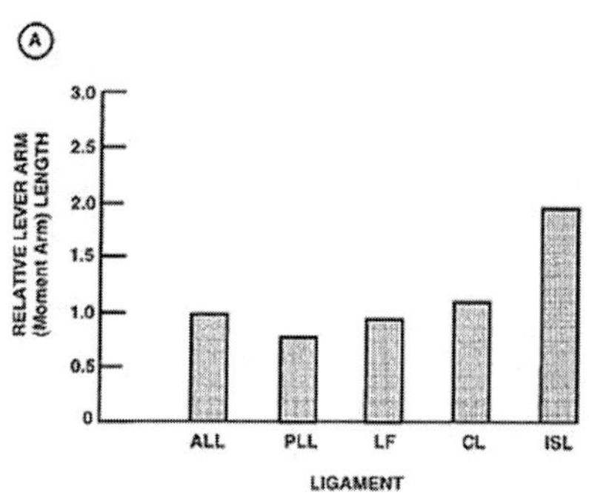

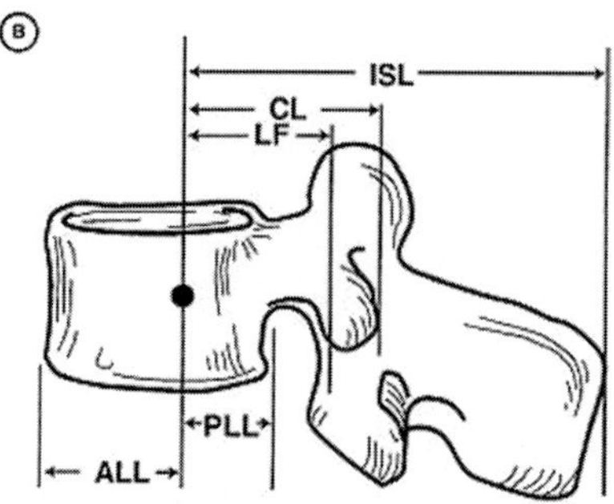

FIG. 7.5 The relative lever arm (moment arm) length of ligaments causing flexion or resisting extension (*A*). The ligaments and their effective moment arms (*B*). Note that this length depends on the location of the IAR. An "average" location is used in this illustration. Dot = IAR; ALL = anterior longitudinal ligament; PL = posterior longitudinal ligament; LF = ligamentum flavum; CL = capsular ligament; ISL = interspinous ligament. [From (1); copyright © 2001 by the American Association of Neurological Surgeons.

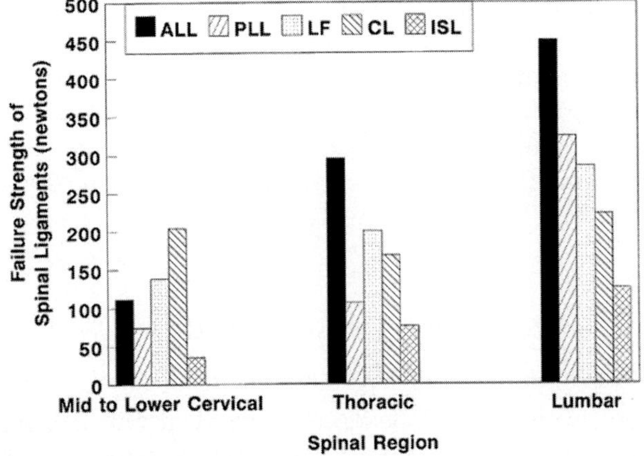

FIG. 7.6 Failure strength of spinal ligaments versus spinal region. ALL = anterior longitudinal ligament; PLL = posterior longitudinal ligament; LF = ligamentum flavum; CL = capsular ligament; ISL = interspinous ligament. [From (1); copyright © 2001 by the American Association of Neurological Surgeons.]

stresses, which stresses are related to an increased bending moment. Thus, the intrinsic configuration of this region of the spine substantially determines the type of spinal column injury that is incurred. The thoracolumbar junction, for example, is the lower terminus of the thoracic kyphosis. It lacks the protective support of the rib cage and does not harbor the excessive support provided by the larger lower lumbar vertebral bodies. This combination fosters vertebral column injury. The intrinsic bending moment allowed by the kyphosis, the lack of intrinsic protection (relative), and the abrupt change in mechanics results in focally increased strain and an increased incidence of compression fractures in this region. The cervical region similarly has a peak incidence of fractures in the midcervical region.

In the lower lumbar region, the more massive vertebral bodies provide substantial support. The intrinsic lumbar lordosis essentially eliminates the bending-moment component of the stresses placed on the spine at the thoracolumbar junction. In the absence of a significant bending moment, pure axial loads are commonly presented to the spine; therefore, burst fractures are more common in this location. Fractures in general, however, are less frequent here than in other regions of the spine.

At the lumbosacral junction, the angle of the sacrum in relation to the L5 vertebral body (the lumbosacral joint angle) may substantially affect pathological processes, both traumatic and degenerative. Furthermore, this joint, which is exposed to significant axial stresses, must resist substantial translational forces. The greater the lumbosacral joint angle, the greater the applied translation forces. The ability to resist these translational forces is diminished by the vertical joint orientation, the orientation of the facet joints, and the strength characteristics of the ligaments. Spondylolisthesis may ensue. Patients with exaggerated lumbar lordoses are particularly prone to the sequelae of these stresses (1).

REGIONAL CHARACTERISTICS

The Upper Cervical Spine and Craniocervical Junction

The upper cervical spine deserves special attention because of its unique anatomic arrangements. C1 has no centrum, and this allows intrusion of the odontoid process of C2 between its two lateral masses. The odontoid process articulates with the dorsal aspect of the ventral portion of the ring of C1 and with the transverse ligament of the atlas by separate synovial joints.

The lateral masses of C1 articulate with the occipital condyles and C2 by kidney-shaped articulations. The superior facet of C1 faces in a rostral and medial direction, whereas the inferior facet faces in a caudal and medial direction. This unique, wedge-like configuration results in a lateral transmission of force vectors resulting from axial loads (C1 burst [Jefferson] fracture). The transverse ligament of the atlas attaches to the tubercles on the medial aspect of the ring of C1. This anatomic arrangement provides for containment of the intruding odontoid process. The short and strong transverse processes allow for the attachment of the rotators of the upper cervical spine. The ventral ring of C1 is strong; that is, it is made up of dense cortical bone. This is important in terms of the integrity of C1 following laminectomy or dorsal arch fractures. A circumferentially intact ring of C1 is not necessary for the attainment of stability.

The C2 ring has many attributes of the more caudal cervical vertebrae. It also, however, has a rostral extension, the odontoid process. The pars interarticularis (not to be confused with the pedicle) is substantial and projects from the lamina in a rostral and ventral direction to attach to the lateral mass. This anatomy is vitally important in terms of transarticular screw fixation techniques. The C2 pars interarticularis attaches to the pedicle, which passes medially to the vertebral body. The transitional nature of this vertebrae ensures a complicated anatomic configuration with an associated variability. The occipital nerve passes dorsally to the atlantoaxial joint. This must be kept in mind during transfacet C1-C2 screw fixation.

The C2 ring is directly connected to the occiput by the alar and apical ligaments and by the tectorial membrane. The C1 ring functions, in a sense, as an intermediate "fulcrum" that regulates movement between the occiput and C2. The atlantooccipital joint allows flexion, extension, and a minimal degree of lateral flexion. Minimal rotation is allowed. The atlantoaxial joint allows some lateral bending, which is coupled with rotation. Most cervical rotation, which occurs about the axis of the dens, is allowed at this joint.

The failure strength of the alar ligament is approximately 200 N, and that of the transverse ligament of the atlas is approximately 350 N. These ligaments are very strong compared to the loads that are placed on them. This explains, in part, the relatively low incidence of failure of the upper cervical ligaments.

Surgery on the upper cervical spine is complicated by the difficulties associated with calvarial fixation by the unique anatomy of the upper cervical vertebrae, vertebral artery relationships, and the substantial spinal movement that is allowed in this region. The anatomic features of the upper cervical spine—especially the articulations of the vertebrae to each other and to the skull—offer little in the way of points of fixation for instrumentation constructs and sites for bony fusion attachment. Furthermore, the unique anatomic arrangement allows movement in all directions, and in rotation as well. Although the movement allowed in the upper cervical region is not manifest in all planes and in rotation at each spinal level, its sum from occiput to C2 is greater than any other region of the spine (1).

The Middle and Lower Cervical Spine

The vertebrae of the middle and lower cervical spine are relatively uniform. This consistency encourages surgical intervention. A unique characteristic of this region is its lordotic posture. This may aid in the prevention of spinal cord injury, because most axial loads are imparted symmetrically to the spine rather than with a significant flexion component, which would cause asymmetric load application. Because the addition of a flexion component to an axial load greatly increases the chance of vertebral body failure and retropulsion of bone and disc fragments into the spinal canal, the lordotic posture also helps to prevent catastrophic injury.

The orientation of the facet joints in the coronal plane does not excessively limit spinal movement in any direction (or in rotation) except extension. With the cervical spine in extension, however, the spine's ability to resist axial loading is greatest. This may be related to the fact that the facet joints can participate in axial load support most effectively in extension and to the fact that, as mentioned above, the likelihood of a flexion component to the injury is small. In this case, the facet joints function in a load-sharing capacity.

The orientation of the facet joints in the cervical spine (in a coronal plane) facilitates spinal instrumentation in certain situations. If the integrity of the facet joints and pedicles in the cervical region has been maintained and the vertebral bodies are able to adequately resist axial loading, translational instability may be effectively managed by the application of a tension-band fixation construct (1).

The cervical vertebrae (C3-C6 and, occasionally, C7) contain bilateral foramina transversaria for the passage of the vertebral artery. This is consistently located laterally to the vertebral body border. There is less room for surgical error in the more rostral segments. Surgical dissection lateral to the vertebral body border may violate the foramina transversaria and the vertebral artery (1).

The Cervicothoracic Junction

The cervicothoracic junction is exposed to unique stresses because of its location and anatomic characteristics. The angle between the facet and intervertebral joints changes significantly between C6 and T1. This, combined with the absence of the protective rib cage, predisposes this region to a susceptibility toward "translational deformation."

The Thoracic Spine

The thoracic spinal cord is shielded from injury by the massive regional paraspinal muscle masses and by the thoracic cage. The narrow regional spinal canal diameter in the upper thoracic region, however, complicates the issue. The former attributes help to protect the neural elements; the latter attribute contributes to neural injury. This may explain the increased incidence of catastrophic neurological injuries associated with spine fractures in this region. The increased paraspinal muscle mass protects the spine from failure, thus causing an all-or-nothing risk of neural injury; that is, significant kinetic energy is required to fracture the upper thoracic spine. If such a fracture occurs, the narrow spinal canal leaves little room to spare for neural element protection. The normal kyphotic posture of the spine, with its associated predisposition to spine fracture, complicates all of these factors.

The Thoracolumbar Junction

The thoracolumbar junction is located at a point of transition that makes it vulnerable to excessive applied force. At this junctional region of the spine, the rib cage no longer provides spinal support, and the kyphotic curvature of the spine predisposes the spine to fracture. Furthermore, the vertebral bodies of the spine have not yet achieved the massive size of the middle to lower lumbar vertebrae (and also lack the middle to lower lumbar vertebrae–associated increased ability to resist deformity). Therefore, an increased incidence of fractures occurs at this junction.

The transverse processes of the lower thoracic region are often diminutive or rudimentary. This presents problems if instrumentation fixation to the transverse processes is desirable; alternate fixation sites are often necessary.

The Upper and Middle Lumbar Spine

The vertebral bodies of the upper and middle lumbar spine are larger and more massive than those of the more rostral spinal levels. Combined with the resumption of a lordotic curvature of the spine in this region, this makes this region of the spine relatively resistant to excessive forces. Furthermore, the transition of the spinal cord into the cauda equina, which is more tolerant of trauma than the spinal cord, makes catastrophic spinal injury from trauma less likely.

The Low Lumbar Spine and Lumbosacral Junction

The caudal end of the spinal column is associated with significant logistical therapeutic dilemmas. A frequently observed inability to obtain substantial points of sacral fixation creates a multitude of surgical problems. Similarly, an appropriate bending moment often is not achieved by the instrumentation construct because of the lack of an adequate length of lever arm below the injury. Furthermore, the relatively steep orientation of the lumbosacral joint exposes the lumbosacral spine to increased risk of translational deformation, whereas facet geometry affects both translational and rotatory deformation (1).

The Sacroiliac Joint

The sacroiliac joint is a complex joint that is a diarthrodial (synovial) joint ventrally and an amphiarthrodial (ligamentous) joint dorsally. Its unique anatomic configuration requires meticulous technique for radiographic assessment. Both anterior-posterior (AP) and oblique views may be necessary. As an aside regarding iliac bone anatomy, the thickest portion of the iliac bone is the iliac tubercle region. This is relevant regarding strategies for iliac crest bone graft harvesting. Considerable sacroiliac joint mobility occurs, even in aged patients.

FUNDAMENTAL BIOMECHANICAL AND PHYSICAL PRINCIPLES

Vectors, Moment Arms, Bending Moments, and Axes of Rotation

Forces applied to the spine can always be broken down into component vectors. A *vector* is defined here as a force that is oriented in a fixed and well-defined direction in three-dimensional space.

A force vector may act on a lever (moment arm), causing a bending moment. The bending moment applied to a point in space causes rotation, or a tendency to rotate, about an axis. This axis is the IAR. To establish an easily defined and reproducible coordinate system, the standard Cartesian coordinate system has historically been applied to the spine. In this system, by definition, three axes exist: the *X*-, *Y*-, and *Z*-axes (*Fig. 7.7*). Rotation and translational movements can occur about these axes. This results in 12 potential movements along or about each axis: two translation movements along (one in each direction) and two rotational movements around (one in each direction) each of the *X*-, *Y*-, and *Z*-axes (1).

The IAR is the axis about which each vertebral segment rotates at any given point in time and is, by definition, the center of the coordinate system (in the plane perpendicular to the IAR) for each motion segment. When a spinal segment moves, there is an axis passing through or close to each vertebral body that does not move—that is, the axis about which the vertebral body rotates (IAR). It usually, but

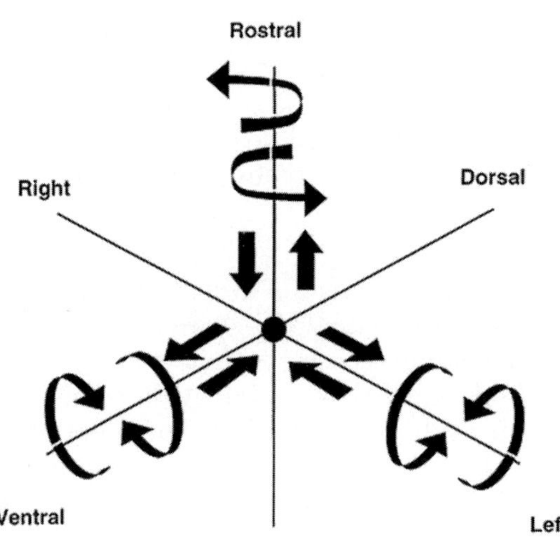

FIG. 7.7 The Cartesian coordinate system with the IAR as the center. Translation and rotation can occur in both of their respective directions about each axis. [From (1); copyright © 2001 by the American Association of Neurological Surgeons.]

not always, passes through the confines of the vertebral body. Multiple factors, such as applied load, degenerative disease, fractures, ligamentous injuries, and instrumentation and/or fusion placement, however, affect the position of the IAR.

The IAR, in a sense, is a fulcrum. For example, if the spine is flexed, then all points ventral to the IAR come closer together, and all points dorsal to the IAR move farther apart.

It is emphasized that the IAR be considered dynamic. As spinal movement occurs, the IAR of each spinal segment moves as well. Indeed, the IAR shifts or moves in response to loads applied, pathology, and spinal instrumentation and fusion (*Fig. 7.8*). The IAR is derived in the clinical situation from dynamic radiographs (flexion and extension radiographs).

The concept of a moment arm and bending moment are critical to an understanding of spinal biomechanics. The moment arm associated with a spinal implant is defined as that "invisible lever" that extends from a point (usually the IAR) to the position of application of force to the spine (perpendicular to the direction of the applied force). This is so regardless of the nature of the force application (e.g., via ligaments, spinal implants, etc.). The bending moment is defined as the product of the force applied to the lever arm and the length of the lever arm:

$$M = F \cdot D$$

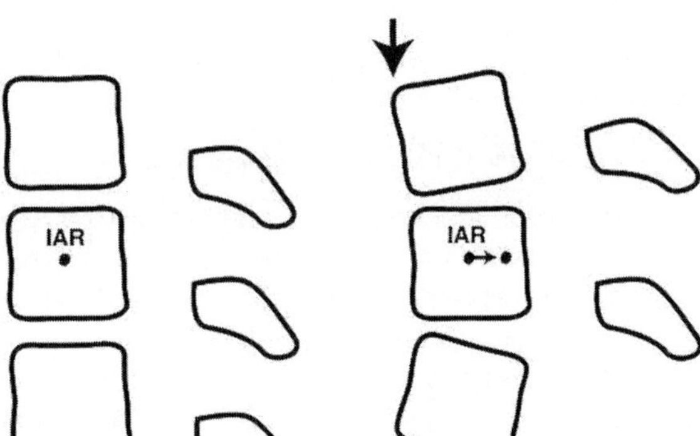

FIG. 7.8 A depiction of an applied bending moment altering the location of the IAR from the preload situation (*A*) to the postload situation (*B*). Because a ventral bending moment was applied, the IAR, as is often the case, moved dorsally. [From (1); copyright © 2001 by the American Association of Neurological Surgeons.]

where M = bending moment, F = applied force, and D = the perpendicular distance from the force vector to the IAR. The bending moment is, effectively, the torque applied by the force (1).

Hooke's Law

No solid is perfectly rigid. When several external forces act on a solid at rest and the resultant net force is zero, the solid remains at rest. Its size or shape, or both, however, will be altered by the external forces; that is, the solid will be deformed. Hooke's law states that for small displacements, the size of the deformation is proportional to the deforming force. This law is of significant importance when one considers the forces applied to the spine by a spinal instrumentation construct (as well as the response of the construct to these forces).

For larger displacements, however, the neutral zone (the component of the physiologic range of motion associated with significant flexibility and minimal stiffness at low loads) is exceeded and the elastic limit is reached. This is the point at which the force departs from the linear relationship between the size of deformation and the deforming force. Exceeding the elastic limit causes the solid to acquire a permanent set, so that if the external forces are removed, the solid does not spring back to its undeformed configuration. The solid will ultimately fail if further forces are applied. This point is termed the *point of failure*. For most materials, the elastic limit occurs close to the point at which a permanent set is produced.

Elastic Modulus

For small deformations, the simple Hooke's law relationship applies and is termed the *elastic modulus*:

$$\text{Elastic Modulus} = \text{Stress/Strain}$$

where the elastic modulus is a constant that is characteristic of a given material. Stress is defined as the force applied to an object (load), and strain is defined as the response of the object to the force (deformation).

Three types of elastic moduli exist: Young's modulus (a measure of the elastic properties of a body that is stretched or compressed), shear modulus (a measure of the shear deformation experienced by a body that is subjected to transverse forces of equal and opposite direction, applied at opposite faces of the body), and bulk modulus (the elastic deformation of a solid when it is squeezed).

Section Modulus and the Moment of Inertia

To understand the properties of spinal implants and instrumentation constructs, two additional concepts are integral: the *section mod-*

ulus (Z) and the *moment of inertia* (I). The section modulus (strength) is an indicator of the strength of an object, such as a rod or screw; the moment of inertia is an indicator of the object's stiffness and is a measure of an object's distribution about its centroid (e.g., the center of the rod). Considering a rod with a diameter D, the section modulus (Z) is defined by the equation

$$Z = \frac{\pi D_3}{32}$$

The moment of inertia (I), which correlates with stiffness, is defined by the equation

$$I = \frac{\pi D_4}{16}$$

It is therefore quite obvious that the diameter of a rod (or the core diameter of a screw) substantially affects their strength (resistance to failure in flexion) and stiffness (to the third and fourth power, respectively).

Stress (θ) is a measurement of the force per unit area applied to a structure and is defined by the equation

$$\theta = \text{Bending moment}/Z$$

Strain is the change in length or angle of a material subjected to a load. Strain may be either normal (linear) or shear (angular) in nature. Normal strain reflects tensile or compressive force–resisting abilities of a material; shear strain reflects angular deformation–resisting abilities of a material. The relationship between stress and failure is graphically depicted in *Figure 7.9*. Fundamentally, implants always fail at the point of maximum stress application. Since the numerator of the stress equation is a linear entity and the denominator is an exponential entity, stress may be maximum at unexpected locations (1) (*Fig. 7.9*).

Coupling

Coupling is the phenomenon whereby a movement of the spine obligates a separate movement about another axis. In the cervical region, for example, lateral bending results in rotation of the spinous processes away from the concave side of the direction of the bend (*Fig. 7.10*). This is due, in part, to the orientation of the facet joints as well as to the presence of the uncovertebral joints. In the lumbar region, however, the coupling movements associated with lateral bending are in the opposite direction, with the spinous processes rotating in the

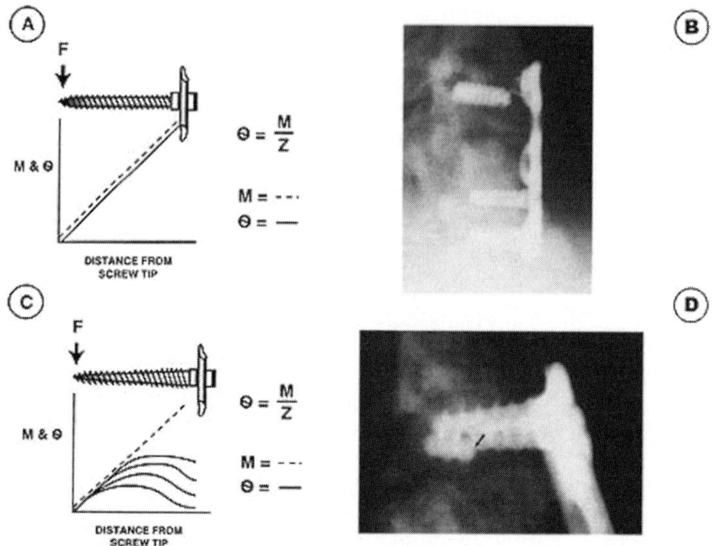

FIG. 7.9 An example of the relationship between stress and the strength of an object (e.g., screw). A screw with a constant inner diameter, attached to a plate in a fixed moment arm cantilevered manner, is exposed to a load as depicted in (*A*). This is associated with a bending moment that linearly increases along the screw from its tip (point of force application) to the plate (dotted line). Because stress (θ) is defined as M/Z ($\theta = M/Z$) and because the inner diameter of the screw (the denominator of the stress equation) is a constant, the stress also increases linearly as one passes along the screw toward the plate (solid line). The stress, therefore, is maximum at its junction with the plate. If the screw were to fracture, it would fracture at this juncture (*B*).

This scenario is altered if the inner diameter of the screw is ramped (conically shaped). This is portrayed in (*C*). The bending moment still increases linearly (dotted line). However, because stress (θ) equals M/Z and Z (i.e., strength) is proportional to the third power of the inner diameter of the screw, the denominator of the equation increases "exponentially" as one passes along the screw. A relatively complex relationship is therefore established between the resultant stress and the location along the screw. This depends on the "rate of change" of the screws inner diameter. A family of curves (solid lines), which is dependent on the extent of the ramp of the inner diameter, is thus generated (*C*). A clinical example of screw failure of a ramped inner diameter screw is depicted (*D*) (arrow designates fracture site). Note that failure occurs between the tip of the screw and its attachment site to the plate. If failure occurs, it occurs at the point of maximum stress application (apex of the curve describing the stress/location relationship for the particular screw; solid line). M = bending moment; Z = section modulus [strength]; θ = stress. [From (1); copyright © 2001 by the American Association of Neurological Surgeons.]

same direction as the concave side of the direction of the bend. The phenomenon of coupling also explains the association of the obligatory rotatory component associated with degenerative scoliosis of the lumbar spine.

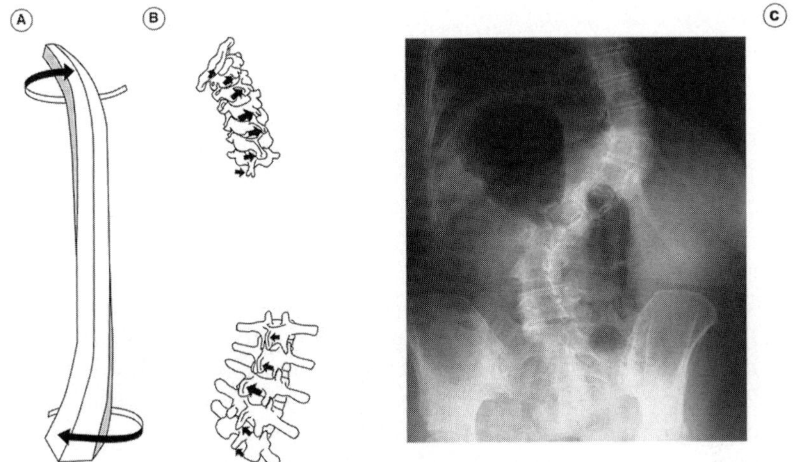

FIG. 7.10 Perhaps the most important manifestation of the coupling phenomenon is the relationship between lateral bending and rotation in the cervical and lumbar regions. This is depicted diagrammatically (*A*) and anatomically (*B*). Note that the coupling phenomenon results in spinal rotation, in opposite directions, in these two regions. A biconcave thoracic and lumbar curve, as depicted in an AP view, illustrates this phenomenon (*C*). Note that the lumbar spinous processes are rotated toward the concave side of the curve. [From (1); copyright © 2001 by the American Association of Neurological Surgeons.]

STABILITY AND INSTABILITY

White and Panjabi (2) define clinical stability of the spine as the ability of the spine under physiologic loads to limit patterns of displacement so as not to damage or irritate the spinal cord or nerve roots and, in addition, to prevent incapacitating deformity or pain caused by structural changes. Spinal stability is a phenomenon of increments ("shades of gray," so to speak); it is not absolutely absent or present. Depending on the circumstances, the spine is expected to provide varying degrees of support (stability). Therefore, spinal stability should be defined according to the circumstances.

The converse of stability, obviously, is instability. Whereas stability is difficult to define, instability is somewhat more easily quantified and assessed. Because instability is possibly more appropriate to consider clinically, it is discussed here. Instability should be defined generally, with specific consideration being given to the type of instability. Instability is the inability to limit excessive or abnormal spinal displacement. The use of the word *excessive* reflects the difficulty of clinical quantitation. This chapter focuses on the understanding of—and how to deal with—the uncertainty associated with the quantitation of instability.

There are two fundamental categories of instability: acute and chronic. Acute instability may be broken down into two subcategories: overt and limited. Chronic instability can likewise be broken down into two subcategories: glacial instability and the instability associated with dysfunctional segmental motion. These subcategories are not distinct from each other (see below).

The Quantification of Acute Instability

One has only to read the voluminous literature on acute spinal instability to appreciate the difficulties associated with the definition process. Many authors have attempted to quantitate the degree or extent of acute instability using a point-system approach. White and Panjabi (2) describe a region-specific point system in which an accumulation of five or more points indicates the presence of an unstable spine. Their regional point system emphasizes differences between the cervical, thoracic and thoracolumbar, and lumbar regions. It is emphasized that these differences are perhaps more theoretical than objective.

White and Panjabi (2) recommend a stretch test for the assessment of acute cervical spine stability. This involves progressive addition of cervical traction weight (to 33% of the patient's weight) with serial radiographic and clinical assessments. A positive test (indicating the presence of instability) shows a disc interspace separation of more than 1.7 mm or a change in angle between vertebrae of more than 7.5° between the prestretch and poststretch conditions. The merits of this test are uncertain. First, it is clearly not without risks, whether those risks be immediately obvious or occult. The risk of tethering the spinal cord over a ventral mass goes without saying, but perhaps the most significant and least immediately recognized risk of such a procedure is the risk of a false-negative test, that is, the seeming presence of stability in an unstable situation. Unfortunately (in the author's opinion), this test has been used as a determinant of eligibility for participation in contact sports. The surgeon must remember that, particularly in athletes, the resistance to stretching by muscle action (voluntary or involuntary) may easily conceal ligamentous deficiencies. Furthermore, physical contact during many sports results in a far greater transmission of force to the spine than that achieved during a stretch test. Finally, the loads are of a different nature (stretch vs axial loading) (2).

Dynamic radiography may provide utility. The surgeon must keep in mind, however, that flexion and extension radiographs may not be helpful, and in fact, following trauma, they may even be misleading. If pathology is observed and iatrogenic injury via the act of flexion and extension is not incurred, they are useful, but they are not without risk if spinal instability is present. Perhaps their greatest risk is that a "normal" flexion-extension radiograph, which implies a safe clinical situation, indeed may not reflect such a situation—that is, the test may be falsely negative. Incomplete patient cooperation and "guarding" against excessive spinal movement because of underlying acute pathology can disguise a pathological process that may lead to catastrophe if treated improperly. If flexion/extension radiographs are used, the surgeon must have a good grasp of the normal flexibility characteristics of the spine. Similar problems have been observed with degenerative disease.

Acknowledgement of the extent of instability is critical for surgical decision making. It is also critical for other reasons, however, such as turning, ambulation, and intubation considerations. The notion that nasal intubation is safer than endotracheal intubation may not be valid, at least regarding the upper cervical spine.

Determination of the presence of more chronic forms of instability should be considered separately. These clinical situations are obviously different, as are the surgeon's expectations and the patient's risks (1).

"Column" Concepts of Spinal Integrity

Many definition schemes for instability use point systems to quantitate the extent of spinal integrity (or loss thereof) and, ultimately, to determine the presence or absence of spinal stability. These schemes are usually based on a "column" concept of spinal structural integrity, such as those described by Louis; by Bailey, Holdsworth, Kelly, and Whitesides; and by Denis (*Fig. 7.11*). The consideration of "columns" in defining the extent of instability is of some value, because it helps the physician to conceptualize and categorize case-specific phenomena. The three-column (one ventral column and two lateral columns) theory of Louis is based on the fact that the spine bears axial loads principally by the acceptance of these loads along the three vertical bony and soft-tissue columns (the vertebral body and intervertebral discs and the two facet joint complexes) at each segmental level (*Fig. 7.11*). Although this is indeed true, the concept of Louis assists in the instability assessment process only when predominantly axial loads are considered. It assesses the bony component of failure much more effectively than the soft-tissue component of failure because of its obvious association with the bony columns of the spine (vertebral body and facet joints). This aspect of stability is easily assessed by radiography and CT. It can be quantitated by assessing the extent of collapse or fracture. Except for the case of significant vertebral body failure, however, a correlation between the extent of bony injury and the presence of overt spinal instability may be tenuous. Furthermore, Louis' three-

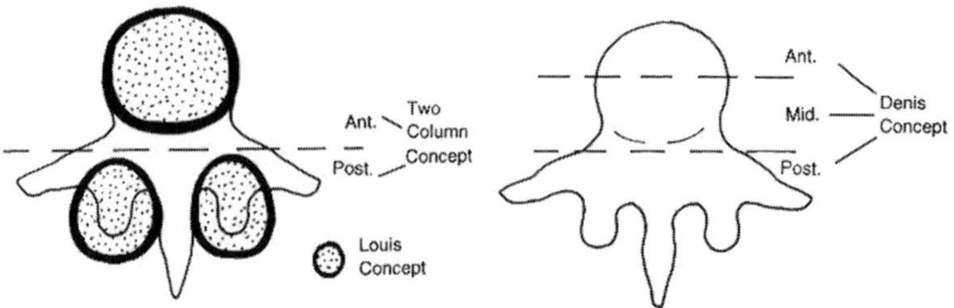

FIG. 7.11 The "column" concepts of spinal stability. The concept described by Louis (*left*) assigns significance to the vertebral body and the facet joint complexes (lateral masses) on either side of the dorsal spine. Denis' three-column concept (*right*) assigns significance to the region of the neural axis and the integrity of the posterior vertebral body wall (the middle column). The two-column construct (*left*) relies on anatomically defined structures, the vertebral body (anterior column), and the posterior elements (posterior column). Louis' three-column concept (*right*) similarly relies on anatomically defined structures. [From (1); copyright © 2001 by the American Association of Neurological Surgeons.]

column theory does not facilitate the assessment of the distraction, flexion, and extension components of the injury (1).

The two- and three-column concepts of Bailey, Holdsworth, Kelly, and Whitesides (two-column) and of Denis (three-column) are more applicable to this situation. They not only assist in assessing the bony collapse associated with axial load-bearing but also offer insight regarding the assessment of the distraction, flexion, and extension components of the injury (injury to the dorsal elements) of the spinal elements of the spinal column. Denis' three-column theory, which adds the concept of a middle column to the two-column theories, allows specific assessment of that component of the spinal column in the region of the neutral axis. The neutral axis is that longitudinal region of the spinal column that bears a significant portion of the axial load and about which spinal element distraction or compression does not excessively occur with flexion or extension. Usually, the neural axis is located in the region of the middorsal aspect of the vertebral body—that is, the middle column of Denis. Usually, the IARs in the sagittal plane are located close to or within the neural axis (1,2).

The three columns of Denis are conceptually useful for determination of the presence or absence of acute instability. The point system used here uses his scheme (1).

Categorization of Instability

To facilitate and understanding of and, therefore, the clinical application of the terms *stability* and *instability* (overt and limited), a more simplistic approach is taken here for the subaxial cervical, thoracic, and lumbar spine. This is done because strict criteria for the universal definition of stability and instability are impossible to derive. Therefore, the surgeon must realize that the clinical decision-making process, as it pertains to the definition of instability, is somewhat tenuous and relies heavily on clinical judgement as well as the surgeon's intuition and "savvy."

Instability is divided here into two categories: acute and chronic. Each is unique; however, neither is clearly defined. Each uses, at least in part, the concepts of each of the column theories discussed above.

Instability, being a phenomenon that is unique to a specific clinical circumstance, is most appropriately defined separately for each category rather than according to the schemes of White and Panjabi (2), which define instability in a global sense but quantitate it on a region-specific basis. The scheme used here for acute instability categorizes instability (overt and limited) with regard to the potential for catastrophe. The scheme used here also differs from that of White and Panjabi (2) by its de-emphasis of region specificity.

Four subcategories of instability are also defined here and are referred to throughout the chapter:

1. Overt instability,
2. Limited instability,
3. Glacial instability, and
4. Instability associated with dysfunctional segmental motion.

The first two are acute, and the second two are chronic. As already mentioned, these categories are not distinct from each other. None are applicable to all clinical situations. Overt and limited instability are applicable to acute posttraumatic situations or cases of spinal involvement by tumor or infection. Therefore, a relatively acute disruption of spinal integrity is implied. Both of these categories of instability may have a chronic component as well. For example, if an overtly unstable spine is not surgically stabilized and does not acquire stability nonoperatively, then the acute overt instability blends into a chronic phase. Similarly, if a spine with acute limited instability does not heal properly, excessive ligamentous laxity may persist and become chronic. The latter may be difficult to differentiate, at times, from glacial instability or dysfunctional segmental motion. Glacial instability and dysfunctional segmental motion are usually manifestations of a process that is more chronic than overt or limited instability. They are usually associated with degenerative disease or the long-term sequelae of trauma, tumor, or infection.

The terms *overt instability* and *limited instability* are applicable to situations in which there is a risk of acute loss of stability. The term *glacial instability* is applicable in more chronic situations. Glacial instability is confirmed by serial assessments or by incriminating evidence (e.g., a translational deformation of the spine in the presence of a pain syndrome consistent with the deformation). The term *dysfunctional segmental motion* is much less objectively defined. It applies to situations in which overt or limited clinical instability is not present but in which pain, combined with abnormal significant spinal motion, is present (1).

A dysfunctional motion segment involves neither the overt disruption of spinal integrity nor deformity progression. The associated instability has been termed *mechanical instability*. The term *dysfunctional segmental motion* is used here, however, because of its less controversial nature and its more accurate reflection of the suspected pathological process involved. It is emphasized that a dysfunctional motion segment is very difficult to define or quantitate (1).

A characteristic pain pattern (deep and agonizing pain that is usually worsened by activity [loading] and improved by inactivity [unloading]) suggests the diagnosis. This pain pattern is similar to that associated with glacial instability. It is akin to the pain described by a patient with a markedly degenerated hip (mechanical pain). When this pain pattern is combined with degenerative disc interspace changes or with tumor or infection involving either the disc interspace, vertebral body, or some other vertebral component, the diagnosis of dysfunctional segmental motion is suggested. The pain pattern implicates an exaggeration of reflex muscle activity that is enlisted to maintain an acceptable amount of stability (implying that adequate intrinsic stability is not provided by the spine proper) (1).

The presence of dysfunctional segmental motion, as ascertained by abnormal segmental movement demonstrated radiographically, or by determination of the IAR or the center of rotation, may aid in this aspect of diagnosis. These types of movement may not be obvious on flexion and extension radiographs.

Dysfunctional segmental motion may be implied by the observation of excessive degenerative changes at a given segmental level. For this degeneration to have occurred, excessive stresses or motion must have been predisposing factors in the disc interspace changes.

It cannot be overemphasized that the lack of objectivity makes the diagnosis of dysfunctional segmental motion often controversial and, simultaneously, subject to abuse. Fusion and instrumentation operations are lucrative for the surgeon. Likewise, the diagnostic algorithm that is used is often lucrative for the diagnostician. These factors, combined with the inability to objectively assess either operative indications or surgical results, enhance the potential for abuse in the establishment of this diagnosis (1).

THE BIOMECHANICS OF SPINAL COLUMN FAILURE

Since tumor and infection often biomechanically affect the spine in a manner similar to that of trauma, spine trauma will be used as the injury paradigm of the spinal column. This is compared and contrasted to the normal situation.

The most common and illustrative spine injury types are presented to portray the associated mechanisms of injury and pathological anatomy. Radiographic diagnosis of instability and pathological anatomy relies heavily on the plain film (AP and lateral radiographs). Computed tomography, however, plays a significant role, particularly when dorsal bony element disruption is in question, and MR imaging may be particularly useful for the definition of soft-tissue injury and neural element compromise. These modalities are referenced herein, when appropriate.

Loss of Structural Integrity of the Upper Cervical Spine

The upper cervical spine is prone to traumatically induced injuries caused by:

1. The unique anatomic arrangement of this region,
2. The substantial spinal movements allowed in this region, and
3. The high incidence of exposure to significant pathological stresses to this region by trauma (usually in association with head trauma).

Previously reported observations indicate that most upper cervical spine injuries are the result of blows to the head. This, however, is not always the case. A deceleration of the torso, combined with a restriction of movement of the cervical spine, creates the application of a flexion/distraction force that can result in an applied bending moment. Spinal involvement with tumor or infection obviously decreases the tolerance to such injuries.

Very violent movements of the head can disrupt the usually stable and protective ligaments of the upper cervical spine. The kinetic energy absorbed by the calvarium in these cases, however, may be sufficient to cause death by head injury. Even so, the spine injury incurred may also be of a fatal nature.

RELEVANT ANATOMY

The C1 vertebrae is essentially a ring with an interconnecting/transecting transverse ligament (transverse ligament of the atlas) and articulating facets (both rostral to the occiput and caudal to the axis) on both sides. A multitude of ligaments secure fixation to surrounding vertebral and cranial bony elements. Failure of these ligaments may occur following excessive load application. The orientation of the articulating facets make the ring of C1 prone to injury from axial loading, and the location of the dorsal arch of C1 make it prone to hyperextension and hyperflexion loading injuries.

The pedicles of C2 are located more ventrally and medially relative to other spinal levels. They essentially form a dorsolateral extension of the vertebral body, connecting the vertebral body proper with its superior articulating process (lateral mass). The pars interarticularis of C2 has a more rostral-caudal orientation. This affects the manner in which loads are transmitted through the occiput-C1-C2 complex and the type of injuries that are sustained when loading to failure occurs; that is, when an axial load is borne, the lateral masses accept the load (1).

FACTORS AFFECTING INJURY TYPE

The orientation of the force vector applied to the cervical spine is the predominant factor dictating the type of injury that results. The applied force vector most commonly arises from a blow to the head, but it may also result from a deceleration injury. The relative intrinsic strengths of C1 and C2 as well as of the surrounding spinal elements (including the adjacent vertebrae, calvarium, and supporting ligaments) secondarily dictate the type of injury by "setting the stage" for dissipating the energy of the applied force vector (*Fig. 7.12*). The kinetic energy imparted predominantly dictates the magnitude of the injury.

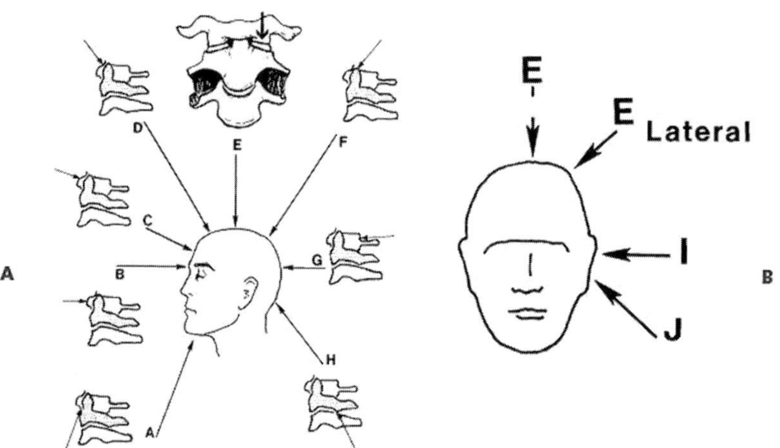

FIG. 7.12 The mechanism of injury (orientation of injury force vector) partly dictates the type of injury incurred. (*A*) Sagittal plain injury. (*B*) Coronal plane injury. [From (1); copyright © 2001 by the American Association of Neurological Surgeons.]

The "stage setting" aspect of the relative intrinsic strengths of the spinal elements is particularly obvious when, theoretically, more than one injury could result from the application of a single force vector. For example, an axially applied load can result in a burst fracture of the atlas, a C2 burst-pedicle fracture, or subaxial cervical spine burst fracture. The relative intrinsic strengths of the ring of C1, the body and pedicles of C2, and the subaxial cervical spine vertebral bodies dictate the type of injury that is incurred if a failure-producing force is, indeed, applied. Usually, the ring of C1 or the subaxial cervical spine vertebral body is the weakest link; thus, the C1 burst fracture (Jefferson fracture) or a subaxial cervical spine fracture is incurred. Occasionally, however, C2 is the weakest link (see below) (1).

APPLIED FORCE VECTORS

The kinetic energy imparted to the upper cervical spine is, in most cases, directed to this region through the odontoid process via the anterior arch of C1 or the transverse ligament of the atlas, unless a true axial load is applied. The direction (orientation) of the applied force vector predominantly dictates the location of the fault line (location of fracture site or ligamentous disruption). The location of the fault line, however, is also dictated by the intrinsic strengths and weaknesses of C1 and C2 and of the surrounding bony and soft-tissue elements.

Although most failure-producing forces applied to the upper cervical spine are applied via the odontoid process, a true axial load injury, in which the superior articulating processes (lateral masses) of C1 and C2 accept the entirety of the load applied to the upper cervical spine, is an exception. If structural failure of the upper cervical spine occurs, a bursting of C1 or, less frequently, of C2 or an occipital condyle fracture may occur.

Loss of Structural Integrity of the Subaxial Cervical, Thoracic, and Lumbar Spine

RELEVANT ANATOMY

The anatomy of the entire subaxial spine is relatively monotonous compared with the significant anatomic variations from level to level observed in the upper cervical spine. Therefore, subaxial injuries are not as varied as the upper cervical injuries in terms of the number of definable injury patterns and types. They are, therefore, grouped together.

FACTORS AFFECTING INJURY TYPE

Denis described several fracture types with accompanying modes of failure for the subaxial spine. This scheme of fracture-type definition is currently the most widely utilized. As opposed to the injury-type definition scheme of Denis, however, the injury types described here are based on mechanism of injury. The difference between the two schemes is subtle, but it is most obvious regarding the differentiation of ventral wedge compression and burst fractures. The presence or absence of retropulsed bone and/or disc fragments in the spinal canal is not used herein as a criteria for fracture-type definition, as is the case with Denis' scheme. Denis' concepts are not to be disregarded, however.

Fundamentally, the manner in which a load is applied affects the bending moment that is applied. This, in turn, alters the stresses placed on a spinal segment.

The fracture pattern is altered by the position of the force application in relation to the IAR. The point of force application directly affects the type and extent of injury by the alteration of the bending moment (not by alteration of the force application). An alteration of the IAR, therefore, can affect the bending moment significantly. In turn, the type and extent of force application and the mode of failure and fracture incurred are altered. A mechanism of injury that not only applies a load to the spine but also alters the bending moment can significantly affect the stresses applied to the spinal elements.

APPLIED FORCE VECTORS

The magnitude and characteristics of the failure-producing force and the resultant configuration of the injured spinal level (as well as the need for spinal decompression) should, in part, dictate the management scheme that is employed. As such, an understanding and appreciation of the aforementioned are essential.

INJURY TYPES AND MECHANISMS OF INJURY

Ventral Wedge Compression Fractures. Ventral wedge compression fractures are the product of an axial load and a ventrally oriented bending moment (to failure); that is, the axial load is eccentrically placed (ventral to the IAR) (*Fig. 7.13*). This results in a flexion deformity of the fractured bone (an asymmetry of vertebral body height in which the ventral height is less than the dorsal height). The cervical spine and the thoracic spine as well as the thoracolumbar junction are prone to such injuries because of the flexibility of the cervical spine and the often-assumed, relatively flexed posture of the cervical and thoracic spine and the thoracolumbar junction at the moment of impact. This often counterbalances the influence of the natural lordotic posture of the cervical spine. If, however, the patient has not assumed a posture of flexion, then the biomechanics of the natural lordotic posture prevail, and

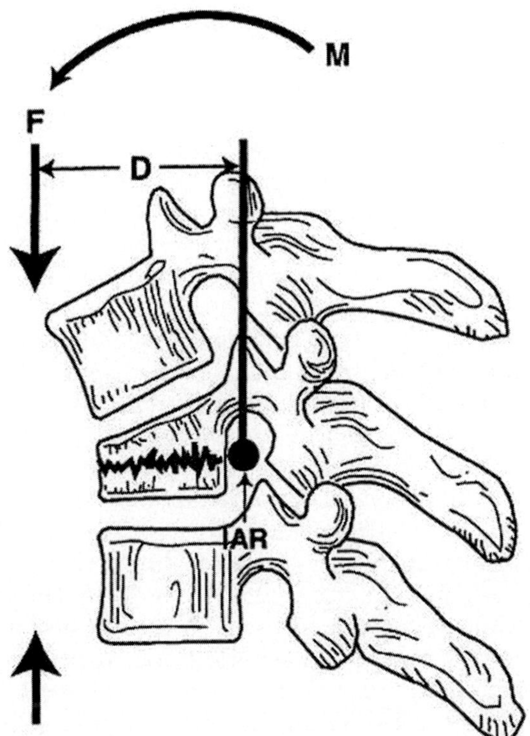

FIG. 7.13 A depiction of the injury force vector causing a ventral wedge compression fracture. *F* = applied force vector; *D* = length of moment arm (from IAR to plane of *F*); *M* = bending moment. [From (1); copyright © 2001 by the American Association of Neurological Surgeons.]

a burst fracture may occur. The thoracic and thoracolumbar spine have a natural kyphotic curvature that, by its nature, exposes the spine to an increased chance for a flexion component of the injury. An eccentric load application to the spine is often encouraged by a flexed posture, whether it be secondary to a "natural" kyphosis or to a superimposed flexion (upon the natural regional spinal lordotic configuration) (1).

Conversely, the mid to low cervical and lumbar spine has an intrinsic lordotic posture. In addition, the lumbar spine, because of the massive size of the vertebral bodies, is simultaneously relatively unyielding. These factors minimize the likelihood of the development of a significant flexion component to the development of a spine fracture in these regions; that is, the bending moment is nil or nearly nil. Therefore, an isolated axial load is often applied to the mid to low cervical and lumbar regions. In the cervical region, however, the assumption of a kyphotic posture during the moment of impact (e.g., during spear tackling) results in a higher incidence of wedge compression fractures in the cervical region than in the lumbar region.

Nevertheless, ventral wedge compression fractures do occur in the mid to low lumbar region. Because of the reasons outlined above, they occur more frequently in the upper limits of the lumbar spine because of the lessening of the natural lordotic curvature that is observed as one ascends the lumbar spine. Retropulsion of bony and/or disc fragments into the spinal canal may or may not occur.

Burst Fractures. If a true axial load (to failure) is applied to the subaxial spine, a wedging (asymmetry of vertebral body height loss) of the resultant vertebral body fracture is unlikely. Thus, a symmetric compression of the vertebral body results and is termed a *burst fracture*. This "pancaking" of the vertebral body often causes a retropulsion of bony fragments into the spinal canal as well as dural sac compression. This retropulsion is a requirement of Denis for his definition of burst fracture. It is a manifestation of an axial load that is not eccentrically placed with regard to the IAR. The latter point is key. It seems appropriate to address it in greater detail here (1).

If a force (an axial load) is transmitted in a rostral-to-caudal direction along the axis of the spine, the vector of the force passes either through or close to the IAR of all the vertebral bodies. Since the axis of rotation of a vertebral body is about the IAR, the location of the IAR dictates the vertebral body's response to the applied force. If a force vector passes precisely through the IAR of a vertebral body that was stressed to failure by the force, a burst fracture will result, because no eccentric component to the force vector is present. Therefore, the moment arm length of this force vector (perpendicular distance from the force vector to the IAR) is zero (*Fig. 7.14*).

If a force vector passes in a plane that is adjacent to the IAR, bending of the spine will occur if the force is less than that required to produce failure. The direction of the bend is such that the concave side of the curvature induced is directed toward the plane and orientation that the force vector assumes in relation to the IAR. If the force applied is sufficient to cause failure, a fracture may result. This fracture will be eccentrically located with respect to the IAR and will result in an eccentric collapse of the vertebral body (wedge compression fracture), the direction of which is dictated by the location of the force vector. Utilizing these biomechanical facts, one can then easily categorize vertebral body fractures by mechanism of injury or, more appropriately (and similarly), by the configuration of the vertebral body following the application of the force to failure (fracture).

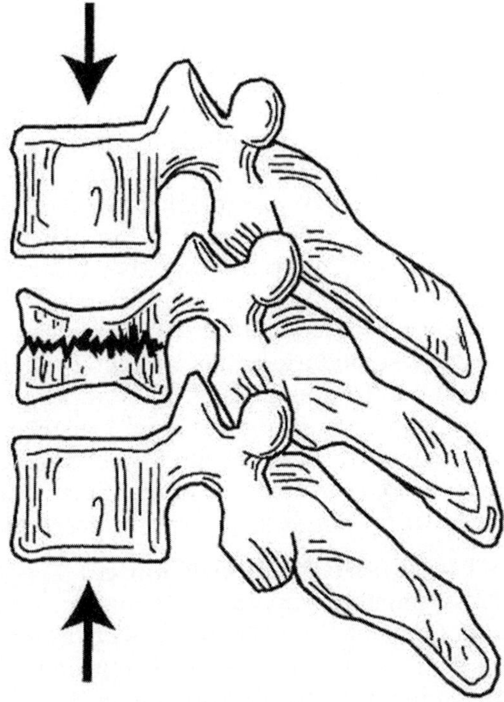

FIG. 7.14 The mechanism of injury of a burst fracture: true axial loading without a bending moment ($D = 0$). [From (1); copyright © 2001 by the American Association of Neurological Surgeons.]

Burst fractures, by virtue of their isolated axial load mechanism of injury requirement (relative), occur most frequently in the upper and mid cervical and lumbar regions. In the case of the lumbar region, this situation is created by the relatively diminished flexibility of the lumbar spine, compared with the cervical spine, as well as by the substantial lordotic posture that is present in the low lumbar spine. In the lower lumbar spine, however, these fractures are less common due to an altered spinal configuration (lordosis) and an increased intrinsic spinal column compression–resisting ability secondary to increased bony and muscle mass in this region. In the cervical region, the flexibility of the spine contributes to an increased incidence of a flexion component to an injury. Therefore, the incidence of wedge compression fractures is greater in this region.

Lateral Wedge Compression Fractures. Most vertebral body fractures are not pure; that is, they are combinations of fracture types that have resulted from multiple injury mechanisms. The two fracture types, wedge compression and burst fractures, are rarely pure. The discussion regarding these two fracture types has centered about the consideration of sagittal plane deformations. Coronal plane deformities, however, often occur simultaneously. Radiograph examinations (AP films) often demonstrate an asymmetric loss of height of the vertebral body (comparing the right and left sides). This being the case, a lateral wedge compression fracture component coexists with the sagittal plane fracture component. They, however, also occur as isolated injuries. These injuries are caused by an axial load that is eccentrically placed relative to the IAR (similar to, but different in location from, the axial load associated with ventral wedge compression fractures).

The mechanism of injury of the lateral wedge compression fracture may be secondary to the "buckling" of the spine that follows the application of an axial load. This buckling results in an "effective" lateral bending moment. An axial load, combined with a lateral bending moment, may result in the same vertebral body deformity as that observed with the axial buckling injury. This buckling may also occur in the sagittal plane, with a resultant compression fracture.

Flexion-Distraction (Chance) Fractures. Axial loading is the most common primary mechanism of spinal column injury. A distraction component uncommonly plays a role, particularly in the subaxial spine, because a distraction component of trauma is rarely applied to the spine. One such circumstance in the subaxial spine, however, occurs when a lap belt is worn without a shoulder harness by a person involved in a deceleration motor vehicle accident. Distraction and flexion of the lumbar spine results. This is secondary to the restriction of pelvic and lumbosacral movement, with accompanying unrestricted distraction and forward flexion of the remainder of the spine (flexion bending moment). This injury was initially described by Chance and, thus, commonly bears his name. It may be broken down into two basic types: a diastases (fracture cleavage) through the pedicles and a fracture through the vertebral end plate. Variations may occur. Regardless of the type of Chance fracture, the mechanism of injury is the same.

Dorsal Element Fractures. Previous discussion has focused on the effects of pure axial loads (force vector passing through the IAR) or predominantly axial loads with a slight eccentric component (force vector passing close to, but not through, the IAR). The majority of the failure-producing axial load force vectors are oriented in a plane anterior or anterolateral to the IAR. If, indeed, they are located dorsal to the IAR (an extension component), then an excessive compressive force is applied to the dorsal elements at the effected spinal level, thus increasing the chance of dorsal element failure.

Dorsal element fractures are not uncommon entities. This is particularly true in the cervical spine, where the spine naturally assumes a lordotic posture and the vertebral segments are small compared with other regions of the spine. The lumbar spine, which also assumes a lordotic posture, has a lesser incidence of posterior element fractures because of the more massive nature of the vertebrae and the somewhat sagittal orientation of the facet joints. In the cervical region, spinal extension thrusts the opposing facet surfaces together, thus subjecting the facets and pars interarticularis to significant stress, while rotation causes them to slide past each other.

Because of the relative lack of flexibility and the vertical orientation of the lumbar facets, their fracture, particularly as isolated entities, is relatively uncommon. A hyperextension injury results in the facet joints sliding past each other because of their vertical orientation. Lamina and pars interarticularis fractures may result. At the same time, the relative restriction of rotation of the lumbar spine minimizes the chances that rotation could result in an injury to the facet joint(s).

Rotatory components may also induce posterior element injuries by forcing opposing inferior and superior articulating facet joints against each other with such force that failure occurs. Often, the forces applied are of such magnitude that vertebral body fracture or disc interspace disruption simultaneously occur. Posterior element lumbar spine fractures are most commonly associated with other injuries to the spinal column complex (compression fractures, rotational injuries, or translational injuries). A violent rotational component of the injury may result in the disruption of posterior elements as well as of the integrity of the ventral axial load–resisting substructure.

Spinous process and laminar fractures may occasionally result from extreme flexion or extension. Similarly, extreme lateral bending may result in transverse process fracture(s) on the convex side of the bend.

Ligamentous Injuries. Ligamentous injuries of the lumbar spine are common, but they are usually associated with other bony injuries. This is as opposed to the cervical spine, where isolated ligamentous injuries are common. This is manifested by the high incidence of positive MR images in the face of negative radiographs or CT scans observed following cervical spine injury. Most useful in this regard are T_2-weighted MR images.

Isolated ligamentous injuries occur more commonly in the cervical region due, in part, to its substantial flexibility. This flexibility allows for a greater strain to be placed on the ligaments. The more massive and less flexible lumbar spine does not rely as heavily as the cervical spine on ligamentous support. In fact, the posterior ligaments, particularly the interspinous and supraspinous ligaments and especially in the low lumbar region, are weak or essentially nonexistent. Therefore, isolated ligamentous injuries occur at a lesser frequency in this region.

Facet Dislocation. Facet dislocation occurs frequently in the cervical and, to a lesser degree, in the upper thoracic region. It is rare in the lumbar region. Occurrence is more common in the cervical and thoracic spine because of the relative coronal orientation of the facet joints in these regions. An exaggerated flexion results in the normal limits of facet joint mobility being exceeded. This, in turn, causes the joints themselves to become dysfunctional by fracture, perching, or locking. Obviously, these deformations affect stability.

The associated force vectors contribute to the complexity of the resultant injury pattern. A true flexion moment application most commonly results in bilateral facet dislocation. A flexion moment, combined with a rotational component, most commonly results in a unilateral facet dislocation. Either of the these mechanisms or hyperextension, combined with an axial load, may result in facet fracture.

Loss of Structural Integrity of the Sacrum and Surrounding Bony Elements

Sacral fractures are uncommon as isolated entities. They are usually associated with disruption of the pelvic ring in at least one additional location. Two basic types of sacral fractures occur: vertical and horizontal. They fundamentally involve three zones of the sacrum and, thus, have been classified as such. Zone 1 injuries involve fractures (usually vertical) through the ala and do not involve the neuroforamina. They usually result from lateral compression forces and, if a significant translational component does not exist, are relatively stable. Zone 2 injuries are generally vertical fractures as well and involve the ventral neuroforamina. Zone 3 injuries are vertical and/or horizontal and involve the sacral spinal canal; thus, neurological injury (particularly bladder dysfunction) often accompanies these fractures.

DEGENERATIVE DISEASE

The management of degenerative and inflammatory spine diseases is complex. The combination of the degenerative alterations of bony spinal integrity and ligamentous instability are the predominant manifestations. Degenerative and inflammatory spine diseases, presented here, include primary degenerative diseases of the spine (e.g., spondylosis and Scheuermann's disease) as well as inflammatory diseases of the spine (e.g., rheumatoid arthritis, ankylosing spondylitis, ossification of the posterior longitudinal ligament [OPLL], ankylosing hyperostosis, and related processes).

The degenerative process involves the disc interspace, facet joints, and intraspinal and paraspinal tissues. Degenerative changes of the intervertebral disc typically involve one, or a combination, of four processes:

1. Loss of disc interspace height,
2. Irregularities in the disc end plate,
3. Sclerosis of the disc interspace in the region of the end plates, and
4. Osteophyte formation.

Soft-tissue proliferation may accompany this process as an associated phenomenon or may be a primary process. Degenerative disc disease is defined by Kramer as biomechanical and pathological conditions of the intervertebral segment caused by degeneration, inflammation, or infection. Like the changes associated with disc interspace degeneration, facet joint degenerative changes are often associated with increased laxity of movement. As the degenerative process proceeds, however, an element of stability is often conferred. This is often referred to as the spine "restabilization" process. Restabilization results from a stiffening of the spine caused by one or more of the four previously mentioned processes.

Intraspinous and paraspinous tissue inflammation, calcification, and hypertrophy are commonly associated with spondylosis (e.g., hypertrophy of the ligamentum flavum), rheumatoid arthritis (e.g., bursa inflammation and pannus formation), and OPLL (e.g., calcification and hypertrophy of the posterior longitudinal ligament). Ankylosing spondylitis is the only inflammatory or degenerative disease not associated with increased stability via diminished motion secondary to ankylosis (fusion).

The pathogenesis of degenerative disc disease varies according to the underlying disease process. Fundamentally, aberrant physiological responses to stresses placed on the spine and accelerated deterioration of the integrity of spinal elements underlie the pathological process, regardless of the disease entity region of the spine that is involved. Before the degenerative process and accompanying pathology can be appreciated, however, the normal physiological processes associated with the disc interspace and related structures must be appreciated (1).

Anatomy and Physiology of the Disc Interspace

The disc interspaces account for approximately 20% of the height of the spine. The disc consists of an outer annulus fibrosus and an inner nucleus pulposus. It is bordered rostrally and caudally by a cartilaginous plate. The latter is part of the vertebral body and is composed of hyaline cartilage. The medullary bone of the vertebral body is connected to the cartilaginous plate and provides it, as well as the disc proper, with nutrients via diffusion through fine pores (laminae cribosae).

The annulus fibrosus is composed of laminated bands of fibrous tissue (predominantly collagen) oriented in opposite directions, with consecutive layers situated in an alternating manner at an approximately 30° angle from the disc interspace. This 30° relationship of the annular fibers to the disc interspace provides a greater resistance to tension (rotation) than to bending. In fact, the rotation-limiting effect is enhanced by distraction of the disc interspace. This may have significant implications regarding torsional instability and even mechanical pain. The inner bands of the annulus are attached to the cartilaginous plate, whereas the marginal zone is attached to the ring epiphysis of the vertebral body and the osseous tissue of the vertebral body. These latter attachments (Sharpey's fibers) are stronger than the more medial (inner) attachments to the cartilaginous plate. The annulus fibrosus is stronger and more abundant ventrally and laterally than it is dorsally. In fact, in youth, the ventral annulus fibrosus merges into nucleus fibrosus. The fact that the dorsal fibers of the annulus fibrosus are weaker contributes to the manifestations of the disc degeneration process (see below).

The nucleus pulposus, a remnant of the notochord, is located in the dorsal portion of the intervertebral disc. It consists of reticular bands of closely packed nuclei surrounded by a liquid mucoid ground substance. It has been implicated as a source of nerve root compression as well as inflammatory irritation. The water content of the nucleus pulposus decreases from approximately 90% at birth to approximately 70% by age 70. The water, however, is not free. It is reversibly bound to macromolecules via their intense hydroscopic properties. In fact, the water content changes from morning to afternoon, which implies changes in response to weight-bearing (see below). In addition, pressure-dependent fluid movement in and out of the intervertebral disc leads to measurable changes in a person's height from the awakening supine position to the late-afternoon erect position. Multiple authors have observed this fact, which is summarized nicely by Kramer (1).

The latter point implies that water escapes and enters the disc through a semipermeable membrane. Other small molecules, such as waste products and nutrients, must also pass through this membrane. Changes in the water content of the disc in response to weight-bearing imply a hydrostatic pressure effect on disc interspace physiology. The hydrostatic pressure within the intervertebral disc in the erect position is many times greater than that within surrounding tissue. For the disc to retain water, fluid movement must occur against this very steep pressure gradient. The mechanism through which this occurs is an osmotic pressure–driven counterforce to the hydrostatic pressure. The macromolecules in the interior of the disc take up fluid on account of their hydroscopic capacity (*Fig. 7.15*). In equilibrium, the following equation is manifest:

Extradiscal hydrostatic pressure + Intradiscal oncotic pressure
= Intradiscal hydrostatic pressure + Extradiscal oncotic pressure

Whenever one side outweighs the other (e.g., because of weight-bearing), equilibrium is disrupted and fluid moves across the semipermeable membrane. Increased weight-bearing causes intradiscal fluid to escape via hydrostatic forces. This increases the concentration of the macromolecules within the disc interspace and results in increased intradiscal oncotic pressure. This, in turn, increases the absorption capacity and nutrients of delivery to the disc. In addition to the biomechanical effects, this fluid movement allows the passage of nutrients and waste products across the membrane. Therefore, the greater the activity of the subject, the more active this form of transport. Traction is an obvious mechanism by which the intradiscal pressure can be reduced, thus causing an increase in intradiscal water content and an increase in disc height.

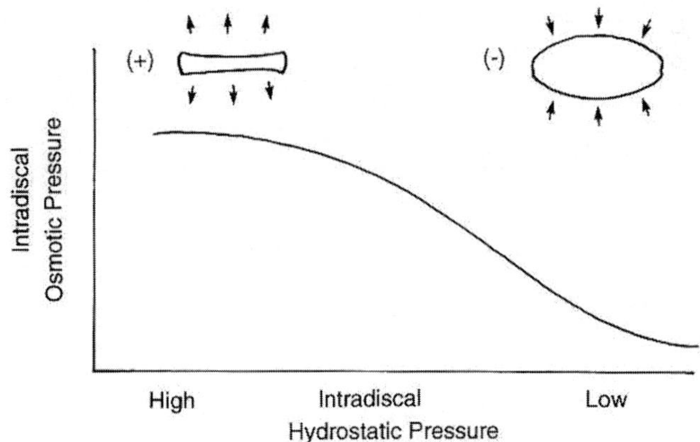

FIG. 7.15 Osmotic and hydrostatic factors affecting the disc interspace (after Kramer). Note that an increased interdiscal pressure, resulting from an increase in weight-bearing, causes fluid to migrate out of the intradiscal space (arrows). This, in turn, increases the concentration of micromolecules and the oncotic pressure within the disc space (+). Hence, the absorption capacity of the disc is increased. Decreasing intradiscal pressure has the opposite effect. [From (1); copyright © 2001 by the American Association of Neurological Surgeons.]

The facet joint, being a synovium-lined diarthrodial joint, is subject to the ravages of inflammatory disease processes (see below). In the strictest sense, the disc interspace is not subject to this type of pathological insult.

Biomechanics of the Intervertebral Motion Segment

During axial loading of a disc interspace, the intradiscal pressures are symmetrically distributed. Eccentrically placed loads, however, result in the asymmetric distribution of pressures within the disc. This, in turn, causes the nucleus pulposus to move within the disc from a region of high pressure (high load) to a region of low pressure (low load); for example, forward flexion results in the dorsal migration of the nucleus pulposus. Conversely, the annulus fibrosus responds to asymmetric force application to the disc interspace by bulging on the side of the disc with the greatest stress applied; that is, the annulus bulges on the side opposite the direction of migration of the nucleus pulposus (*Fig. 7.16*).

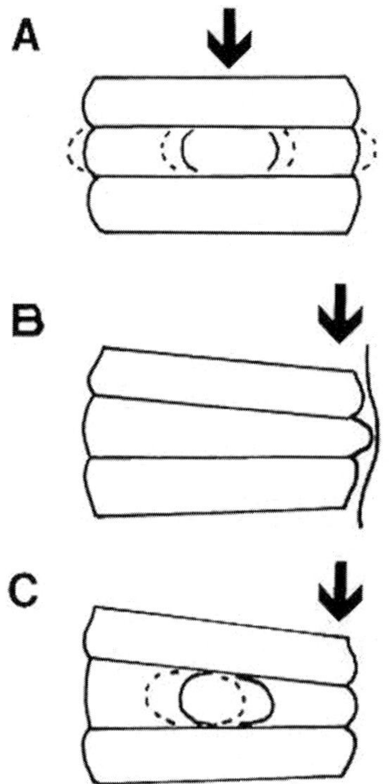

FIG. 7.16 An axial load causes an equally distributed force application to the disc (*A*). An eccentric force application results in annulus fibrosus bulging on the side of the greatest force application (i.e., the concave side of the bend) (*B*). The nucleus pulposus moves in the opposite direction. Dashed lines indicate the positions of structures during force application (*C*). [From (1); copyright © 2001 by the American Association of Neurological Surgeons.]

Pathophysiology of Disc Degeneration and the Degenerative Process

Spondylosis is defined as "vertebral osteophytosis secondary to degenerative disc disease." Spondylosis is not to be confused with inflammatory processes that are associated with osteophyte formation. These inflammatory processes are associated with osteophyte formation and are grouped together as arthritides. The osteophytes of spondylosis are associated with degeneration of the intervertebral disc, which is an amphiarthrodial joint (one with is no synovial membrane). Arthritis, on the other hand, classically involves the synovial membranes of diarthrodial joints (joints lined with synovium; e.g., the facet joints). The presence of spondylosis is defined, therefore, by the presence of noninflammatory disc degeneration. The process of disc degeneration is complex and involves many alterations of normal physiology as well as the process of aging. It is often preceded by mild segmental instability.

INTRADISCAL HYDROSTATIC AND ONCOTIC PRESSURE

Persistent elevation of intradiscal pressures causes narrowing of the disc interspace. This results in annulus fibrosus and facet joint capsule distortion and stretching, with acceleration of the degeneration process. It appears that end-plate damage further accelerates this process. The degeneration process itself should be considered to be simply a manifestation of the normal aging process, but its pathological acceleration, or the deterrence of the same, is of obvious clinical significance.

The water content of the disc interspace, as previously mentioned, decreases gradually throughout life. In addition, the vascularity of the disc also decreases, ranging from a well-vascularized disc at birth to essentially no vascular supply by age 30. This and other factors contribute to changes in the chemical and anatomic makeup of the disc. Fibroblasts produce inferior-quality fibers and ground substance. The disc becomes desiccated and less able to function as cushion. Fissures occur in the cartilaginous plates with defects resulting in internal herniations (Schmorl's nodes). Gas accumulates in the disc (vacuum phenomenon). Mucoid degeneration results in instability. This, in turn, can lead to further degeneration and other sequelae, such as annulus fibrosus bulging and torsional instability.

DISC DEFORMATION

The bulging of the annulus fibrosus causes the periosteum of the adjacent vertebral bodies to be elevated at the attachment site of Sharpey's fibers. Bony reactions (subperiosteal bone formation) occur, resulting in spondylotic ridge (osteophyte) formation (*Fig. 7.17*). This process most commonly results in spinal canal encroachment in the cervical and lumbar regions, relatively sparing the thoracic region. This is caused by the natural lordosis in the cervical and lumbar regions, which results in a dorsally oriented concavity of the spinal curvature (lordosis) and, hence, the tendency of annular bulging toward the spinal canal. The spondylotic process is lessened by fusion or immobilization (1).

Regarding a lateral bending deformity (scoliotic curvature), osteophyte formation occurs predominantly *on the concave side of a curve*, where annulus fibrosus bulging is similarly most pronounced. The concave side of the spinal curvature, however, is usually not the side of the spine that harbors the predisposition for disc herniation. This discrepancy warrants further attention.

As mentioned previously, many factors play roles in inducing disc degeneration and dorsolateral disc herniation. These include the migratory tendencies of the nucleus pulposus, the relatively weak lateral portion of the posterior longitudinal ligament, the thin dorsal portion of the annulus fibrosus, and the morphology of the iliolumbar ligament. A familial predisposition has, in fact, been suggested. Most disc herniations do not occur (or, to put it more correctly, do not become manifest) immediately following trauma. Laboratory investigations that attempt to determine the mechanism of disc herniation are lacking—a fact that has hampered investigations in this area for years.

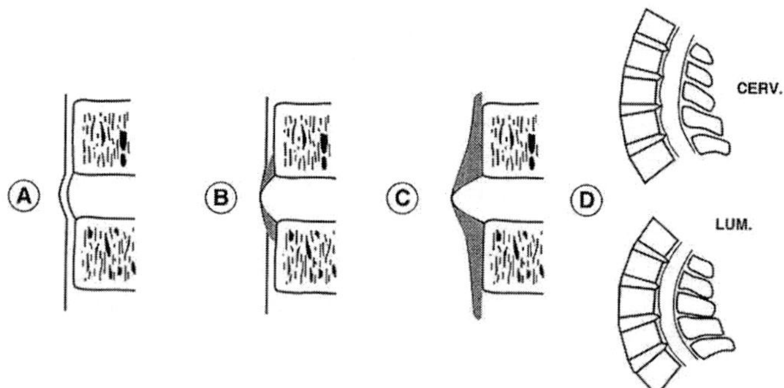

FIG. 7.17 Osteophyte formation results from subperiosteal bone formation, which results from elevation of the periosteum by disc bulging (*A*). A spondylotic ridge then develops (*B* and *C*). This commonly encroaches on the spinal canal in the cervical and lumbar regions, because the lordotic spinal curvature causes the disc bulging and osteophyte formation to occur toward the spinal canal (*D*). This is less common in the thoracic region, because the concavity is oriented away from the spinal canal. [From (1); copyright © 2001 by the American Association of Neurological Surgeons.]

Adams and Hutton, however, determined that a high percentage of lumbar discs in the laboratory could be encouraged to herniate if, first, the disc was degenerated and, second, a specific force pattern was delivered acutely to the motion segment. This force pattern includes:

1. Flexion (causing posterior nucleus pulposus migration),
2. Lateral bending away from the side of disc herniation (causing lateral nucleus pulposus migration), and
3. Application of an axial load (causing an increase in intradiscal pressure).

This complex loading pattern causes:

1. The application of tension to the weakest portion of the annulus fibrosus (dorsolateral position [the location of the herniation]),
2. migration of the nucleus pulposus toward this position, and
3. an asymmetric increase in intradiscal pressure.

A degenerated disc is a requisite for the occurrence of this process. These factors, in general, have been corroborated by others. These factors, plus the increasing frequency of annulus fibrosus tears with age and observation of peak nucleus fibrosus pressures in 35- to 55-year-olds, are among the factors giving rise to an increased incidence of disc herniation in this age group (*Fig. 7.18*). Of note is that disc resorption occasionally occurs. The progression of the "degenerative restabilization" process during the aging process and the factors affecting it are, perhaps, most appropriately portrayed pictorially (*Fig. 7.19*).

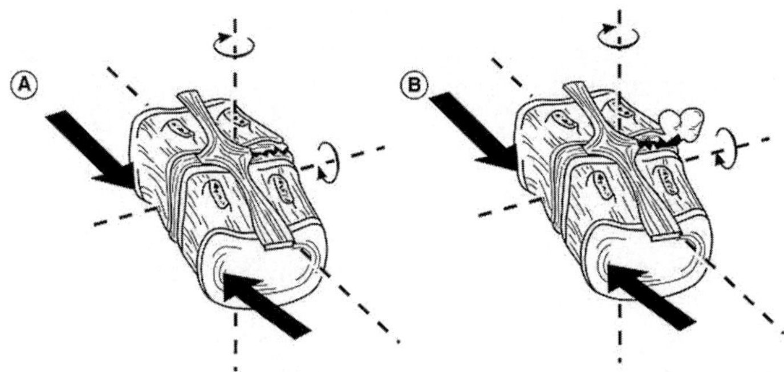

FIG. 7.18 The application of an axial load, lateral bending, and flexion causes the nucleus pulposus to migrate in the direction of the region of the annulus fibrosus that is under tension and prone to tearing (*A*). This may result in disc herniation in the dorsal paramedian location if the disc is degenerated (and, thus, is predisposed to pathological migration) (*B*). [From (1); copyright © 2001 by the American Association of Neurological Surgeons.]

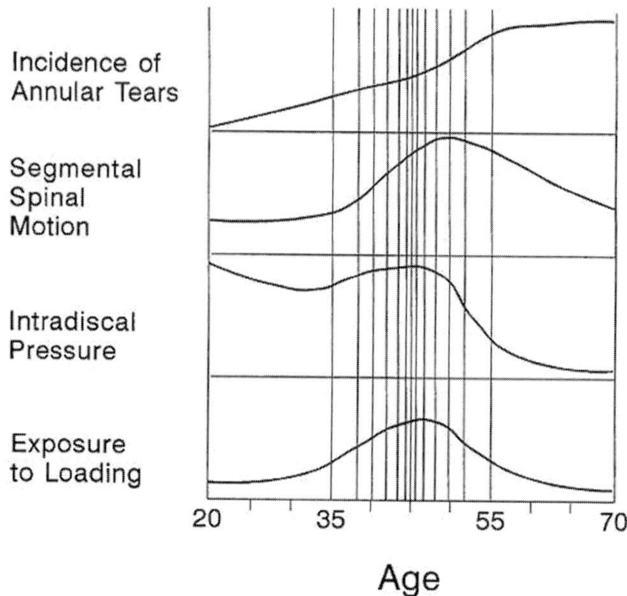

FIG. 7.19 The age-related factors associated with disc herniation. The densities of the vertical lines correlate with the incidence of disc herniation. [From (1); copyright © 2001 by the American Association of Neurological Surgeons.]

Controversy exists regarding decompression. It has been suggested that decompression via discectomy is effective, even in high-risk patients. Effectiveness is enhanced in patients with positive attitudes. This evidence, however, does not exist for spondylosis, nor does it exist for fusion. Structural findings may be more significant than the patient's symptoms in this regard.

The cauda equina syndrome, secondary to lumbar disc herniation, is obviously an outlier in the aforementioned regard. Urgent surgery is clearly indicated in this patient population. Finally, controversy also exists regarding the necessity of the routine pathological examination of the operatively resected degenerated disc. The surgeon must weigh carefully the cost and advantage to the patient of submitting disc specimens for pathological examination. It appears that unless the surgeon suspects an atypical process on the basis of clinical history, examination, or gross inspection at the time of surgery, the routine examination of surgically resected intervertebral disc specimens is not warranted. This is corroborated by the observation that no correlation has been found between histology and clinical findings (1).

REGIONAL VARIATIONS

Variations

Degenerative diseases that involve the cervical spine include spondylosis, rheumatoid arthritis, ankylosing spondylitis, and OPLL. Because of the relative ease of access to the cervical spinal cord from both the ventral and dorsal directions, surgical management of cervical spine degenerative diseases is common.

Degenerative diseases of the thoracic spine, although uncommon, deserve serious attention. They include many of the processes affecting the cervical spine, ankylosing hyperostosis, and Scheuermann's disease. The surgical approach to these problems is often complicated by the need for decompression of the ventral aspect of the thoracic spine. Surgical considerations differ from those in the cervical spine (cervical lordosis and thoracic kyphosis).

Surgical considerations in the lumbar spine also differ substantially from those in the cervical and thoracic regions. Although the intrinsic curvature of the lumbar spine is lordotic, the massive size of the vertebral bodies and the forces they resist make the lumbar spine unique. The often-near-vertical orientation of the lumbosacral joint space is an additional confounding factor. The sagittal orientation of the facet joints and the usual manner of progression of facet joints and of facet joint degenerative changes also differentiate lumbar degenerative processes from thoracic and cervical ones.

Spinal Configuration

CERVICAL SPINE

The surgical approaches for both decompression and stabilization of the degenerative diseases of the spine often include a combination of decompression, fusion, and instrumentation performed from either a ventral exposure, a dorsal exposure, or both. The surgical approach used for any given spinal disorder, including the application of an instrumentation construct, should be determined, at least in part, by the intrinsic curvature of the spine.

Because the assessment of the curvature of the spine is imperative to sound decision making, a relatively precise definition of curvature types is necessary. An "effective" cervical kyphosis is a configuration of the cervical spine in which any part of the dorsal aspect of any of the vertebral bodies C3 through C7 crosses a line drawn in the midsagittal plane (on a lateral cervical spine tomogram, myelogram, or MR image) from the dorsocaudal aspect of the vertebral body of C7. Conversely, an "effective" cervical lordosis is a configuration of the cervical spine in which no part of the dorsal aspect of any of the vertebral bodies C3 through C7 crosses this line. The definition of this imaginary line is associated with a zone of uncertainty ("gray zone") within which the surgeon's bias and clinical judgment together determine whether lordosis or kyphosis is the predominant spinal configuration in the midsagittal section. If, in the opinion of the surgeon, no "gray zone" exists—that is, if only an "effective" kyphosis or an "effective" lordosis is possible—then surgical decision making is simpler. On the other hand, if the surgeon discerns a "gray zone," then the decision-making process is more complex. Perhaps patients whose spinal configuration falls in the "gray zone" should be defined as having a "straightened" spine (1) (*Fig. 7.20*).

The surgical indications for myelopathy associated with degenerative diseases vary. Both ventral and dorsal decompressive approaches are potentially useful for degenerative and inflammatory diseases of the spine; in a given case, the choice should be for the approach that seems to carry the higher probability of success. Spinal geometry is emphasized as an important determinant of the appropriateness of either the ventral or the dorsal approach in individual situations. An "effective" lordosis may be a relative indication for a dorsal approach,

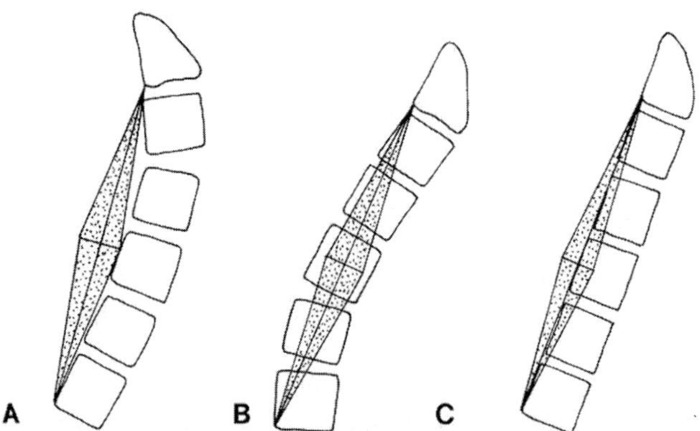

FIG. 7.20 A midsagittal section of a cervical spine (as observed by MR imaging or angiography) configured in lordotic postures ("effective" cervical lordosis). A line has been drawn from the dorsocaudal aspect of the vertebral body of C2 to the dorsocaudal aspect of the vertebral body of C7 (solid line). The "gray zone" is outlined by the other lines (*A*). A midsagittal section of a cervical spine configured in kyphosis ("effective" cervical kyphosis). Note that portions of the vertebral bodies are located dorsally to the gray zone (*B*). A midsagittal section of a "straightened" cervical spine is also shown (*C*). Note that the most dorsal aspect of a cervical vertebral body is located within, but not dorsal to, the gray zone. [From (1); copyright © 2001 by the American Association of Neurological Surgeons.]

whereas an "effective" kyphosis may be relative indication for a ventral approach. A straightened spine may be approached either ventrally or dorsally. The surgeon must also, however, consider the propensity of the spine for deformity progression, which is greatest in the kyphotic and least in the lordotic spine. A straight spine with a moderate tendency to deformity progression becomes more likely to kyphose if the dorsal tension band has been removed by laminectomy. In these situations, a laminectomy accompanied by a fusion, or a ventral procedure (with fusion), should, perhaps, be considered.

Spinal deformity should be corrected if practical and safe. Persistent deformity not only permits persistent neural compression but also causes eccentric disc interspace loading and subsequent end-fusion accelerated degenerative changes.

THORACIC SPINE

In the thoracic spine, disc height loss (predominantly ventral disc height loss) results in progression of the kyphotic deformity. This, however, is superimposed on a preexisting kyphotic deformity, thus exaggerating or enhancing the chance of deformity progression. This tends to occur in Scheuermann's disease.

The rib cage, however, substantially adds to the stability of the thoracic spine. This stability is predominantly related to the rib's attachment to the vertebral and costovertebral joints and the sternum. The attachment of the rib to the sternum is crucial to the rib's contribution to stability. The stability conferred by the rib cage minimizes progression of the thoracic kyphosis caused by degenerative changes.

LUMBAR SPINE

The lumbar spine is not protected by the rib cage. Furthermore, the coupling response to movements is different from that observed in the cervical region. This is attributed to the absence of the uncovertebral joints and the different orientation of the facet joints. These factors contribute to the progression of lateral bending deformities in the lumbar spine rather than to kyphotic deformities, as observed in the cervical and thoracic spine. An asymmetric loss of height of the lumbar intervertebral disc may progress to an asymmetrical collapse of the vertebral body. If this lateral bending (scoliotic deformity) occurs and progresses, it is associated with an obligatory rotation of the spine that is caused by the coupling characteristics of the lumbar spine. The osteophytes occur, as previously depicted, on the concave side of the curvature.

This obligatory association of a rotatory deformity with a lateral bending deformity (coupling) makes lumbar spinal instrumentation surgery in these patients more difficult and dangerous. Lateral transverse process dissection can result in nerve root injury because of their relatively dorsal location with respect to the transverse processes. Deformity correction by the distraction of the concave side of the spine may result in stretching of shortened and tethered nerve roots. Proximal (intradural) nerve roots are much less tolerant of stretching than their more peripheral nerve counterparts because of their lack of perineurium. This type of deformation can also affect the side of disc herniation.

SPINAL FUSION

Ultimately, the bone graft and the resulting bony fusion are the components that lend stability to the spine. No matter how secure an internal fixation device may appear to be, it will eventually fail unless bony fusion and stability are achieved. There is a proverbial "race" between the failure of the implant and the acquisition of bony fusion. After fusion, the implant and its interface with bone become progressively weaker, and the bony union (assuming the fusion process is proceeding satisfactorily) usually becomes stronger (*Fig. 7.21*). Therefore, most internal fixation techniques should be applied in conjunction with a bone graft.

Ventral interbody bone grafts provide superior ultimate strength characteristics. They are placed in the weight-bearing region of the spine along the axis of the IAR. Weight-bearing itself promotes healing and bony fusion. Care must be taken, however, to prevent progressive deformation following the placement of a ventral interbody fusion. Stauffer and Kelly have reported a high incidence of angular deformities following ventral fusions for cervical spine trauma. Dorsal stabilization procedures may be necessary (either alone or in combination with a ventral decompression and fusion) to achieve acceptable stability and neural element decompression. Ventral plating techniques, likewise, may be used for this purpose. Their use for this purpose, without dorsal stability augmentation, must be considered carefully, however, because their ability to resist flexion is much less than their ability to resist extension.

Dorsal bone grafts generally are not, by themselves, weight-bearing. Spine flexion, which causes flexion ventral to the IAR, causes distraction of the segments to be fused (dorsal to the IAR). Unless ventral axial load–resisting support is provided (i.e., by an anterior intervertebral bone strut graft) or already exists (e.g., in patients with cervical locked facets without vertebral body fracture), dorsal bone grafts should be avoided unless an accompanying instrumentation con-

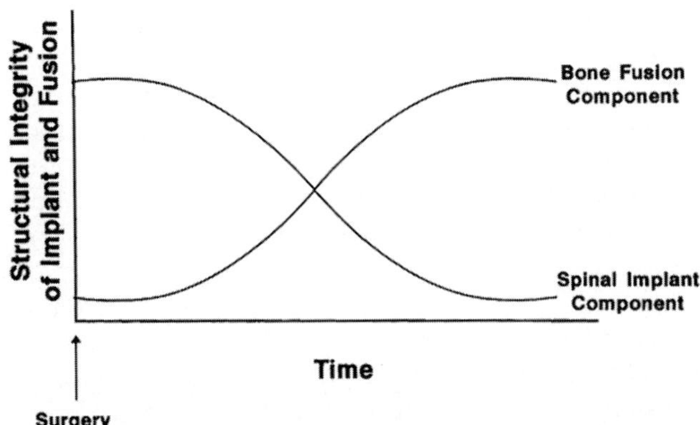

FIG. 7.21 After surgery, the relationship between bone fusion acquisition and spinal implant integrity changes with time. [From (1); copyright © 2001 by the American Association of Neurological Surgeons.]

struct provides the needed support. If the bone graft is applied in association with a tension-band fixation-in-flexion construct (e.g., with interspinous wiring), ventral support must be provided if ventral weight-bearing ability is suspect.

Frequently, stabilization procedures are performed after decompressive operations. The reduction of a ventral mass impinging on the spinal cord, therefore, frequently requires an operative approach in addition to that used to place the dorsal instrumentation device. Furthermore, so that the dural sac is decompressed before spinal manipulation, the ventral (decompression) aspect of the operation should be performed first (before placement of the dorsal instrumentation device). For situations in which spinal distraction is the desired mode of application, the interbody bone graft should not be placed until the dorsal instrumentation devices have been applied (for fear of adversely altering spinal biomechanics by loosening the already placed bone graft). Theoretically, in this case, the most appropriate order of procedures should be decompression of neural elements and loosening of the spine (by discectomy and corpectomy; e.g., a relaxing procedure) first and then placement of the ventral bone graft. If spinal compression is the desired mode of application, however, then it may be desirable to place the interbody bone graft strut first (1).

Load Bearing and Load Sharing

The concepts of load-bearing and load-sharing should be considered whenever a spinal implant is used. This may be no more evident than for the thoracolumbar fractures treated with short-segment (pedicle screw) fixation with or without an interbody fusion. Neutral implants, in the truest sense, do not exist. This has already been emphasized. When weight is borne by the torso, a spinal implant is exposed to myriad forces (load-bearing). This occurs inevitably, even in cases when an implant is initially placed in a neutral mode.

It may be instructive to consider a hypothetical situation that emphasizes the concepts of load-bearing and load-sharing. For the purposes of discussion, it is relevant to consider isolated axial loads and force applications. The clinical situation, however, is often quite different, with myriad forces applied by the torso to the implant (and by the implant to the torso). Nevertheless, the bearing of a load by the torso during the assumption of the upright posture causes a spinal implant to absorb at least a portion of the axial load. The important concepts with regard to load-bearing and load-sharing are well illustrated when considering an L1 fracture that is treated with dorsal short-segment pedicle screw fixation, with or without a ventral interbody strut. If the implant is placed in a neutral mode (no distraction or compression and no surgical load-bearing) and without an interbody strut, the axial load that is borne by the implant changes from zero (the load borne by the implant at the time of surgery) to roughly the weight of the torso positioned above the implant after the assumption of the upright position. This may or may not cause the implant to fail, either at the screw-bone interface or via screw fracture. The implant bears a significant load, although it shares the load minimally with ventral structures.

If the implant is placed in a distraction mode at the time of surgery and, similarly, without an interbody strut, the axial load that is borne by the implant when the patient assumes the upright posture is the sum of the load borne at the time of surgery (surgical load-bearing) and the weight of the torso above the implant. This load most certainly is associated with a significant chance of failure, either at the screw-bone interface or by means of a screw fracture. The load is borne solely by the implant (totally load-bearing); no load sharing occurs in this situation. This, perhaps, contributes to the recent demonstration of a lack of success (compared to uninstrumented fusion) of instrumented dorsal-lateral lumbar fusions.

The placement of an implant in a compression mode at the time of surgery alters the forces considerably. In the hypothetical situation in which only axial loads are considered, the placement of an implant in a compression mode after performing a corpectomy and the placement of an interbody strut results in a negative surgical load-bearing. If an axial load is subsequently borne by the assumption of the upright posture, the surgical compression load is effectively diminished, and the net load approaches zero. Thus, a spinal implant placed in a compression mode can share the loads applied by the weight of the torso above the fracture by allowing some of the axial load to be borne by the existing spinal axis or an interbody strut.

In addition to its load-sharing advantage, compression also provides enhancing stresses in terms of bone healing. Grafts under compression heal better and faster than those under tension. This is an application of Wolff's law. Wolff published his *Das Gestz der Transformation der Knochen* (*The Law of Transformation of Bone*) in 1892. He explained the functional adaptation of bone tissue; that is, that every change in the function of a bone is followed by certain definite changes in internal architecture and external conformation in accordance with mathematical laws. This effect also has an electrophysiological connection.

SPINAL INSTRUMENTATION

Component-Component Interfaces

A variety of implant components may be affixed to each other by a variety of techniques. It is appropriate to define these components and then to describe the mechanisms by which they are attached to each other. An implant is a device used to stabilize the spine via the connection of two or more spine components (segments). A construct is the combination of the implant and the spine segments encompassed by the implant. An assembly is the collection of components that together make up the implant. A longitudinal member (e.g., rods or plates) connects two or more anchors. An anchor affixes to the bone and the longitudinal member (e.g., screws, wires, or hooks). A cross-fixator affixes two (usually parallel) longitudinal members to each other. The mechanism by which longitudinal members, anchors, and cross-fixators are affixed to each other is the topic of this section.

The locking mechanism used between components of a spinal implant system (construct) is essential for the establishment of construct integrity. For the most part, two types of longitudinal members are used clinically: rods and plates. The longitudinal member is connected to other implant components by one, or by a combination of seven, commonly used fundamental types of locking mechanisms (*Fig. 7.22*):

1. Three-point shear clamps,
2. Lock screw connectors,
3. Circumferential grip connectors,
4. Constrained bolt-plate connectors,
5. Constrained screw-plate connectors,
6. Semiconstrained screw-plate connectors, and
7. Semiconstrained component-rod connectors.

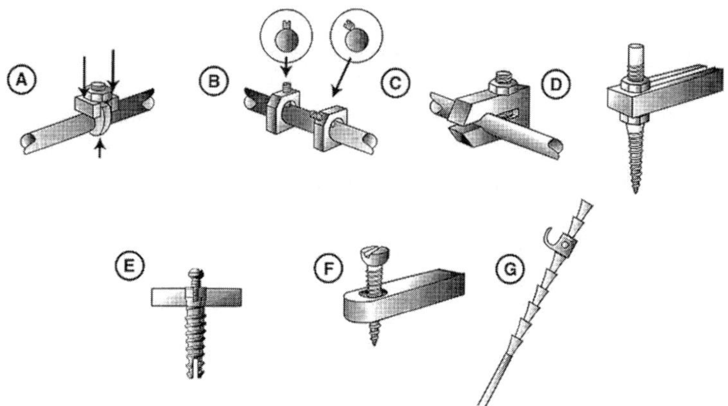

FIG. 7.22 The seven fundamental component-component locking mechanisms. (*A*) Three-point shear clamp. (*B*) Lock screw, end-on (*left*) and tangential (*right*). (*C*) Circumferential grip. (*D*) Constrained bolt-plate. (*E*) Constrained screw plate. (*F*) Semiconstrained screw plate. (*G*) Semiconstrained component-rod. [From (1); copyright © 2001 by the American Association of Neurological Surgeons.]

Usually, a combination of two of these locking mechanisms, working in opposition to each other, is used at each component-component interface. This provides a pincer-like action to grip the rod or plate on opposite sides. For example, a circumferential grip connector may be used with a lock screw connector at opposing sides of a rod. Interface friction may be enhanced by providing knurled surfaces, which allow seating of lock screws (e.g., Cotrel-Dubousset), or by providing a grid-on-grid surface (see below) (1).

Constrained (rigid) screw-plate interfaces, such as constrained bolt-plate connectors (e.g., the Steffee plate), generally are stronger than most hook-rod or hook-screw interfaces. Other factors, however, must be considered in the implant selection process.

IMPLANT SURFACE CHARACTERISTICS

All locking mechanism types rely on friction between the components to minimize or prevent failure at the component-component interface. Therefore, implant surface characteristics are a critical aspect of component-component interface considerations. Compatibility (or lack thereof) between the surfaces of the interfacing components is also critical. Some component-component interfaces rely mainly on torque or other forces being applied; others rely more on friction between components to secure the desired interface integrity. All, however, rely on both to one degree or another. Component-component interfaces are assessed by the American Society for the Testing of Materials criteria.

In general, friction between the components must be enhanced to achieve maximal torsional or axial push strength. An analogy to contact between automobile tires and terrain is appropriate here: A mud tire has deep treads with a knobby surface. It matches well the surface of the terrain for which it is designed. A drag-racing slick is smooth and wide. It, too, matches well the surface of the terrain for which it is designed. In the former case, a rough surface is matched to a rough surface (as in a grid-on-grid interface; see below). In the latter case, two relatively smooth surfaces are matched, with maximum surface-to-surface contact (as in a circumferential grip connection). Mixing of the two systems may result in less friction. For example, a knurled surface (off-road terrain, or half of a grid-on-grid interface) will not allow significant friction at the interface with a smooth surface (drag slick, or circumferential-grip half of a pincer). The surface area of contact is diminished; thus, the desired interface friction is not achieved (*Fig. 7.23*). Of perhaps greater importance is the fact that the surface textures changed. This alters the coefficient of friction (see next paragraph).

Other factors also play roles in this process. Friction between two surfaces is affected not only by the surface characteristics but also by the coefficient of friction and the force that is applied. If the surgeon were to diminish the surface area of contact between two surfaces but maintain the same force, the force/area of contact would increase, but the surface area of contact would decrease. These changes would neutralize each other, resulting in no net change in friction (friction is independent of the surface area of contact). These relationships are described by the equation

$$f = \mu \cdot N$$

where f = friction force, μ = coefficient of friction, and N = force applied to the surfaces.

Cross-Fixation

Cross-fixation is defined herein as the rigid fixation of bilaterally placed dorsal fixation devices to each other in a rigid or semirigid manner to make the construct effectively a quadrilateral frame. This technique has been used for some time with wire and acrylic cross-fixation of Harrington distraction rods and other dorsal rigid devices.

Cross-fixation provides substantially greater stiffness and stability than that achieved without cross-fixation. This is especially advantageous with longer systems. The increase in stability is obvious at surgery and warrants the use of cross-fixation with long instrumentation systems whenever possible. Short pedicle screw systems can also use

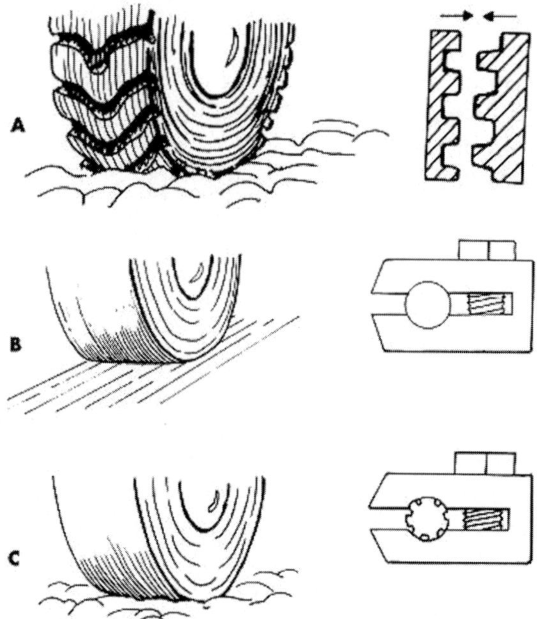

FIG. 7.23 The two opposing surfaces of a component-component interface must match if the security of fixation is to be optimized. In each portion of this figure, an analogy to tire-versus-terrain is depicted (*left*), and the component-component relationship is also depicted (*right*). (*A*) A mud tire on off-road terrain and grid-grid interface is shown. Note the meshing of the two surfaces. (*B*) A racing slick on an asphalt road, and a circumferential grip connector on a smooth road. In (*A*) and (*B*), the surfaces are matched, and contact between surfaces is optimal. If a mismatch of surfaces exists, surface area of contact is diminished. (*C*) This is depicted with a racing slick interfacing with an off-road terrain and a knurled rod interfacing with a smooth component. [From (1); copyright © 2001 by the American Association of Neurological Surgeons.]

cross-fixation to their advantage by using the triangulation effect. The rigid cross-fixation of the two sides of a system, in which the screws are toed in, provides substantial pullout resistance as well as a resistance to sagittal plane translation or subluxation.

Implant-Bone Interfaces

Interfaces between bone and surgically applied implants are used clinically. In spine surgery, there are five fundamental types of implant-bone interface:

1. Abutting (e.g., interbody bone or interbody acrylic),
2. Penetrating (e.g., nail, staple, or screw),
3. Gripping (e.g., hook or wire),

4. Conforming (e.g., acrylic), and
5. Osseointegration (e.g. titanium or ceramics).

Within these categories are subcategories and implant variations. The biomechanical principles involve range from the very simple, as with the abutting interbody implants, to the very complex nuances of screw-bone interfaces. Each category is considered separately, with accompanying theoretical and biomechanical information.

ABUTTING IMPLANT-BONE INTERFACES

The predominant location for the placement of abutting implants is the interbody region. Their application elsewhere, on or within the vertebra, makes little sense. For an abutting construct to be effective, it must bear a load. Because the interbody region is the approximate region of the neutral axis and most of the axial load is borne in this region, the interbody location is the most appropriate region for placement of abutting implants.

Abutting implants, by their nature, distribute loads over a relatively large surface area. A surgeon would not usually select a slender interbody implant, because it would likely knife its way through the relatively soft cancellous bone of the vertebral body. The placement of an interbody implant in close approximation to the end plate (where bone is more compact and, thus, more able to resist compression) may be desirable.

Specific information on the biomechanics of such implants is lacking. All other factors being constant, however, the larger the surface area of the contact between the implant and the bone, the more effective the implant's resistance to axial loads. The axial load-resisting capacity is, in theory, directly proportional to the surface area of contact. The larger the circumference of the interbody abutting implant—be it bone, acrylic, or a metal implant—the more effective it is in achieving one of its most important goals—to resist applied axial loads—but the less surface area is provided for ultimate bony fusion.

There are two types of cage interfaces with the vertebral body end plate: flat-faced and round-faced. The former presents a relatively large surface area of contact to the end plate. This effectively resists the pistoning of the implant into the vertebral body. Round-faced cages (e.g., threaded interbody fusion cages) present a round surface to the end plate. Because the end plate is only 1- to 2-mm thick and the round-faced cage penetrates the end plate somewhat, the rounded surface of the cage only "sees" a small portion of the end plate (*Fig. 7.24*).

The wall (cortex) of the vertebral body buttresses interbody implants better than the center of the vertebral body. This is akin to the edge

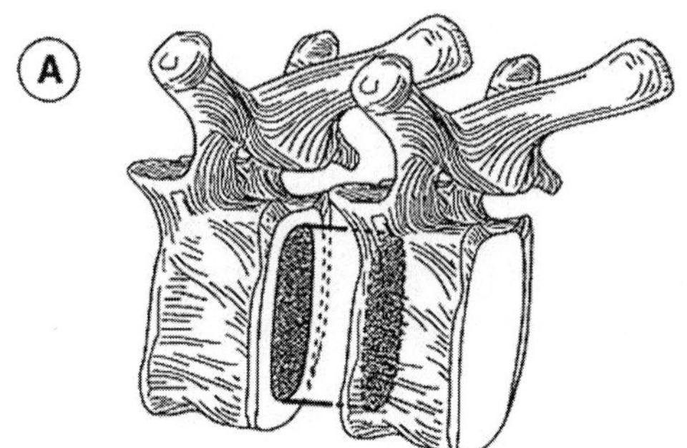

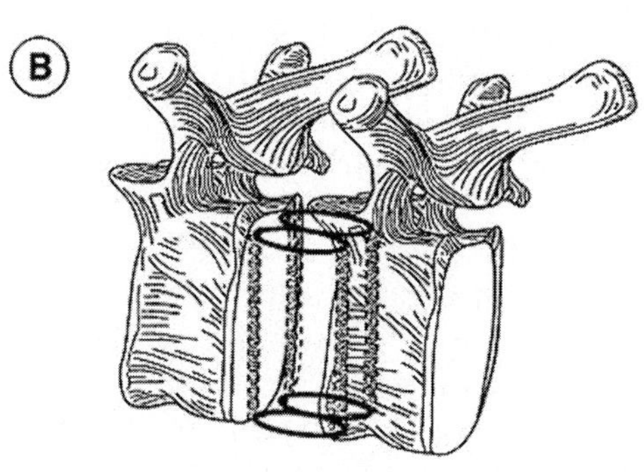

FIG. 7.24 Flat-faced cages present a flat surface to the end-plate region (*A*) compared to a round-faced cage (TIFC) (*B*). [From (1); copyright © 2001 by the American Association of Neurological Surgeons.]

of a tin can being better able to bear loads than the center of the can. One can take advantage of this concept clinically via the use of a fin that abuts the end plate in the region of the cortical margin (1) (*Fig. 7.25*).

PENETRATING IMPLANT-BONE INTERFACES

Penetrating implant-bone interfaces are of two fundamental types: those without pullout-resistance attributes and those with pullout-resistance attributes. The former type includes nails, spikes, and staples. The penetrating adjuncts of the abutting implant-bone interface implants are examples of this type. The latter type includes screws and penetrating implants that change configuration on placement into bone (e.g., expanding tip screws).

PENETRATING IMPLANT-BONE INTERFACES WITHOUT PULLOUT RESISTANCE (POSTS)

Nails, spikes, and staples are seldom used as sole methods of implant-bone interface in clinical practice. This is due, in part, to their relative inability to resist dislodgement; their pullout-resistance ca-

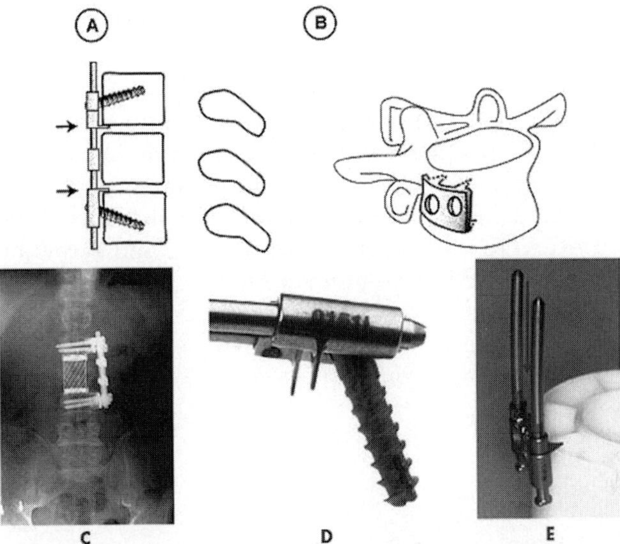

FIG. 7.25 A buttress using a fin applied at the end plate in the region of the ventral vertebral body cortex (*A*) or a spike placed into a vertebral body (*B* and *C*) provides "extra" points of fixation and, hence, security. A small (short) fin or spike is all that is required. A fin or spike need only pass through the fin of a DOC system (Depuy Acromed, Raynham, MA) moving "just past" the cortical edges of the vertebral body in the region of the end plate, thus taking advantage of the "boundary effect." This allows the device to more effectively bear axial loads (arrows) (*D* and *E*). [From (1); copyright © 2001 by the American Association of Neurological Surgeons.]

pabilities are nearly nil. They usually function as adjuncts (stabilizers) for implants (e.g., as adjuncts for interbody axial load–bearing implants); as the cantilever components of rigid, constrained implant systems for axial load bearing (fixed moment arm cantilever beam); or as the cantilever components of terminal three-point bending constructs (posts).

PENETRATING IMPLANT-BONE INTERFACES WITH PULLOUT RESISTANCE—IMPLANTS THAT CHANGE CONFIGURATION AFTER INSERTION

Implants that change configuration after insertion into bone have the capacity to resist pullout. They are not, however, commonly used in clinical practice; therefore, little biomechanical information is available. The available information suggests that expanding tip screws effectively increase pullout resistance, particularly in osteoporotic bone. Adding a nut on the opposite side of a bicortical vertebral body screw significantly increases pullout resistance.

PENETRATING IMPLANT-BONE INTERFACES WITH PULLOUT-RESISTANT SCREWS

Most of the information available on implant-bone interfaces is about screws. This parallels the frequency of their clinical use. In fact, the screw, whether alone or as a component of a more complex spinal implant, is used clinically with increasing frequency and through increasingly broader applications. A relatively thorough knowledge of screw anatomy, screw interactions with bone, and screw biomechanics is mandatory for effective and safe use of screws.

Screws

A screw has four basic components:

1. The head,
2. The core,
3. The thread, and
4. The tip.

Each component can be altered to achieve a specific desired clinical effect (*Fig. 7.26*).

THE HEAD

The head of the screw resists the translational force created by the rotation of the thread through the bone at the termination of screw tightening. The screw head, therefore, should be designed to optimally abut the underlying surface. If this surface is medullary cancellous bone, a wide head is necessary to minimize the chance of pullthrough. A smaller diameter is required for cortical bone. If the underlying surface is metal, as with a dynamic or semiconstrained screw plate system, then the undersurface of the screw head should conform to the trough in the plate; that is, it should have a rounded undersurface. This usually allows toggling. On the other hand, if toggling is not desired, a flat undersurface that abuts the flat surface of the plate may be desirable. Obviously, because of the significant deformation resistance of metal compared with bone, the head diameter can be smaller

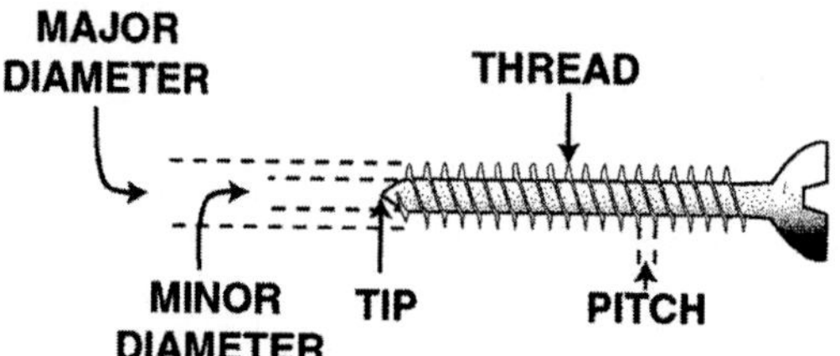

FIG. 7.26 Screw core (minor) and outside (major) diameters, thread depth, and screw pitch. [From (1); copyright © 2001 by the American Association of Neurological Surgeons.]

with metal-on-metal applications than it can with metal-on-bone applications.

Once the screw head has come into contact with the underlying surface during tightening, one or a combination of two sequelae will result from further tightening of the screw: screw thread-bone interface failure (stripping or pullout) and deformation of the underlying surface against the undersurface of the screw head.

THE CORE

The core (inner diameter) gives the screw most of its fracture resistance, in the form of resistance to cantilever bending and torsion. In clinical practice, the torsional strength of the screw is relatively insignificant. Frequently, however, screws are required to bear substantial cantilevered loads (loads oriented perpendicular to the long axis of the screw); hence, bending strength is of considerable importance. Bending strength is proportional to the section modulus (Z) and is defined by the equation

$$Z = \frac{\pi D^3}{32}$$

in which D = core diameter. Therefore, screw (or rod) strength is proportional to the cube of the core diameter. As the core diameter rises, the strength of the screw rises exponentially. This is especially significant for the core diameters that are commonly used clinically. Note that the difference in strength between a 5.0-mm and a 6.0-mm core diameter screw is nearly twofold (125 vs 216). Hence, the largest screw diameter allowed by the local bony anatomy should be used so that the likelihood of screw failure (fracture) can be minimized. This principle is difficult to apply when the pedicles are narrow, as is usually the case in the thoracolumbar region. This underscores, in part, the biomechanical and clinical problems associated with pedicle fixation in this region. In view of the simplicity of the mathematical relationship between screw diameter and screw strength, it is not surprising that most implant systems have similar attributes.

Stress reduction osteoporosis results from stress shielding associated with the use of very rigid implant systems. It is intuitive that shielding of bone from applied loads may result in demineralization. This, indeed, occurs, but the stiffness and stability imparted to the spine by the implant more than compensates for this phenomenon. With less rigid systems, movement at the screw-bone interface may occur. Movement at the screw-bone interface causes the screw to become enveloped with fibrous tissue. This parallels the degradation of the screw-bone interface.

THREAD AND TIP

Screw core diameter (minor diameter) is proportional to strength. Outside (outer) diameter (major diameter), on the other hand, is more important as a determinant of screw pullout resistance. The depth of the thread may be even more important in this regard.

Three types of screws are used in spinal surgery:

1. Machine screws (cortical screws),
2. Self-tapping machine screws, and
3. Wood screws (cancellous screws).

Cortical screws are used in hard, relatively incompressible bone. Their shallow threads minimize bone compression during screw insertion. The problem of pathological bone compression by the screw during insertion is eased by pretapping the hole for the screw. For a cortical screw to provide maximal pullout resistance, pretapping is optimal. Tapping carves threads into the wall of the bone. The cutting edges of the tap screw perform this task.

Two characteristics of a screw tap are fundamental to its success: a tapered tip and a full-length flute. The tapered tip helps to align the screw in the desired direction by directing it down the predrilled hole. The full-length flute gathers bone debris carved from the wall of the drill hole by the tap screw. This is facilitated by periodic loosening of the screw by an approximately one-quarter to one-half turn during tightening, which allows the bone debris to collect in the flute. Tapping has been shown to decrease pullout resistance in osteoporotic bone. It is less relevant in nonosteoporotic bone.

Self-tapping screws obviate the need for this multistep process. A leading-edge flute is built into the tip, allowing debris to accumulate within its confines. The shorter flute of self-tapping screws cannot accommodate all the debris created (*Fig. 7.27*). Thus, the drill holes should be larger with self-tapping screws (slightly larger than the core diameter of the screw) to facilitate debris accumulation around the threads.

Pretapped nonself-tapping and self-tapping screws, if used properly, provide similar pullout strengths. Furthermore, the pullout strength of both pretapped nonself-tapping screws and self-tapping screws is not significantly affected by multiple insertions and removals in cortical bone.

Cancellous (wood) screws are used in softer material—that is, in cancellous bone. Compression of cancellous bone by the screw during insertion increases its density and, thus, its pullout resistance. With cortical bone, compression during screw insertion causes microfractures that decrease bone integrity. Although pretapping is desirable in cortical bone, it is less desirable in cancellous bone. *In fact, in cancellous bone, tapping weakens the implant-bone interface.*

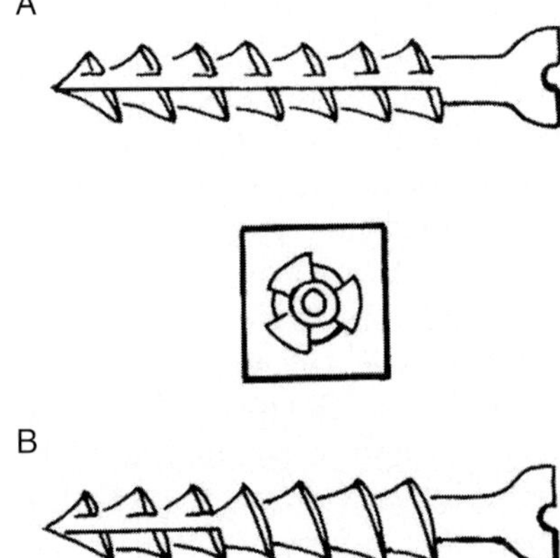

FIG. 7.27 (*A*) A screw tap. Note the tapered tip and the full-length flute. (*B*) A self-tapping screw. Note the leading-edge flute that does not extend the length of the screw. (Insert) An end-on view of the tip. [From (1); copyright © 2001 by the American Association of Neurological Surgeons.]

Pedicle screws rarely obtain cortical purchase within the pedicle. Because tapping weakens the implant-bone interface in cancellous bone, the tapping of pedicle screw holes is of questionable value. In cortical bone, however, bone microcracking around screw threads is greater with untapped than with tapped screws. Therefore, in cortical bone, untapped screws loosen more frequently than tapped screws. Pretapping is, thus, desirable in cortical bone.

PULLOUT RESISTANCE

Pullout resistance correlates with insertional torque. This has been defined by the equation

$$y = (x/1{,}142) + 0.02$$

in which y = insertion torque in newton-meters and x = pullout resistance in newtons. Insertional torque is increased by employing conical inner diameter screws. As mentioned above, the main determinants of screw pullout resistance are major screw diameter and thread depth. Other important facts are extent of cortical purchase, depth of screw penetration, and thread design. The several treads nearest the screw's head bear most of the load that is transferred from bone during pullout stressing. Therefore, proximal cortical "purchase" is very important regarding pullout resistance. Of secondary importance is the depth of penetration of the screw within the bone. In addition, opposite cortical purchase seems to be even less important in this regard. This last point is understandable in view of the fact that the greatest load is transferred by the most superficial threads.

Thread design also plays a role in screw pullout resistance. Two factors dominate this aspect of screw mechanics: thread pitch and thread shape. Thread pitch is the distance from any point on a screw thread to the corresponding point on the next thread. This is equal to the distance a screw advances axially in one turn (the lead). A fundamental rule of thumb for screw biomechanics is that pullout resistance is proportional to the volume of bone between the threads. This, however, is a significant generality (see below). As previously mentioned, increasing thread depth increases pullout resistance. Thread depth is obviously proportional to bone volume between threads. Similarly, the pitch of the thread is proportional to the volume of bone between threads and thus to pullout resistance.

Alteration of the shape of the thread can increase or decrease the interthread volume. For example, flattening or reversing the angle of the following edge of the thread further increases interthread volume (by decreasing metal volume) and results in an even greater increase in pullout resistance. Screw toe-in (triangulation) also contributes to pullout resistance if the two sides of the construct are rigidly affixed to each other by a cross-member.

The factors that determine screw pullout resistance are obviously complex. Chapman and coworkers have attempted to quantify these factors objectively by the equation

$$F_s = S + A_s = \{S \cdot L \cdot \pi \cdot D_{major}\} \cdot TSF$$

where F_s = predicted shear failure force (N), S = material ultimate shear stress (MPa), A_s = thread shear area (mm^2), L = length of thread engagement in material, D_{major} = major diameter (mm), TSF = thread shape factor (dimensionless). The TSF is calculated as

$$TSF = (0.5 + 0.57735\ d/p)$$

where d = thread depth (mm) = $(D_{major} - D_{minor})/2D_{minor}$ = minor (root) diameter (mm) and p = thread pitch (mm). The equation for F_s, however, does not entirely define the relationship between bone, screw geometry, and pullout resistance, as is evident from the study of clinically employed screws. This is further complicated by screw hole preparation. Both cortex overdrill and pilot hole overdrill adversely affect pullout resistance, as does as tapping. Bicortical purchase increases pullout resistance. The use of an awl that compresses and compacts cancellous bone should theoretically enhance screw purchase over that observed with holes prepared by drilling. Finally, in this regard, expandable tip screws and acrylics have been shown to increase pullout resistance (1) (*Fig. 7.28*).[1]

Security of the implant-bone interface can be problematic. This commonly occurs in patients with osteoporosis. Mineral density of bone has been shown to correlate inversely with pullout resistance. In pa-

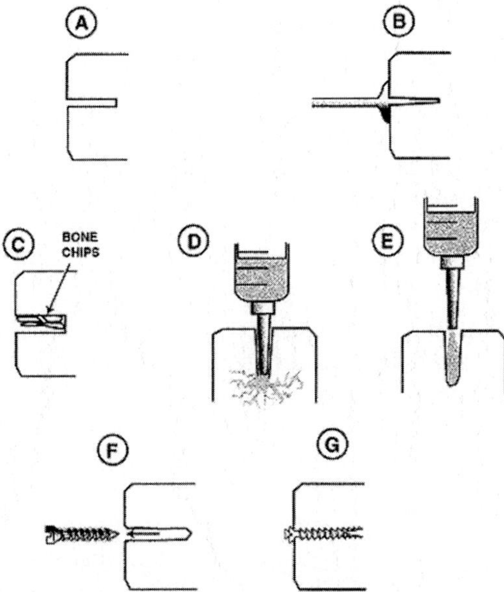

FIG. 7.28 The integrity of a screw-bone interface in medullary bone can be enhanced by drilling and not tapping (*A*) or, in fact, by using an awl instead of a drill (*B*). This strategy causes compression of the soft medullary bone, which strengthens it; as opposed to removing the bone debris using a drill. Bone chip(s) placed into a hole can increase bone compression and screw-bone interface integrity (*C*). Pressurized polymethylmethacrylate injection can force acrylic into the interstices of the bone (arrows) (*D*). This increases pullout resistance. The use of nonpressurized polymethylmethacrylate does not cause this degree of penetration into the medullary bone (*E*). It therefore does not augment but, in fact, may diminish pullout resistance by diminishing thread purchase in bone (*F*). Expanding tip screws may also be used to increase pullout resistance (*G*). [From (1); copyright © 2001 by the American Association of Neurological Surgeons.]

tients with severe osteopenia, screw pullout resistance may be diminished so much that screw fixation may be a suboptimal choice. This can be assessed preoperatively.

Closeness of fit between a screw and bone plays a role regarding strength and stiffness. This is most relevant with screw-pedicle fit in nonosteoporotic bone (the use of wider screws increases fixation stiffness).

For cases in which screw hole stripping or cutout has occurred intraoperatively, injection of polymethylmethacrylate into the screw hole before screw insertion should be considered. Zindrick and coworkers showed this to be a viable option only when the polymethylmethacrylate is injected under pressure. In this case, the acrylic most likely is forced into the interstices of the medullary bone, thus providing an equivalent, of sorts, of increased thread depth.

TRIANGULATION

Screw-bone interface failure may be minimized by paying scrupulous attention to screw trajectory and configuration. Rigidly connected diverging or converging screws (triangulation) provide increased pullout resistance. The triangulation effect is optimal with screws placed at an approximately 90° angle with respect to each other. The minimization of compression stress at the screw-bone interface during tightening via the use of triangulated screws provides adequate fixation without excessive bone resorption.

Screw pullout resistance may be enhanced by using pressurized polymethylmethacrylate injection into the screw hole before placing the screw. This poses risk to juxtaposed structures if extrusion occurs. Nonpressurized injection is less effective. It does not cause penetration of the polymethylmethacrylate into the bony interstices, as does pressurized injection. Its efficacy without pressurization, however, is not insignificant. Apatite cement and bone slivers may also be used.

Herein, the term *toe-in* is defined as the utilization of paired converging and cross-fixed fixed moment arm screws, whereas the term *toe-out* is defined as the utilization of paired diverging and cross-fixed fixed moment arm screws. In both situations, the screws are rigidly affixed to the same platform or implant. They can function in their proscribed manner (toed-in or toed-out) in any plane (e.g., sagittal or axial), thus creating what is termed a *triangulation effect*, which is defined here as resistance to screw pullout that is created by the convergence or divergence of fixed moment arm screws connected by a platform (cross-fixed). The triangulation effect is proportional to the area that is defined by the triangle below the screw. The triangulation effect is always accompanied by the rigid fixation of one screw to another (e.g., cross-fixation). Cross-fixation, in addition to enabling the triangulation effect, helps to stabilize the construct, thus minimizing the chance that other types of failure (other than pullout) will occur. When pullout does occur, significant portions of bone must be extracted with the implant.

Triangulation is affected by:

1. The orientation of the load(s) resisted,
2. The *consistency* of the bone into which the screws are placed, and
3. The limitations created by the geometry of the structure into which the implant is placed.

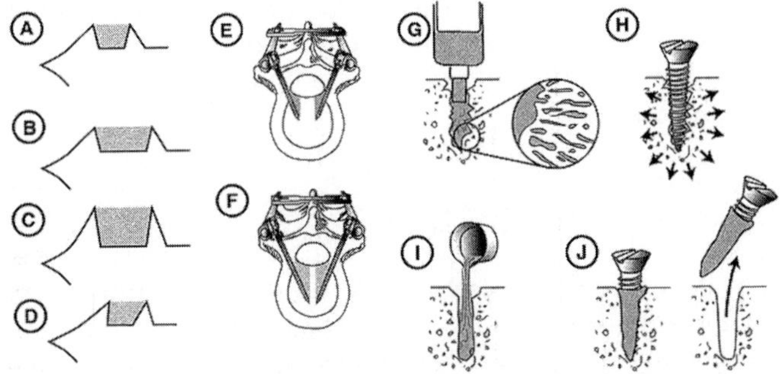

FIG. 7.29 Methods of minimizing screw pullout. Screw pullout resistance is mainly a function of the volume of bone (shaded area) between screw threads (*A*). Thread pitch affects this by altering interthread distance (*B*). Thread depth affects this by altering thread penetration into bone (*C*). Thread shape affects this by altering the amount of bone volume directly. If the pitch and depth are unchanged, the only factor that can affect bone volume is screw thread volume (metal volume) Decreasing screw thread volume (metal volume) increases bone volume (*D*). The triangulation of pedicle screws provides additional resistance to pullout. Pullout resistance is proportional not only to volume of bone between screw threads but also to the triangular area defined by the screw, the perpendicular, and the dorsal vertebral body surface (shaded area) (*E*). Whereas screw length does not routinely contribute significantly to pullout resistance, it contributes significantly when screws are rigidly triangulated (*F*). Note the increase in shaded area. Increasing the screw angle (e.g., toe-in) also increases the size of the shaded area and, thus, pullout resistance. The pressurized injection of polymethylmethacrylate into the screw hole causes the acrylic to penetrate into the bony interstices (*G*). This effectively increases the diameter of the screw (*H*). If a nonpressurized injection is used (*I*), the penetration of the acrylic into the interstices of the bone does not occur. In fact, the acrylic may clump around the screw, thus decreasing its efficiency (*J*). [From (1); copyright © 2001 by the American Association of Neurological Surgeons.]

All three factors must be considered when designing and using such implants. Other screw-bone interface strategies (e.g., acrylic augmentation) are also of biomechanical significant (*Fig. 7.29*).

BICORTICAL PURCHASE

Bicortical purchase improves pullout resistance. Furthermore, angling the vertebral screws toward the end plate (corner of the vertebral body) provides longer screw paths and exposure to bone of greater density. Thus, forces applied to the screws are more effectively resisted.

SCREW TURNOUT

Screw turnout (the elective loosening of a screw) theoretically decreases bone interface integrity by simple motion (wear and tear) at the screw-bone interface and by leaving a gap. The latter effect is most significant when a tapered inner diameter screw is used. The clinical significance of this is not proven, but it has been shown to be of significance biomechanically.

LAG EFFECT

Three conditions must be met for a screw to function as a lag:

1. The near surface of the bone hole must allow the unthreaded screw shaft to glide freely,
2. The far surface of the bone-screw interface must be able to provide purchase for the screw, and
3. When the screw is tightened, its head must contact the near surface to halt progression of the screw's longitudinal movement.

The tension within the screw causes compression between bone fragments.

QUALITATIVE ATTRIBUTES OF SPINAL IMPLANTS

Spinal implants are either predominantly rigid (constrained) or dynamic (semirigid or semiconstrained) and impart distractive, compressive, or neutral axial forces to the spine. Rigid implants are used to achieve a rigid fixation of the spine. Dynamic implants allow for some intersegmental movement, which eases (offloads) stresses placed elsewhere in the system (usually at the implant-bone interface). These factors are the determinants of the mode of application.

Most spinal implants apply forces to the spine in a complex manner. The complex nature of their force application is simplified by considering the six mechanisms of implant:

1. Simple distraction,
2. Three-point bending,
3. Tension-band fixation,
4. Fixed moment arm cantilever beam fixation,
5. Nonfixed moment arm cantilever beam fixation, and
6. Applied moment arm cantilever beam fixation.

It is important to recognize that no truly neutral spinal implant exists. For example, if an implant is placed in a neutral mode at the time of surgery, its characteristics soon change when the spine is loaded (e.g., via the assumption of an upright posture after surgery). Stated differently, implants are loaded differently and alter the mechanism by which they apply and resist loads under different loading conditions. This is universally true.

Thus, many spinal implants that are initially placed in a neutral mode eventually bear axial loads; that is, they function as a distraction device when axial loads are applied. For the purpose of consistency, and with this in mind, neutral devices are considered herein as those that are placed in a neutral mode at the time of surgery—that is, without distraction, compression, three-point bending, or cantilevered force application.

A discussion follows of the "desired axial forces applied" by the spine surgeon using spinal implants. The "axial components" of these desired forces can be broken down into ten clinically used categories. They include both dorsal and ventral techniques (five varieties of each) for spinal instrumentation. The dorsal categories are:

1. Rigid distraction (with or without three-point bending),
2. Rigid neutral,
3. Rigid compression (including most tension-band fixation constructs),
4. Dynamic neutral fixation (including most cantilever bending constructs with nonfixed moment arms), and
5. Dynamic compression (including some tension-band fixation constructs; i.e., springs).

The ventral categories are:

1. Rigid distraction (simple distraction or interbody buttressing),
2. Rigid neutral (cantilever bending constructs with fixed and nonfixed moment arms),
3. Rigid compression,
4. Dynamic neutral fixation (interbody strut placed without distraction), and
5. Dynamic compression.

No true dynamic distraction devices (ventral or dorsal) are readily available for clinical use.

A "clean" separation of these desired axial force applications into their respective categories is often impossible. The attempt to categorize here, therefore, is somewhat artificial. This material is presented to facilitate an understanding of spinal implants and to foster matching of what the surgeon expects from the implant (desired force application) to what is actually achieved (achieved force application).

Dynamic spinal instrumentation allows varying degrees of intersegmental movement. Although excessive movement suppresses bony fusion, minimal intersegmental movement (compression) increases the chance for bone healing via the augmentation of bone healing–enhancing forces. The major advantage of this type of fixation is that the minimal intersegmental movement allowed by the implant absorbs some of the movement that would normally be absorbed at the hook-bone interface or the screw-plate interfaces of more rigid implants. This markedly decreases the chance of failure at the metal-bone interface. It is emphasized that dorsal dynamic compression fixation devices must be applied in conjunction with a solid ventral intervertebral strut or in the presence of existing intact spinal elements so that ventral axial load–bearing ability is present. Following axial loading, excessive flexion will result if this cardinal rule is violated.

Special Considerations

Knowledge of the mechanism of injury may help to determine the most appropriate construct-induced force vector application technique. For example, a hangman's fracture, which usually results from excessive capital extension, requires a capital flexion vector, with accompanying distraction and true neck extension, to assist with reduction; the force application is akin to that used for reduction of a Colles fracture of the wrist. Similarly, for a Chance fracture, a ventral neural decompression, followed by the application of dorsal compression, is an appropriate treatment plan. The stabilization techniques in these two examples use forces that are, for the most part, opposite in orientation to those that caused the injuries.

Fracture type and location obviously dictate, to a significant degree, the type of reduction and fixation technique to be used. Substantial translational injuries may be best reduced and fixated with rigid distraction and three-point bending techniques. In these cases, segmental fixation substantially augments stability. Other complex fractures may require long dorsal rigid neutral rod fixation techniques with multiple-level fixation. Rigid distraction or compression techniques, when combined with a three-point bending force application, should, at least in part, correct scoliotic deformities. They also provide stable constructs for kyphotic deformities when applied with multiple segmental fixation. Rigid distraction, using accompanying multiple segmental fixation and cross-fixation, may provide a strong construct for complex fractures in the low lumbar region. This provides an alternative to pedicle fixation techniques.

The extent of neurological injury obviously plays a major role in the operation selection process. There are two indications for surgery after spine trauma: neural element decompression and spine stabilization. Either may stand alone as an indication for surgery. Obviously, a more "cavalier" approach to spine reduction and fixation may be undertaken when the patient manifests a complete myelopathic injury.

Only minimal hope for neurological recovery, other than nerve root function, exists in these patients, even following dural sac decompression.

Conversely, if any neurological function distal to the injury is present preoperatively, a chance for neurological recovery exists. Therefore, great care should be taken to prevent neurological deterioration and to promote neurological recovery. Aggressive surgery for spinal canal decompression should be considered when appropriate.

Effective Use of Intrinsic Spinal Anatomy

Several anatomic features of the spine can be effectively used by the spine surgeon during the application of instrumentation. The orientation of the facet joints may provide a substantial biomechanical advantage regarding the application of tension-band fixation constructs in the cervical region. The orientation of the cervical facets joints is predominantly in the coronal plane. This orientation does not lend itself well to the resistance of rotation, flexion, or dorsal translation. Ventral translation without flexion is resisted well, provided there is an intact facet joint complex. If an element of cervical instability in flexion is present, with an accompanying disruption of the disc space, then the facet joint cannot function in the capacity as a resister of ventral translational deformation. This is seen during situations in which dorsal interspinous ligamentous instability has been incurred. The repair of an interspinous ligament disruption injury by the application of a tension-band fixation construct provides reduction of the deformity and the prevention of further ventral translation by "locking" the intact facet joints against each other (facet engagement). Longer constructs may occasionally be required.

Although not of biomechanical significance, the imaging characteristics of spinal implants is of significant clinical concern. In general, all metal implants obscure radiographs, CT scans, and MR images to one degree or another. Stainless-steel performs poorly in this regard, particularly with CT and MR imaging. Titanium performs relatively well with both MR imaging and CT, whereas tantalum performs well with MR imaging but not with CT.

QUANTITATIVE ATTRIBUTES OF SPINAL IMPLANTS

A thorough understanding of the forces applied to the spine by spinal implants is mandatory. These applied forces are often extremely complex. If they are broken down into components, however, then the component force vectors may be quantitated and better understood.

The force vector of a simple compression instrumentation construct is usually applied at a finite distance from the IAR and is perpendicular to the long axis of the spine, thus creating a bending moment that is proportional to the perpendicular distance from the point of application of that force to the IAR—that is, proportional to the lever arm or moment arm).

The use of distraction as an isolated force to the dorsal aspect of the spine is uncommon; however, distraction may be applied in the interbody region. Thus, the distraction is applied "in line" with the IARs in the region of the neutral axis. A distraction force that is applied "in line" with the IAR does not result in an applied bending moment, whereas a distraction force applied at a perpendicular distance from the IAR creates a bending moment that is proportional to the length of the lever arm.

Of course, most spinal implants can be placed in a neutral mode; that is, they apply no forces of any type to the spinal column at the time of surgery. The application of an implant so that it never applies (or bears) a load (force), however, is impossible. Even if the implant is placed in a neutral mode at the time of surgery, any movement or change in body position after surgery presents stresses to the construct that alter its neutral-mode characteristic. Hence, an implant placed in a neutral mode resists compression when the patient assumes an upright posture. Thus, this implant, in a sense, is placed in a distraction mode. This same implant resists forces applied, to one degree or another, in all planes. In so doing, it may function as a distraction device, tension-band fixator, a cantilever, and so forth. Implants seldom function by only one biomechanical mechanism. In other words, the mechanism of load-bearing varies, depending on the loading conditions.

Conversely, a spinal implant placed in a compression mode may be used to "share" the load with an accompanying interbody strut. If a cantilever beam is placed in a distraction mode, it bears all of the load. If placed in a compression mode, it shares the load with intrinsic vertebral components or interbody struts. Such an implant placed in compression might even be nonweight-bearing in the upright position (zero weight-bearing; see below). These points must always be considered during the clinical decision-making process.

All spinal instrumentation techniques apply forces to the spine via one or a combination of six basic mechanisms:

1. Simple distraction,
2. Three-point bending,
3. Tension-band fixation,
4. Fixed moment arm cantilever beam fixation,

5. Nonfixed moment arm cantilever beam fixation, and
6. Applied moment arm cantilever beam fixation.

The biomechanical principles involved with each of these techniques are discussed separately. These strategies may be employed via a ventral, a lateral, or a dorsal approach (1).

Simple Distraction Fixation

Simple distraction fixation can be applied from either a ventral interbody or a dorsal approach. Ventral distraction constructs generally apply forces that are in line with the IAR (in the interbody region). This allows the ventral distraction implant to effectively resist axial loads without applying a bending moment (*Fig. 7.30*). Ventral interbody distraction can cause extension of the spine if the distraction forces are applied ventral to the IAR (ventral to the neutral axis). Application of a dorsal distraction force as an isolated entity is uncommon because of its propensity to pathologically exaggerate or cause a kyphotic deformity. The location of the point of force application dorsal to the IAR creates a bending moment that results in flexion. The combination of distraction and three-point bending instrumentation

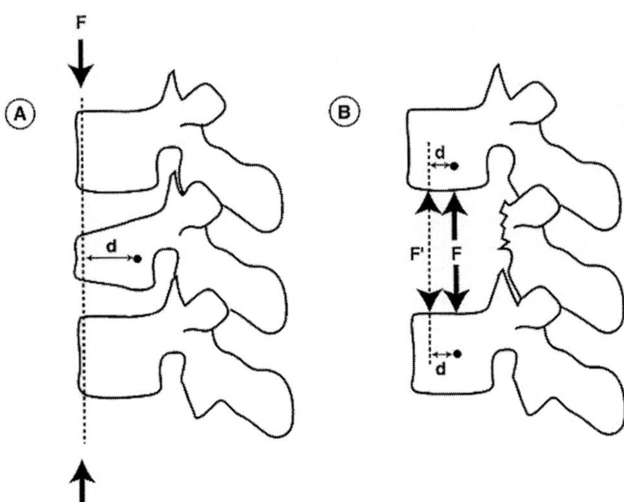

FIG. 7.30 (*A*) A compressive force (F) that is applied at a finite distance (d) from the IAR (dot). (*B*) A distraction force (*F*) that is applied "in line" with the IAR (in the neutral axis) does not result in bending moment application. A distraction for (*F'*) that is applied at some distance (*d*) from the neutral axis causes a bending moment, the magnitude of which is dictated by the perpendicular distance (*d*) from the IAR. [From (1); copyright © 2001 by the American Association of Neurological Surgeons.]

application eliminates this pathological situation by applying a ventrally directed force at the fulcrum (1).

Distraction applied to the spine at a finite perpendicular distance from the IAR results in a force application similar (but opposite in direction) to that achieved with tension-band (compression) fixation. This distraction force application might be termed *tension-band (distraction) fixation*.

Three-Point Bending Fixation

A springboard is a common example of a three-point bending force application. It consists of a fulcrum that directs a force vector opposite the direction of the terminal force vectors (*Fig. 7.31*). Three-point bending spinal instrumentation constructs apply similar force vectors. They are usually applied with an accompanying distraction or com-

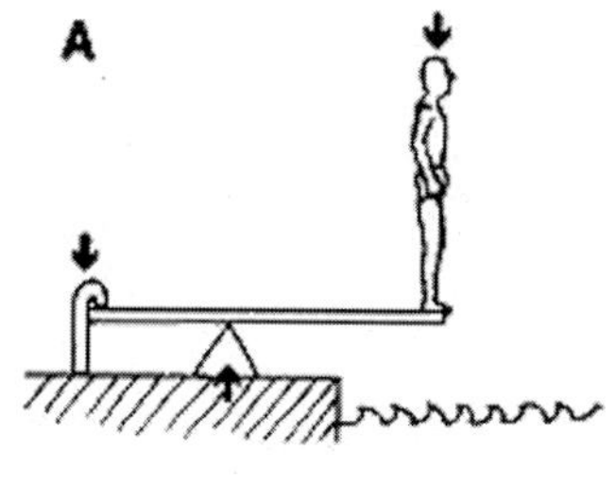

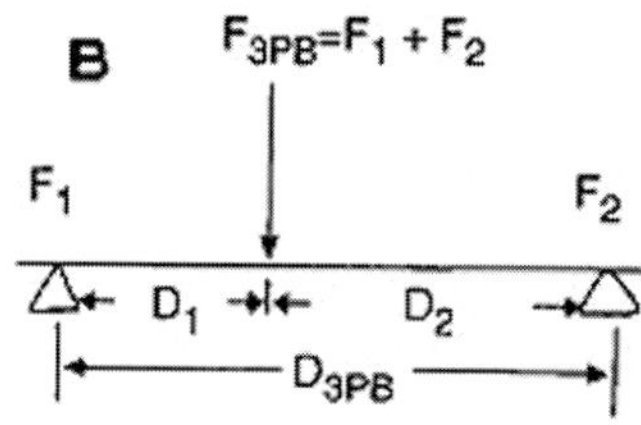

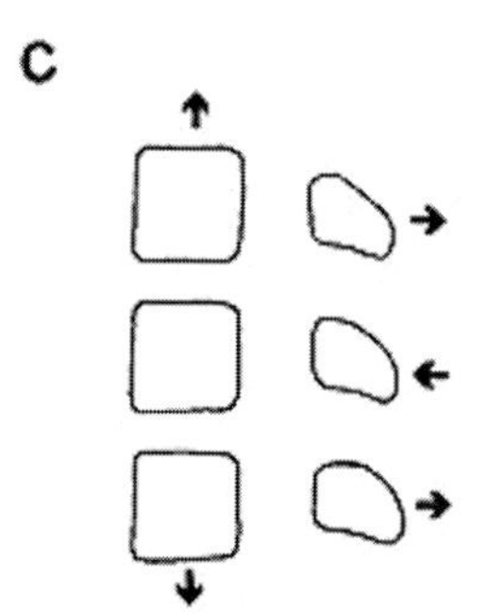

FIG. 7.31 (A) The force vectors are at work when a person is standing on the end of a springboard. (*B*) These three-point bending forces are defined by the equation $M = D_1D_2 \cdot F_{3pb}/D_{3pb}$, in which D_1 and D_2 are the distances from the fulcrum to the terminal book-bone interfaces, D_{3pb} is the sum of D_1 and D_2, and F_{3pb} is the ventrally directed force applied at the fulcrum. (*C*) Spinal three-point bending constructs (horizontal arrows) are usually applied in combination with another force vector complex; commonly, distraction (vertical arrows). [From (1); copyright © 2001 by the American Association of Neurological Surgeons.]

pression force application (e.g., by Harrington distraction rods) or by universal spinal instrumentation techniques applied in a distraction (or compression) mode. Three-point bending constructs commonly involve instrumentation application over multiple spinal segments (five or more spinal segments) with accompanying, dorsally directed forces at the upper and lower construct-bone interfaces and a ventrally directed force at the fulcrum that is equal to the sum of the two dorsally directed forces. This technique can be used to decompress the ventral dural sac following trauma by distracting the posterior longitudinal ligament (ligamentotaxis or annulotaxis). The desired resultant force is the pushing of the offending bone and/or disc fragments ventrally and away from the dural sac. Because of the relative weakness of the posterior longitudinal ligament and/or the fixed nature of the retropulsed fragments, however, this technique may not always succeed (1).

Dorsal distraction force vector application is rarely "pure." It is frequently used in combination with the application of a three-point bending force to the spine. The application of sufficient dorsal distraction so that the implant makes contact with the spine at the level of the site of pathology (at an intermediate point along the construct; i.e., at a fulcrum) results in three-point bending force application. The application of a distraction force between two adjacent spinal levels where a fulcrum is not present is an exception (e.g., the use of a Knodt rod in distraction that spans only one motion segment). In this case, no intermediate point of fixation at a fulcrum is available. With longer constructs, flexion occurs before engagement of the fulcrum because of the application of the distraction force at points dorsal to the IAR. This is most common in the lumbar region, where a lordotic posture is present (*Fig. 7.32*).

The bending moment at the site of pathology from three-point bending construct application is defined mathematically by the equation

$$M = \frac{D_1 \cdot D_2 \cdot F_{3pb}}{D_{3pb}}$$

in which M = the bending moment, D_1 and D_2 = e the distances from the fulcrum to the terminal hook-bone interfaces, D_{3pb} = the sum of D_1 and D_2, and F_{3pb} = the ventrally directed force applied at the fulcrum (1).

TERMINAL THREE-POINT BENDING FIXATION

A three-point bending construct can be used to correct a deformity near the termini of the construct, as opposed to the more common midportion of the construct. This is termed *terminal three-point bending*

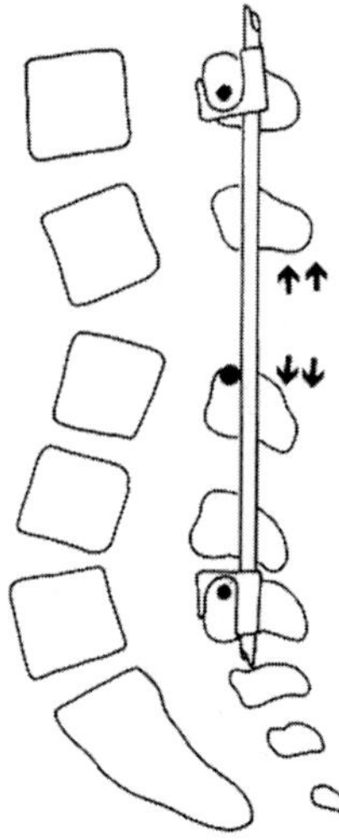

FIG. 7.32 The application of dorsal distraction forces to a lordotic spine may result in inadvertent flexion. [From (1); copyright © 2001 by the American Association of Neurological Surgeons.]

fixation. Usually, the implant is positioned so that the sagittal deformation is at the rostral end of the construct (if ventral subluxation is present).

In reality, terminal three-point bending fixation is simply a three-point bending construct in which the fulcrum is situated near one end of the construct; that is, D_1 is short and D_2 is relatively long. In light of this, the springboard discussed above is more appropriately considered as a terminal three-point bending structure. Of note is that the moment arm attained by a terminal three-point bending construct is less than what is attained if similar ventrally and dorsally directed forces are applied when the fulcrum is the midportion of the construct. This must be taken into consideration clinically.

Tension-Band Fixation

Dorsal spinal compression (tension-band fixation) is usually applied by wires, clamps, springs, or rigid constructs, such as Knodt rods in compression, Harrington compression rods, or universal spinal instrumentation techniques applied in compression. These techniques apply spinal compression forces at their dorsal application sites. Ventral tension-band fixation constructs, however, may also be applied (1) (*Fig. 7.33*).

It is reemphasized that implants function differently under different loading conditions. A ventral cervical fixed moment arm cantilever (i.e., constrained plate) functions as a cantilever if an axial load is ap-

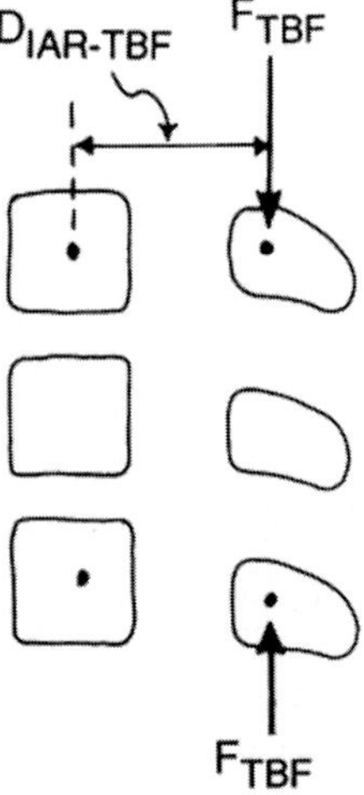

FIG. 7.33 The forces applied by a tension-band fixation construct are described by the equation $M_{tbf} = F_{tbf}D_{iar\text{-}tbf}$, where M_{tbf} is the bending moment, F_{tbf} is the compression force applied at the upper and lower termini of the construct at the instrument-bone interface, and $D_{iar\text{-}tbf}$ is the perpendicular distance from the IAR to the tension-band fixation applied-force vector. [From (1); copyright © 2001 by the American Association of Neurological Surgeons.]

plied. If, however, the patient extends the neck, the implant will limit extension at the instrumented segment via a tension-band fixation (in extension) mechanism. Tension-band fixation applies compression forces at a perpendicular distance from the IAR (e.g., from the plate to the IAR).

By the nature of the tension-band fixation construct, an extension (dorsal) or flexion (ventral) bending moment is applied to the spinal segments that are "compressed." For tension-band fixation techniques, the bending moment applied at the site of pathology is defined mathematically by the equation

$$M_{tbf} = F_{tbf} \cdot D_{iar\text{-}tbf}$$

in which M_{tbf} = the bending moment, F_{tbf} = the compression force applied at the upper and lower termini of the construct at the instrument-bone interface, and $D_{iar\text{-}tbf}$ = the perpendicular distance from the IAR to the applied force.

Ventrally positioned extradural masses (bone and/or disc fragments) might be thrust dorsally into the spinal canal during the application of dorsal compression forces. Therefore, ventral decompression procedures may be appropriate before the application of dorsal instrumentation constructs, particularly if ventral compression via retropulsed bone and/or disc fragments exists. Additionally, tension-band fixators do not, in and of themselves, bear axial loads; they simply apply compression via a tension-band. Therefore, if axial load–bearing ability is inadequate, it must be restored (*Fig. 7.34*).

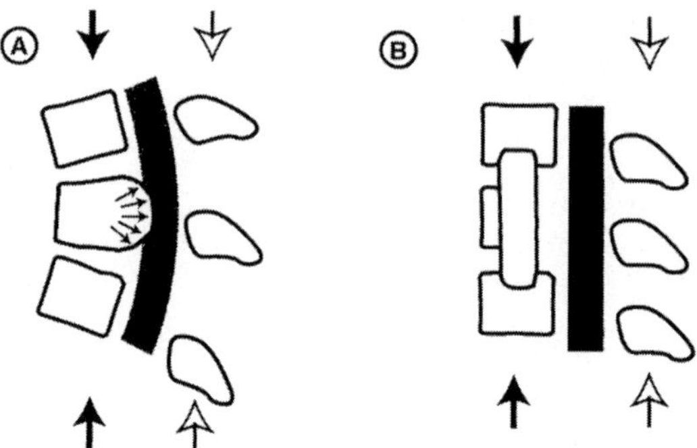

FIG. 7.34 (*A*) The application of dorsal compression (hollow arrows) may result in the retropulsion of ventral disc or bone into the spinal canal. (*B*) Decompression and the restoration of axial load-bearing ability will prevent this. Tension-band fixators (hollow arrows) do not, in and of themselves, bear axial loads. If axial load-bearing ability is not present, it must be restored. [From (1); copyright © 2001 by the American Association of Neurological Surgeons.]

Comparing Distraction and Compression

The concepts of load-bearing and load-sharing should be considered each time a spinal implant is used. As mentioned, neutral implants do not exist in the truest sense. When weight is borne by the torso, the implant is exposed to a myriad of forces (load-bearing). This inevitably occurs, even among cases in which an implant is initially placed in a neutral mode. In fact, if the negative surgical load is equal to the weight of the torso positioned above the implant, the load borne by the implant during the assumption of an upright posture is zero; that is, the surgical load is equal, and opposite in direction, to the weight of the torso positioned above the implant.

For the purposes of discussion, isolated axial loads and force applications are considered. This, however, is quite different from the clinical situation in which a myriad of forces are applied by the torso to the implant and by the implant to the torso. The bearing of a load by the torso, while assuming an upright posture, causes a spinal implant to absorb an axial load. If the implant was placed in a neutral mode, the axial load that is borne changes from zero (the load borne by the implant at the time of surgery; i.e., surgical load bearing = 0) to roughly the weight of the torso positioned above the implant. If the implant was placed in a distraction mode, the additional axial load that is borne by the implant with the patient assuming the upright posture is the sum of that initially borne at the time of surgery (surgical load-bearing) plus the weight of the torso above the implant. The placement of an implant in a compression mode alters the forces considerably. For the hypothetical situation in which only axial forces are considered, the placement of an implant in a compression mode results in a negative surgical load-bearing force. If an axial load is subsequently borne by the patient assuming an upright posture, the surgical compression load is effectively diminished, and the net load approaches or surpasses zero. A spinal implant placed in a compression mode thus allows the implant to share a portion of the load that is applied by the torso with the spine proper. This occurs via existing spinal axial load–bearing capabilities or by an interbody strut graft.

Comparing Three-Point Bending and Tension-Band Fixation

Three-point bending and tension-band fixation constructs differ substantially. Three-point bending fixation techniques require the use of long constructs to optimize efficacy of the construct; the bending moment associated with a three-point bending construct is proportional the length of the construct. The bending moment applied by a tension-band fixation construct is independent of construct length. Therefore, three-point bending constructs are usually employed over more spinal segments than tension-band fixation constructs.

The bending moment that is applied at the fracture site by three-point bending fixation techniques is defined mathematically by the equation depicted. The bending moment applied by tension-band fixation techniques, however, is defined mathematically by the equation portrayed in *Figure 7.33*.

Long three-point bending constructs allow for the application of two widely spaced bending moments at the termini of the construct (terminal bending moments). This encourages the development of an exaggerated extension deformity.

If the bending moment applied at the fracture site is the same for three-point bending and tension-band fixation techniques, the two equations may be simultaneously solved. This implies that to achieve an equal bending moment, the two instrumentation constructs utilize a fourfold difference in moment arm length.

It is reemphasized that these moment arms are not equivalent with regard to orientation. The moment arm of a tension-band fixation construct refers to a lever arm that is perpendicular to the long axis of the spine (and the instrumentation construct), whereas the moment arm of a three-point bending construct refers to a lever arm that is parallel to the long axis of the spine (and the instrumentation construct). Nevertheless, a three-point bending technique requires a longer construct than in the tension-band fixation technique to achieve the same bending moment at the fracture site with similar applied forces.

Since the bending moment at the fracture site is unchanged by the length of a tension-band fixation construct and the ventrally directed effective force diminishes as the construct length is increased, short tension-band constructs may often be more desirable. Conversely, longer three-point bending constructs offer greater stability (better deformity progression prevention and deformity correction biomechanical advantages). Therefore, if substantial axial loading, rotational, and/or translation resisting characteristics are desired, long three-point bending constructs (more than five spinal segments) may be most appropriate.

Three-point bending fixation techniques most often utilize additional, superimposed forces applied in distraction at the terminal (and intermediate) construct-bone interfaces. This adds to the stresses applied to the bone (by adding a distraction component). It, however, does not alter the bending moment if the ventrally directed force at the fulcrum is not changed. Three-point bending and distraction force applications should be considered as independent of each other. Some authors have advocated the exaggeration of such forces to accomplish spinal column reduction and spinal canal decompression. This, however, has not always met with success.

Application of the terminology associated with biomechanics and physics in the spine surgery literature has often been confusing. Specifically, much of the confusion has been associated with the biomechanics of injury and instrumentation. The concept of the bending moment has been misrepresented and, thus, poorly understood.

In this regard, the bending moment associated with instrumentation application is often greatest at the level of the deformity (particularly with regard to three-point bending techniques). This is fortuitous regarding deformity reduction because of the requirement for torque application at the deformity site to achieve spinal deformity reduction. The maximum bending moment applied at the deformity site is located at the center of the circle defined by the arc of the force causing the bending moment.

Fixed Moment Arm Cantilever Beam Fixation

A cantilever is a bracket or a beam that projects from an immobile object. It is supported at one end only (*Fig. 7.35*). A cantilever is usually designed to bear a load over a space in which support cannot be provided or is not desired. There are three types of cantilever beams:

1. Fixed moment arm,
2. Nonfixed moment arm, and
3. Applied moment arm.

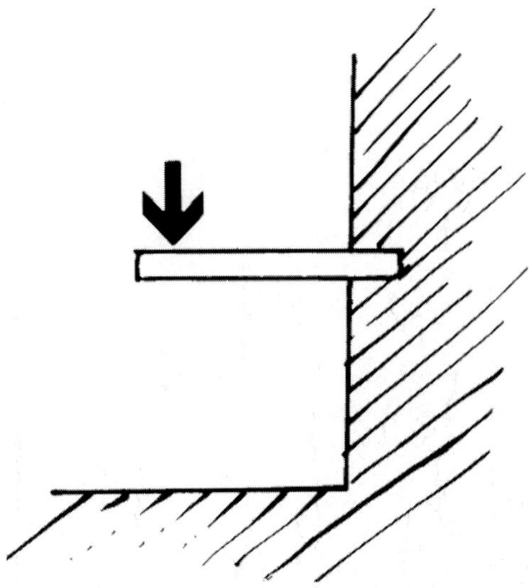

FIG. 7.35 A fixed moment arm cantilever beam. In this case, the cantilever beam is rigidly affixed to the wall. Note the lack of need for an accompanying applied force vector during the bearing of a load (arrow). [From (1); copyright © 2001 by the American Association of Neurological Surgeons.]

A characteristic example of this type of structure among spinal instrumentation constructs is the rigid (constrained) pedicle fixator. Rigid pedicle fixation techniques (e.g., rigid plate or screw-rod combinations) may compensate for a short moment arm by providing a fixed moment arm cantilever beam configuration for structural support. Although the initial application of such a construct may be in a neutral mode (no distraction, rotation, compression, or translational forces applied) during the assumption of an erect posture, the construct resists the axial loads by virtue of it intrinsic fixed moment arm cantilever beam characteristics (by rigidly buttressing the spine). Worthy of note is its lack of need for a ventrally directed force at the midportion of the implant, as is the case with three-point bending fixation. This causes a significant stress to be applied to the implant, commonly at the screw-plate or screw-rod interface. This stress may be excessive, resulting in screw fracture (an infrequently observed phenomenon with modern construct designs). Biomechanical studies have confirmed this (1).

Nonfixed Moment Arm Cantilever Beam Fixation

A nonfixed moment arm cantilever beam does not effectively bear an axial load without the assistance of other structures (e.g., vertebral body, bone graft, and so on); however, it assists the already-present axial load-supporting structures to do so (*Fig. 7.36*). Nonfixed moment arm cantilever beam constructs do not apply substantial axial load–resisting forces to the spine. The toggling of the screw on the

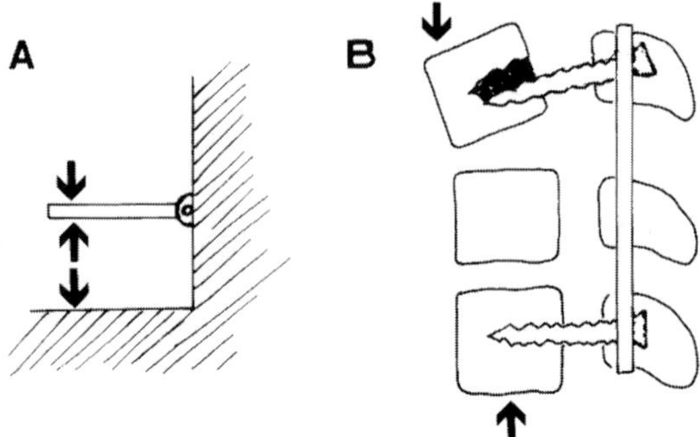

FIG. 7.36 A nonfixed moment arm cantilever beam. (*A*) In this case, the cantilever beam is fixed by a hinge to the wall. Note the requirement for an accompanying applied force vector (opposed arrows) during the bearing of a load (single arrow). (*B*) Nonfixed moment arm cantilever beam constructs may fail by screw pullout. [From (1); copyright © 2001 by the American Association of Neurological Surgeons.]

plate allowed by this technique dictates that little, if any, bending moment is applied to the spine or is resisted by the implant during axial loading. If three or more segments are affixed, however, then a nonfixed moment arm cantilever beam fixator can apply a three-point or four-point bending moment that resists kyphotic deformation. These techniques are appropriately used only when axial load–resisting capabilities of the spine are present. Because of their biomechanical characteristics, their ability to resist screw pullout is diminished.

The application of nonfixed moment arm cantilever beam constructs in the cervical spine via lateral mass screw-plate systems or in the lumbar spine via transpedicular screw-plate or screw-rod systems may create situations in which they function, at least in part, as tension-band fixation constructs. In this situation, they resist flexion, thus functioning as a tension-band fixator in flexion. They also function as three-point bending constructs, especially if used in predominantly cortical bone, with its relatively good screw pullout resistance. Finally, they augment stability by pulling the bone to the underside of the plate (see below). In the end, the construct-type categories cannot be completely and cleanly separated (1).

Applied Moment Arm Cantilever Beam Fixation

Finally, cantilever beam fixation can be applied with either a flexion moment or an extension moment (*Fig. 7.37*) to the applied moment arm. These constructs usually are rigid and are used to reduce deformities. Extension moment arm application is the most common clinical use at present.

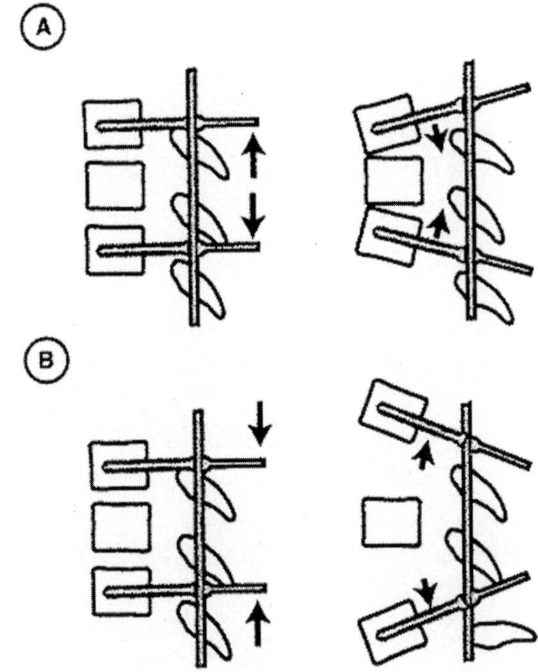

FIG. 7.37 (*A*) Applied moment arm cantilever beam construct using a flexion moment. (*B*) Applied moment arm cantilever beam construct using an extension moment. [From (1); copyright © 2001 by the American Association of Neurological Surgeons.]

Dynamic Fixation (Controlled Axially Dynamic Fixation)

Dynamic fixation is a unique and separate concept from that of the aforementioned six forms of fixation. It applies some of their selected attributes. In addition, it does not involve the application of a bending moment to the spine (related to its dynamic nature). A nonfixed moment arm cantilever beam is, in some respects, a dynamic implant. Axially dynamic implants are, in the purest sense, the only true dynamic implants. They permit axial subsidence and, hence, do not apply or resist axial loads (*Fig. 7.38*). They employ the aforementioned types of fixation to resist or apply loads on other planes.

Dynamic spine fixation is predominately employed in the ventral cervical spine. Its evolution as a viable alternative to rigid fixation has been a long and circuitous process. This process has been complicated by nomenclature issues: Implants that permit the toggling of screws on a plate as the only mechanism to achieve subsidence are not truly axially dynamic implants. They do not permit telescoping of the spine (axial subsidence) except by failure at the screw-bone interface via the toggling process (windshield wipering).

Controlled axially dynamic implants, which permit screw movement along a plate within a slot or permit the screws and a platform to slide

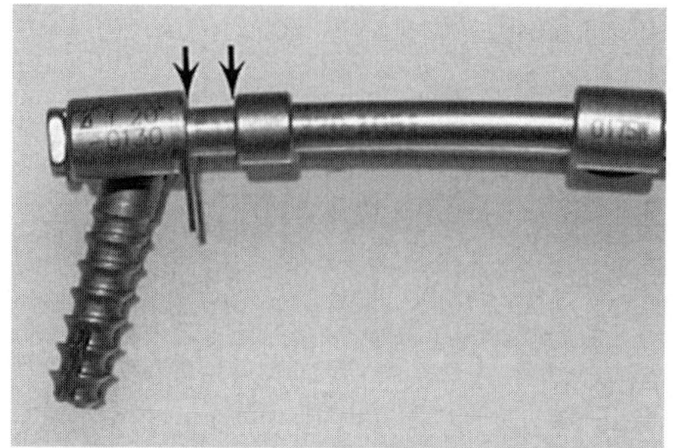

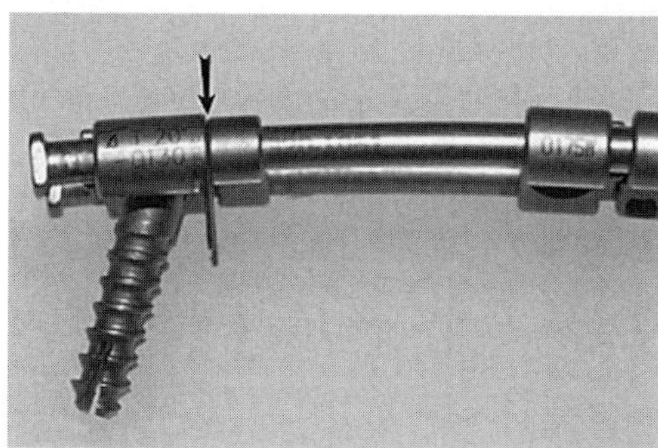

FIG. 7.38 The DOC ventral cervical spine system (DePuy Acromed, Raynham, MA) allows axial subsidence without screw toggling (fixed moment arm cantilever screws) (*A* and *B*). Note movement of platform on rods (arrows). [From (1); copyright © 2001 by the American Association of Neurological Surgeons.]

along rods, are the two clinical strategies currently employed for the attainment of true axial subsidence. This type of subsidence (via an axially dynamic implant) controls the axis along which the subsidence occurs (by the surgeon-determined sagittal contour of the implant) as well as the extent of axial subsidence (by the length of slots, the location of the placement of the screws with the slots, and the placement of "blockers" [i.e., cross-fixators] that limit platform "travel"). Hence, this type of fixation is perhaps best termed *controlled axially dynamic fixation*. The implant type that permits subsidence via the screw toggling within a plate or a platform is best described or defined by the term that defines its quantitative effect—for example, *nonfixed moment arm cantilever beam fixation*.

Dynamic spine fixation, as defined above, facilitates:

1. Bone fusion via the augmentation of bone healing enhancing forces (compression, ala Wolff's law),
2. Minimization of axial implant loading due to offloading of the implant and the loading of the interbody bone graft,
3. Facilitation of spine subsidence along an axis conceived and created by the surgeon (via the surgeon's predetermined curvature of the implant), and

4. Provision of multiple intermediate points of fixation (to maximize bony fusion union rate and construct minimize failure rate).

CONSTRUCT FAILURE AND FAILURE PREVENTION

Constructs can fail because of failure of the implant (e.g., by fracture of a plate), failure of the bone at the implant-bone interface, or failure at the component-component juncture. Each of these mechanisms of failure is addressed in the following discussion.

Implant Failure

Implants always fail at points of maximum stress (θ) application. Stress is a function of bending moment (M) and the section modulus (Z). Stress (θ) is defined by the equation

$$\theta = M/Z$$

Section modulus (Z) defines the ability of an object such as a screw or rod to resist bending. It is proportional to the third power of the diameter of a rod or the third power of the inner diameter of a screw. Examples of two scenarios regarding fixed moment arm cantilevered screws, with a constant inner diameter and a "ramped" ("tapered" or conical) inner diameter, are portrayed in *Figure 7.39*. The point of failure of a fixed inner diameter fixed moment arm cantilever beam screw is usually at the screw-plate juncture (point of maximum stress). The point of failure of a ramped inner diameter screw is somewhere between the tip of the screw and the plate. In the example depicted in *Figure 7.41*, the bending moment increases linearly along the screw (dotted line). The solid lines depict the section modulus, which is unchanged along the length of the screw for a fixed inner diameter screw but rises exponentially (to the third power) for a tapered inner diameter screw.

The longitudinal member (plate) itself can fail. Long moment arms and bending moments that are applied to regions of an implant with a relatively small section modulus (Z), result in the application of significant stress ($\theta = M/Z$). This has been shown to be the case with the Harrington distraction rod system (Zimmer, Warsaw, IN).

Nonfixed moment arm cantilever beam screws also fail at points of maximum stress. Nonfixed moment arm cantilever beam screws, however, are often exposed to different forces than those to which the fixed moment arm counterparts are exposed. Fixed moment arm screws are exposed to fixed moment arm cantilevered loads and moment arms that are perpendicular to the screw, in addition to their associated stresses, although nonfixed moment arm cantilever beam screws are exposed predominantly to three-point bending forces and stresses. As

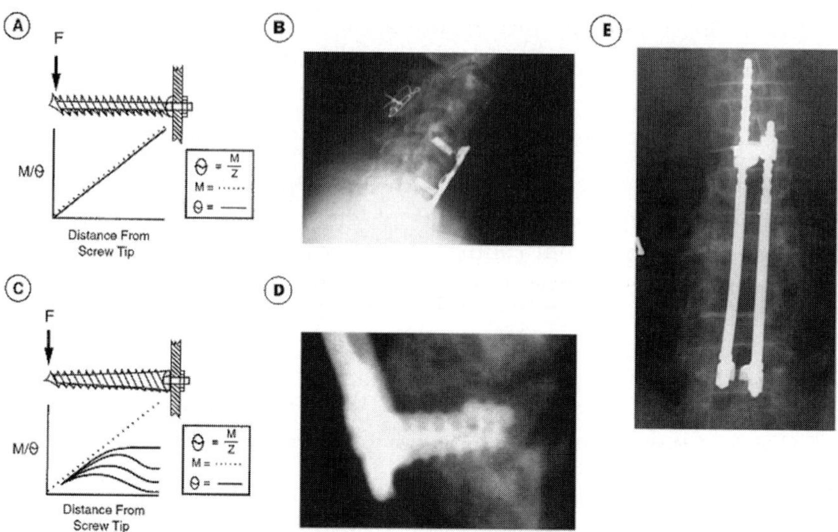

FIG. 7.39 A fixed moment arm cantilever beam fixed inner diameter screw is more likely to fracture at the screw-plate junction, and a conical inner diameter screw is more likely to fracture in midshaft if transverse loads are applied to the tip of the screw. This is so because the stress applied is maximum at the point of fracture, as depicted by line drawings in (*A*) and (*C*) and radiographically in (*B*) and (*D*). The dotted lines represent the bending moment (*M*). The solid line(s) represent the strength (Z = section modulus). For tapered screws, a family of curves is depicted. The shape of the curve depends on the extent of taper of the screw's inner diameter (*C*).

A radiograph of a patient with a 7-ratchet and 11-ratchet Harrington distraction rod is also shown (*E*). The 11-ratchet rod is associated with a significant failure rate at the proximal ratchet as a result of the significant moment arm and, hence, stress applied at this juncture. [From (1); copyright © 2001 by the American Association of Neurological Surgeons.]

an axial load is applied to a nonfixed moment arm cantilever beam screw-plate construct, the screw "sees" different force vectors (both in magnitude and direction) at various points along the screw (*Fig. 7.40*). These are usually three or four in number and relate to both the loads applied and the varying consistencies and integrities of the materials through which the screw passes. The latter varies from the metal of a plate to cancellous bone. These can cause a "shear" effect and a three- or four-point bending force application. This results in a bending moment that stresses a fixed moment arm cantilever beam screw with a fixed inner diameter maximally at the point of maximum bending moment application.

The toggling of a nonfixed moment arm cantilever beam screw in bone degrades the integrity of the bone as well as of the screw-bone

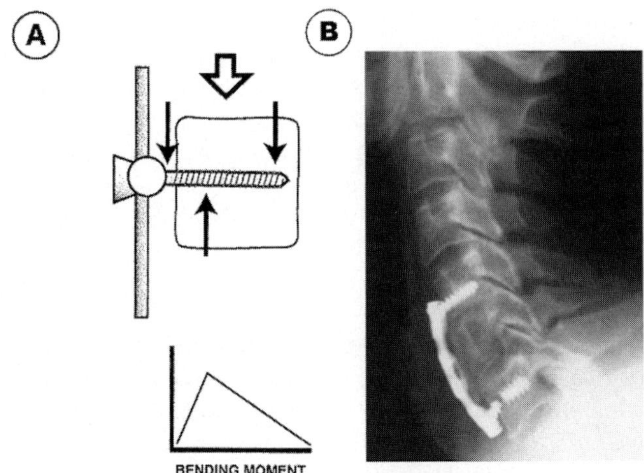

FIG. 7.40 The three-point bending forces applied to a nonfixed moment arm screw cantilever beam (solid arrows) exposed to axial loads (hollow arrow). These forces are applied in opposing directions. This is related to the differences in integrity of the materials through which the screw passes (e.g., cortical bone, cancellous bone, metal, etc.) and the resistance to the loads applied (*A*). The bending moment (depicted below the line drawing) is maximum at the fulcrum. A screw fracture resulting from such a mechanism is shown (*B*). [From (1); copyright © 2001 by the American Association of Neurological Surgeons.]

interface by its "windshield wipering" (sweeping) motion. It may result in the screw itself abutting the end of the bone graft, thus obliterating a portion of the surface area of contact between the bone graft and vertebral body.

The strength characteristics of plates are defined, in part, by their section modulus (Z). With plates, the section modulus is a function of cross-sectional area and geometry. Although a plate may appear to be bulky, it is no stronger than its weakest link. As with screws or rods, plates fail at the point of maximum stress application ($\theta = M/Z$). This is the point at which the ratio of the applied bending moment and the section modulus (M/Z) are maximum. A plate, screw, or rod is most vulnerable at the point of maximum bending moment application. If the section modulus (Z) is not adequate, fracture will occur.

Rigid (fixed moment arm) multisegmental fixation constructs tend to load the caudal screws more than the rostral screws. This can cause failure of the caudal screws. Long fixed moment arm cantilever beam screw implants, in general, are associated with a high failure rate. In this situation, use of a shorter implant (if clinically appropriate) is associated with a shorter bending moment applied to the screws, thus decreasing the chance of failure. A corollary of this phenomenon is observed in the low cervical spine and the cervicothoracic junction, in which the regional anatomy and geometry apply additional stresses to the caudal screw-bone interface.

Screw fracture may pose unique problems related to extraction. A variety of strategies have been employed for this purpose. It should be remembered that screw extraction may be difficult and is often not necessary (1).

Implant-Bone Interface Failure

Implant-bone interface failure can be obviated by not employing implants. In the cervical spine, this has been shown to be relatively prudent in selected circumstances. Newer clinical strategies, however, may reverse this "philosophy." Ultimately, decreasing the range of motion by means of an implant has a positive effect on fusion.

The integrity of the implant-bone interface can be optimized in many ways. The ability of the implant to resist failure is, in part, related to its ability to distribute loads (load-sharing) so that no single portion of the implant or spine bears an excessive portion of the load (load-bearing). In other words, it is optimal if applied loads are distributed over multiple implant components and multiple points of contact with the spine (load-sharing). This can be accomplished by:

1. Improving the integrity of the existing implant-bone interfaces,
2. Providing additional implant-bone interfaces,
3. Improving the integrity of the bone, and
4. Normalizing geometry.

Additionally, any strategy that offloads the implant obviously minimizes the chance of implant failure. This has been accomplished via the use of dynamic implants.

IMPROVING THE INTEGRITY OF EXISTING IMPLANT-BONE INTERFACES

Screw geometry can be altered so that pullout resistance is enhanced. Similarly, the concept of triangulation can be used to an advantage. Spine configuration must also be taken into account. For example, cervical spine lordosis causes ventral cervicothoracic junction screw-bone interfaces to be exposed to loads that increase the chance of failure. Additional innovative strategies include expanding the screw tip (e.g., like a molly bolt or drywall screw), employing vertebral body margin buttressing strategies (see below), and employing screw hole augmentation strategies (e.g., bone chips or polymethylmethacrylate). An appreciation of the changing angular relationships of the lower cervical spine at the cervicothoracic junction is imperative. This causes significant loading of the caudal screw-bone junction and often leads to failure. This is related, in part, to the high failure rate that is observed at the caudal end of long ventral cervical constructs. It is also, however, related to the angle of the screw in relation to the axis that is perpendicular to the floor (see below).

PROVISION OF ADDITIONAL IMPLANT-BONE INTERFACES

The provision of additional fixation points provide a biomechanical advantage via two mechanisms: the provision of additional points of fixation and the provision of the ability to resist deformation in more than one plane and by more than one mechanism. Regarding the former, the integrity of fixation is proportional to the number "high-quality" fixation points (load-sharing). The ability to resist spinal deformation in more than one plane and by more than one mechanism is illustrated in *Figure 7.41*. In this example, a rigid ventral construct acts as a fixed moment arm cantilever. For this situation, in which two screws are used at each termini of the implant, axial loads are borne relatively well. Implants and implant-bone interfaces, however, rarely fail following simple unidimensional loading. They usually fail following repetitive loading (fatigue). This has been shown to occur with regard to implants that are applied without intermediate points of fixation to a "parent vertebral body." Furthermore, the loads are usually applied from a variety of angles and orientations. This includes transverse and shear loads. The implant depicted in *Figure 7.41* bears axial loads effectively but does not effectively resist translational or rotational loads. This may cause degradation of the screw-bone interface and, ultimately, failure as a result of axial loading. The longer the implant, the more prone to these effects it becomes. The addition of intermediate points of fixation allows the implant to resist these translational loads via the addition of a third fixation point and the use of three-point bending mechanical strategies. Thus, the additional fixation points not only permit axial loads to be borne more effectively but also increase the resistance of translation and shear forces as well. This has been shown to be the case in the lumbar spine with the employment of pedicle screws.

Stability is not enhanced by adding an intermediate point of fixation to a bony strut; it actually is lessened. The flexibility-related bowing of the implant is not impeded by this strategy. Instead, it causes harmful ventral and dorsal loads to be applied to the strut. Finally, when instrumentation is not used, multiple-level discectomies are associated with a high failure rate. This observation further underscores the importance of multiple level fixation.

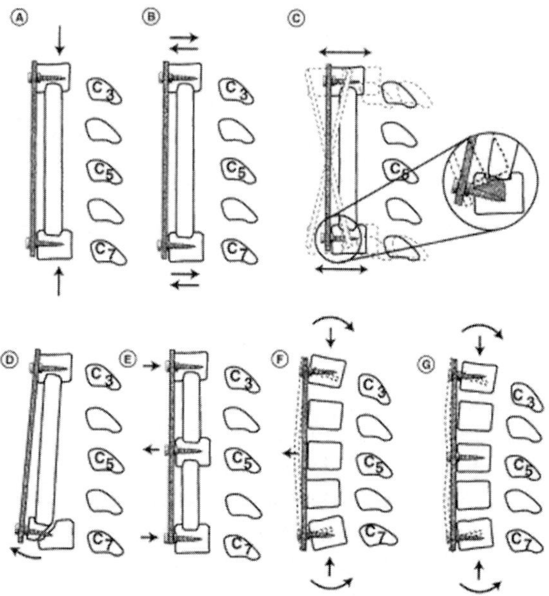

FIG. 7.41 A rigid fixed moment cantilever beam implant with two screws at each end. This is a bridging implant. This construction resist axial loads (vertical arrows) well (*A*). However, loads are usually applied from a variety of orientations. Shear loads (horizontal arrows) can cause translation (*B*). This may cause the screw-bone interface to degrade (shaded areas) (*C*) and, ultimately, to fail, usually as a result of axial loading (*D*). The addition of a third (intermediate) point of fixation causes the implant to more effectively resist these loads (e.g., translation) via a three-point bending mechanism (arrows) (*E*). The three-point bending effect resists shear-producing loads in multiple planes.

Axial loads can also be resisted more effectively by using an intermediate fixation point. The flexibility of an implant bearing an axial load (*F*) is significantly diminished by using an additional intermediate point of fixation (*G*). The intermediate fixation point minimizes flexibility (as depicted by the dashed implant in *F* and *G*). [From (1); copyright © 2001 by the American Association of Neurological Surgeons.]

In the case of a long ventral corpectomy decompression operation, attaining an intermediate point of fixation to the parent spine may be achieved in the cervical spine by "leaving" an intermediate vertebral body. For example, if one could "leave" the C5 vertebral body intact for a C4-C6 decompression and a C3-C7 fusion, then C5 could be used as an intermediate point of fixation, thus employing C3-C5 and C5-C7 interbody fusions instead of a single C3-C7 interbody fusion (*Fig. 7.42*). This, perhaps, may (and probably does) offset the disadvantages associated with the increased number of fusion interfaces that must heal. Another method of achieving the same biomechanical advantage

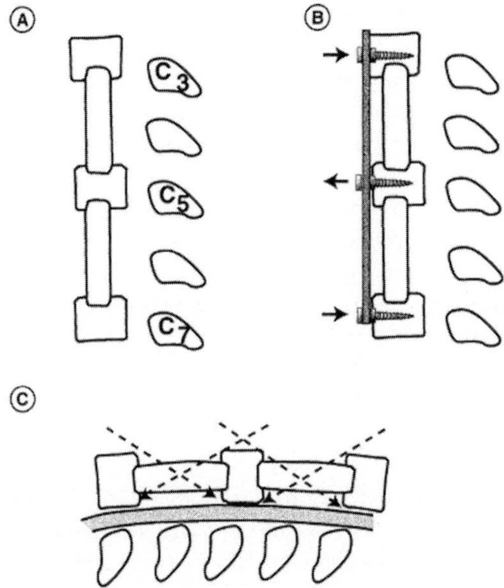

FIG. 7.42 A long cervical decompression (C4-C6 inclusively) can be accomplished with a C4 and C6 corpectomy and a C3-C5 and a C5-C7 interbody fusion (*A*). This provides a solid vertebral body site (C5) for intermediate screw fixation (*B*) while also providing adequate visualization for dural sac decompression (dashed arrows) (*C*). [From (1); copyright © 2001 by the American Association of Neurological Surgeons.]

(intermediate points of fixation) is to employ a ventral and a dorsal operation (ventral corpectomies plus dorsal lateral mass fixation). The lateral mass fixation points, however, are not as solid as ventral intermediate vertebral body. A second operation is also required. Nevertheless, three-level (or greater) corpectomies with strut graft fusion may be effectively augmented by adding a dorsal implant that provides intermediate points of fixation and, thus, both resists and applies three-point bending forces that resist translation and rotation.

Other fixation points include the spikes (e.g., the tetra spike of the Kaneda system) and the provision of a buttress point of fixation (e.g., using fins) at the end plate in the region of the cortical margin.

The use of additional vertebral body screws (three instead of two) may provide a theoretical biomechanical advantage. The volume of bone displaced by the metal and its effect on bony purchase and bone integrity, however, must also be considered. Finally, the surgeon must ensure that optimal implant-bone contact is achieved, lest suboptimal implant-bone interface contact results.

Intermediate points of fixation may also be provided by use of the interference screw technique. Passing a screw between an interbody strut graft and the parent vertebral body remnant (following performance of a corpectomy) may provide a surface for solid contact of the screw with the parent vertebral body following cervical corpectomy. The latter can be "gripped" by the interference screw, which is simply a screw that captures two separate but juxtaposed bony surfaces. In this case, it captures the bone graft and the remnant of the parent vertebral body. Although the former provides little support via the "capture" of the bone graft, the latter may provide a significant advantage regarding an intermediate point of solid fixation with the parent spine. Furthermore, the bone graft may be forced or wedged against the contralateral (to the interference screw) corpectomy wall, thus increasing stability (1).

IMPROVING BONE INTEGRITY

Improving bone integrity is obviously of value. Vitamin D, calcium, and hormonal manipulation strategies can be used. Bone augmentation with acrylics and other materials have found utility as well.

NORMALIZING GEOMETRY

Deformity correction (and prevention) causes less stress to be applied to implants, implant-bone interfaces, and bone-bone interfaces. This decreases the chance of failure. Therefore, significant attention should be paid to deformity correction as a clinical strategy (see below).

BONE-BONE INTERFACE FAILURE

The interface between the bone graft (interbody) and the vertebral body is prone to failure. Subsidence and nonunion are encouraged by a poor fit between the bone graft and the vertebral body. Small (in cross-sectional area) bone grafts subside more than larger grafts. Grafts that are positioned in the center of the vertebral body will piston more than grafts positioned more laterally. Wider grafts that abut the cortical margins circumferentially are very stable in this regard. Finally, fins may be used to augment vertebral body cortex region purchase via the boundary effect (*Fig. 7.43*).

Lateral abutment (close lateral fit) using the remaining portion of the parent vertebral body is also important both for lateral stability augmentation via buttressing and for bone healing at each segmental level. If the diameter of the bone graft is small, it will be suspended between the lateral margins of the corpectomy trough, thus negating both effects. Care must be taken with excessively wide approaches from a vascular injury (vertebral artery injury) perspective as well as from the aforementioned biomechanical perspective (1).

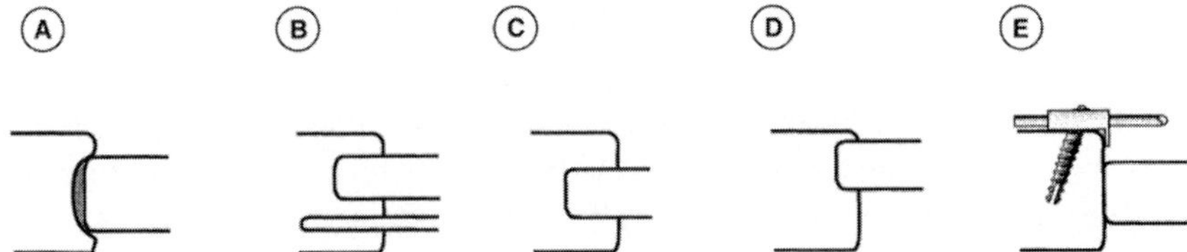

FIG. 7.43 Interbody bone-bone interface failure can be minimized by considering factors that predispose to subsidence. "Fit" is important. A careful consideration of mortise geometry and precise "carpentry" should minimize gap formation (shaded area) (*A*). Small cross-sectional area grafts piston more than large cross-sectional area grafts (*B*). Grafts positioned in the center of the vertebral body piston more than those positioned at the edge, nearer the cortical margin (*C* and *D*). This is a manifestation of the boundary effect. In fact, grafts that are wide and abut the cortical margin circumferentially are optimal. Fins (e.g., as with the DOC system [Depuy Acromed, Raynham, MA]) may assist in resisting subsidence by taking advantage of the boundary effect (*E*). [From (1); copyright © 2001 by the American Association of Neurological Surgeons.]

Other Complications

INFECTION

Implant integrity-related complications are common, but other complications also exist. Heading this list is infection. Traditionally, spinal infection in patients with spinal implants were treated, in part, by removal of the implant. Recently, however, implant salvage strategies have been developed, thus significantly advancing the field.

PSEUDOARTHROSIS

Fusion failure (pseudarthrosis) following long ventral decompression is not positively affected by ventral plating. This has been corroborated by multiple studies, although conflicting information exists, particularly for single-level disc surgery. Of note is that uninstrumented multiple-level discectomy with fusion compares poorly with uninstrumented corpectomy and fusion. Of final note in this regard, fusion is impeded by agents that adversely affect healing (e.g., corticosteroids).

END-FUSION ACCELERATED DEGENERATIVE CHANGES

Accelerated end-fusion degenerative changes (transition syndrome) are common. This phenomenon is related to the length of the fusion and the configuration of the spine after fusion. The loss of normal spinal alignment (loss of sagittal balance) significantly affects this process (see *Adjacent Segment Deformity* below). Spinal implant stiffness, as was traditionally thought, does *not* appear to substantially affect this process.

SUBOPTIMAL IMPLANT-BONE INTERFACE INTEGRITY

The integrity of bone may be enhanced—or, rather, the loss of integrity may be diminished—by several factors. Tapping cortical bone improves the integrity of the screw-bone interface, although tapping cancellous bone weakens it. Simply drilling cancellous bone, without tapping, provides greater pullout resistance than is achieved with tapping. Similarly, using an awl for the preparation of the hole compresses the "areolar" cancellous bone, thus improving its integrity, as opposed to drilling and removing the bone debris. Placing bone chips in the hole or using pressurized polymethylmethacrylate can augment integrity as well. Nonpressurized polymethylmethacrylate does not confer an increase in integrity; in fact, it may lessen it. Expanding tip screws have been shown to augment pullout resistance. Of note, an oxygen deprivation anode, which may theoretically be harmful to the bone at the implant-bone interface, can result from coating the tip of the screw with acrylic. This effect, however, is most certainly negligible. Finally, materials other than polymethylmethacrylate may provide additional advantages. Such materials include ceramics and biological glasses.

These materials may osteointegrate with bone (polymethylmethacrylate does not). This creates a positive load-sharing and load-distribution environment.

COMPONENT-COMPONENT INTERFACE FAILURE

Component-component interface failure can occur as a result of:

1. Improper surgical techniques (e.g., improper implant installation),
2. Acute failure of a properly installed implant, or
3. Failure by fatigue of a properly installed implant.

All, to one degree or another, are surgeon-related failures. Either the surgeon improperly installed the implant, or the surgeon asked too much of the implant-bone interface. It is, indeed, the surgeon's responsibility to understand what to expect from the implant.

ADJACENT SEGMENT DEFORMITY

The effect of spine deformity and fusion on further deformity and deformity progression, as well as degenerative changes, is substantial. This, in part, is related to the effect of the deformity and moment arm length on adjacent motion segments.

LAMINOPLASTY

The effect of laminoplasty on spinal integrity has not been adequately investigated. Although spinal stiffness may be increased (compared to that with laminectomy), deformity progression may not be impeded, particularly if a kyphosis is present preoperatively. Deformity progression is expected on the basis of the bending moment created by the kyphosis.

INFREQUENTLY CONSIDERED PRINCIPLES

Spinal implants may be loaded in ways that are not intuitively obvious and that may have undesirable consequences. Furthermore, implants are loaded differently under differing loading conditions. The importance of these two facts/principles cannot be overemphasized. The placement of a long fixed moment arm cantilever beam implant (*Fig. 7.44*), following the placement of a multiple-level cervical corpectomy, is associated with a high incidence of structural failure. The addition of an intermediate point of fixation permits the application of three-point bending forces to the spine. This alone causes the construct (implant plus bone) to move as a unit. This, in turn, minimizes fatiguing of the implant (screw)-bond interface. Even though the implant may ultimately "kick out", its mode of failure was most likely related to the aforementioned fatiguing at the screw-bone interface. (This was discussed above and illustrated in *Figs. 7.41* and *7.42*.)

A long bridging implant, such as that depicted in *Figure 7.44*, also is associated with an environment that induces excessive loading and unloading of the bone graft. This has been studied and documented

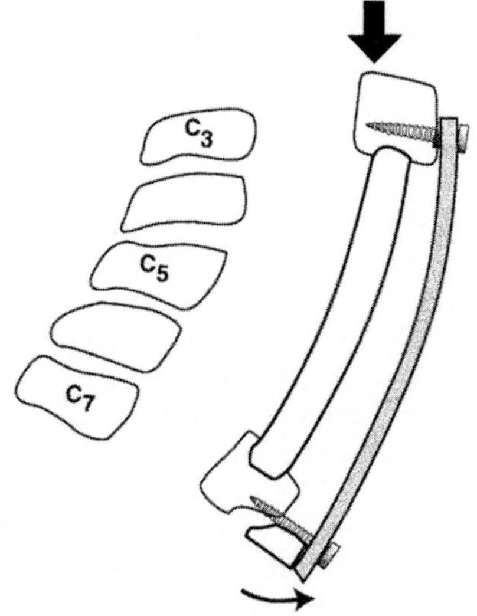

FIG. 7.44 The lordotic curvature of the cervical spine causes axial loads to impinge on the rostral ventral corner of the caudal vertebral body of the construct. This may lead to failure, as depicted. [From (1); copyright © 2001 by the American Association of Neurological Surgeons.]

by DiAngelo and Foley. In extension, the bone graft is loaded, and in flexion, the bone graft is unloaded. This is because placement of the implant causes the IAR to migrate toward the implant. Therefore, in extension, all points dorsal to the implant (IAR) come closer together. The converse is true for flexion. This causes the loading and unloading of the implant. Interestingly, this phenomenon is buffered significantly by an axially dynamic implant, thus underscoring an additional biomechanical advantage of such axially dynamic implants. Finally, this process is even further aggravated by the fact that the caudal aspect of the implant is positioned in such a manner that it is exposed to significant shear stresses (1) (*Fig. 7.44*).

FINAL COMMENTS

Although a fixed moment arm cantilever beam can be applied in a distraction mode, the buttressing effect of this construct clearly separates it biomechanically from a simple distraction construct. Simple distraction can apply a torque to the IAR if it is applied at a perpendicular distance from the IAR, whereas the cantilever beam technique applies no effective torque unless an applied moment is used.

Pedicle fixation devices may fail to effectively bear axial loads because of a lateral parallelogram-like translational deformation. A simple toe-ing in of the screws should prevent this mechanism of construct failure. A rigid cross-fixation of the rod or plate on each side to its counterpart would have similarly prevented this complication. The IAR, however, is dependent upon the method of determination. In the context utilized herein, the IAR is theoretical. In the unloaded and nonpathological spine, it is assumed to be located within the vertebral body confines in the sagittal plane. This assumes that the vertebral body pivots about a point within, ventral, or dorsal to its confines.

The ability of a cantilever beam construct to resist translation may be limited; particularly with regard to those constructs that employ a nonfixed moment arm. In this situation, a parallelogram-like effect may occur in the sagittal plane, particularly if only one motion segment is included in the construct. If a more rigid construct is used (fixed moment arm cantilever beam construct) or a longer (e.g., a nonfixed or a fixed moment arm cantilever beam construct) is used over more motion segments, sagittal translational deformation is more effectively resisted. In the former, the rigidity of the construct does not allow translation unless screw pullout occurs. With the latter system, the increased length of the lever arm with at least three points of attachment to the spine creates a substantial biomechanical advantage (three-point bending).

Dynamic fixation techniques provide an alternative to the more rigid (e.g., fixed moment and cantilever beam) techniques that have been conventionally available. Such techniques, in selected ventral cervical spine applications, may improve fusion rates through the application of the fundamental principles associated with Wolff's law, as well as the prevention of deformity, the optimization of deformity correction, the offloading of the implant, and the axial loading of the interbody bone graft.

Finally, the importance of bone graft and mortise preparation cannot be overestimated. The proverbial race between bone fusion, depicted in *Figure 7.21*, is lost by the patient and surgeon if a fusion does not transpire, no matter how solid or well-placed the spinal implant (1).

REFERENCES

1. Benzel EC: **Biomechanics of Spine Stabilization**, 2nd ed. Rolling Meadows, IL: AANS Press, 2001.
2. White AA, Panjabi MM: *Clinical Biomechanics of the Spine*, 2nd ed. Philadelphia: JB Lippincott, 1990.

CHAPTER

8

Honored Guest Presentation: Leading the Future of Spinal Surgery

VOLKER K.H. SONNTAG, M.D., AND NICHOLAS THEODORE, M.D.

> [T]he existence of the operating specialist, as contrasted to the general surgeon, is justified only if the former takes advantage of his opportunities to contribute to the knowledge of the disorders he specially treats. When progress ceases to be made, through intensive studies which the smaller field of work permits, there is every reason why the vagrant specialty should be called back under the wing of its parent, general surgery, from whom under no circumstances should it ever be permitted to wander too far.
>
> Cushing

When Harvey Cushing made this statement in his *Consecratio Medici and Other Papers* (45) in 1928, it is doubtful that even a visionary such as himself could have predicted the exponential growth that neurosurgery would experience in the next 75 years. Cushing was concerned with the specialty of neurosurgery surviving as its own discipline. During Cushing's time, and until at least the 1970s, more interest and attention were directed toward cranial surgery than toward spinal disorders. If Henry Schwartz's description of neurosurgery (163) at the time was that of a "mistress . . . brazen hussy . . . [who] kept intimate company with those of us who are older while continuing to lure younger men into amorous liaison," then surely spinal surgery would have been a one-night stand. The appeal of being a "brain surgeon" during this period seemed to be infinitely more fascinating than handling the comparatively mundane issues of the spine. In 1958, Martin (116) probably spoke for most neurosurgeons when he stated in his article, "Recent trends in neurosurgery," that the "spinal cord continues to arouse much less interest, both as to pathology and physiology, than do the intracranial contents, and much of the literature concerning the cord has to do with case histories."

Since then, the field of neurosurgery has blossomed, and it continues to grow exponentially. Examining the current state of spinal surgery as a subspecialty of neurosurgery provides a glimpse of what the future has to offer in terms of training, research, and therapeutics. Advances in molecular biology, nanotechnology, and genetics will forever change the complexion of neurosurgery in general and of spinal surgery in particular.

HISTORICAL PERSPECTIVES

The contemporary era of neurosurgery began with Macewen's treatise on *Pyogenic Infective Diseases of the Brain and Spinal Cord* in 1893 (122) and with the appointment of Sir Victor Horsley as surgeon to the National Hospital for the Paralyzed and Epileptic in Queen Square in 1896. From the very beginning, neurosurgeons have been involved in caring for patients with spinal disorders (178). Horsley was the first major contributor to modern spinal surgery, with his report of removing a spinal tumor in 1888 (65, 136). The next major advance in the first half of the twentieth century was the description of the origin of ruptured discs. Although Dandy (46) first accurately described this entity and its ability to cause a cauda equina syndrome, Mixter and Barr more clearly associated a ruptured disc with the far more common unilateral sciatica.

The "dynasty of the disk," as it has been called, that followed Mixter and Barr's report began the exponential growth of the field of spinal surgery. From the 1950s to the present, spinal surgery has been on a fast track, with new information becoming available almost daily. Milestones of the past 50 years include descriptions of lumbar stenosis by Verbiest (182), of central cord syndrome by Schneider et al. (162), and of spondylolisthesis by multiple individuals (63, 124, 177, 185). The many surgical advances during this period include anterior cervical discectomy with fusion, as described by Robinson and Smith (157) and by Cloward (40); the posterolateral and transthoracic approaches to the spine (32, 90, 132, 143); and endoscopic approaches as well as minimally invasive techniques (23, 26, 43, 50, 51, 121, 137, 142, 153–155, 172, 191).

Other innovations followed the development of CT in 1972 and MR imaging in 1976, the latter of which was not readily available for several more years. It is hard to underestimate the effect of these images on the practice of spinal surgery (42, 89, 92, 132). The introduction of the microscope was another welcome addition to the armamentarium of the spinal surgeon (33, 75, 156, 187).

Since the introduction of the first widely available spinal fixation system devised by Harrington (76, 77), the growth of spinal instrumentation during the last 30 years has been unprecedented. These events opened the door for the countless systems and techniques, ranging from anterolateral thoracolumbar plates to occipitocervical fusion devices and interbody cages, that are now available. Perhaps one of the most monumental discoveries was the characterization of bone morphogenetic proteins (BMPs) by Urist in the 1960s (180). This singular discovery will likely forever change the practice of spinal surgery as we know it today.

These are but a few of the most significant advances in spinal surgery during the past century. The tremendous advances in the scientific arena also have been associated with a plethora of changes in the politics and organization of spinal surgery. These changes have come as the specialty has evolved from its infancy in the era of Mixter and Barr (with orthopedic and neurosurgeons collaborating) to its current state of precocious puberty, with daily advances in molecular biology and genetics.

Historically, the average neurosurgeon (with some noted exceptions; e.g., Ralph Cloward) was relegated to the decompressive part of a spinal operation and had little or nothing to do with the arthrodesis that occurred afterward (if one was indicated). Not until the 1970s did neurosurgical pioneers such as Sanford Larson begin to work seriously with arthrodesis of complex spinal anomalies (104, 105). The progression, however, was natural for neurosurgeons, who had been doing spinal surgery since the days of Horsley.

The 1980s were difficult times. In Phoenix during this period, for example, when the senior author began doing thoracolumbar instrumentation, the orthopedic surgeons fought this trend. The latter saw this evolution as an infringement on their specialty. Only after extensive scrutiny by outside reviewers was the issue settled. Similar stories could be heard across the nation as neurosurgeons began to assert their independence as "complete" spinal surgeons. Ultimately, issues such as the pedicle screw litigation helped to foster an atmosphere of camaraderie with our orthopedic colleagues. Civility has now returned to the arena of spinal surgery with neurosurgeons and orthopedic surgeons united to fight their common enemy—disorders of the spine.

TRAINING AND CERTIFICATION OF NEUROSURGEONS IN SPINAL SURGERY

The path of neurosurgical training has been one of constant evolution. It would have been hard to conceive that the preceptorships in neurosurgery, common during Cushing's time, would have evolved into distinct residency programs in neurosurgery. This evolution formally began in 1933 with the first officially recognized training program in neurosurgery at the Medical College of Virginia in Richmond, under the direction of Claude Coleman. By 1934, six approved programs existed, and by 1940, this number had risen to 18. In 1942, the American Board of Neurological Surgeons published the requirements for certification, which included a 1-year surgical internship and at least 3 years of study in neurological surgery. In 1950, the Board required "progressive responsibility for trainees," which prompted some training programs to become associated with "charity" hospitals (150). Today, there are just over 90 accredited programs in the United States, each charged with training residents to provide comprehensive neurosurgical care.

Residency Training

Guidelines exist concerning the amount of time spent on "clinical neurosurgery." Certifying organizations such as the Residency Review Committee and the American Board of Neurological Surgery, however, have stopped short of requiring set numbers of cases in each subspecialty of neurosurgery to accommodate variations among programs. Spinal surgery has been part of the neurosurgical residency curriculum since its inception, but as times have changed and techniques have expanded, the role of education in spinal surgery has increased. The most current *Resident Curriculum Guidelines for Neurosurgery*, published by the Congress of Neurological Surgeons (CNS) Education Committee, outlines competency-based knowledge and performance objectives that begin at the craniocervical junction, extend to the sacral region, and cover everything in between (85, 179). Given the list of subjects for which neurosurgical residents are responsible, all neurosurgery residents are spinal surgeons, by definition, even if they ultimately migrate to another subspecialty.

Residency training programs have kept apace with the latest advances in spinal surgery. This task, however, is daunting, because neurosurgeons are expected to be facile with all aspects of both cranial and spinal surgery. In a special commentary in *Neurosurgery*, Kelly (99) pointed out that "neurosurgeons are the only spinal surgeons who can be trained in their residency." He argues that neurosurgeons are uniquely suited to lead the future of spinal surgery given "our surgical approach to the tissues of and surrounding the nervous system."

Fellowship Training

The explosive growth in spinal surgery has been associated with a significant expansion in the number of spinal surgery fellowships. What began as a handful of programs in the 1980s has burgeoned during the past few years. One of the first recognized neurosurgical fellowships in spinal surgery was under the direction of Sanford Larson at the University of Wisconsin. The fellowship at the Barrow Neurological Institute began in 1988, and Ian Kalfas was the first fellow. Today, more than 90 fellowships are available in spinal surgery each year in the United States.

How did this evolution occur? Subspecialty fellowships in neurosurgery are a relatively new addition to an otherwise cumbersome training scheme. Although the number of individuals pursuing fellowship training has increased sharply during the past few years, the path is better defined in specialties such as orthopedic surgery. Of the almost 620 residents who complete orthopedic training programs each year in the United States, more than 60% pursue a fellowship of some kind (62). In 1990, the American Council of Graduate Medical Education approved "spinal surgery" as an official subspecialty in orthopedic surgery. This event has pressured organized neurosurgery to at least consider subspecialty certification. This topic has been debated hotly among practicing neurosurgeons, most of whom may be "opposed to formalization and accreditation of neurosurgery subspecialty training owing to the fear (real or imagined) that a proliferation of accredited subspecialty programs may fragment our relatively small specialty" (144).

In 1991, the first guidelines for neurosurgical spine fellowships were developed under the auspices of the Senior Society of Neurological Surgeons. These guidelines were endorsed by the CNS, the American Association of Neurological Surgeons (AANS), the Joint Section of Disorders of the Spine and Peripheral Nerves, and the then-existing Spine Task Force. These guidelines outlined the suggested content of fellowship training in spinal surgery, but certification or accreditation was not recommended. In fact, organized neurosurgery wanted to avoid falling into the trap of "certificamania," a term coined by Robert Petersdorf, a past president of the American Association of Medical Colleges, who was commenting on the trend in the late 1980s to issue more and more certificates of special or added competence (130).

When just a handful of spinal fellowships existed, their eventual proliferation was never imagined. They primarily existed to offer specialized training to individuals who intended to practice in large academic centers. The thought that they would become an economic tool was almost certainly never considered.

With the rampant growth of medical knowledge, however, comes the need for subspecialization. Given the large percentage of orthopedic residency graduates who enroll in fellowship training, it may be surprising for neurosurgeons to consider that in a recent survey (106), 84.6% of neurosurgical residents had considered fellowship training. The most popular fellowships were spine (25.6%), pediatric (16.5%), and vascular (16.1%). The top three reasons cited by neurosurgery residents for pursuing a fellowship were "personal interest and knowledge," "job market demand," and "academic prestige." A small percentage of respondents cited "inadequate training during residency," but this response typically reflected residents pursuing fellowship training in the fields of endovascular, peripheral nerve, and skull base programs. These findings suggest that most residents feel they have received adequate training in spinal surgery during their residency.

Much has been written about the need for fellowship training in neurosurgery in general and in spinal surgery in particular (85, 130, 144, 174). The consensus is that fellowships should not be designed to overcome substandard training during residency; should not interfere and, in fact, should enhance the training of residents at a particular institution; should provide broad exposure to the depth and breadth of spinal surgery; should provide exposure to the multidisciplinary approach needed to enhance the subspecialty; and should produce leaders and stimulate research in spinal surgery, thus strengthening the subspecialty as a whole.

As the field of spinal surgery expands, fellowship training is likely to remain. The Society of Neurological Surgeons (SNS) was given the task of accrediting all neurosurgical fellowships. In May 2002, the Spinal Fellowships Programs (Barrow Neurological Institute and University of Florida) were given accreditation by the SNS. Although daunting, this step is necessary in recognizing fellowships as a legitimate part of neurosurgical training and in ensuring excellence in these programs.

Recertification

Another issue confronting organized neurosurgery is adoption of a recertification program for practicing neurosurgeons. Of the 24 specialties approved by the American Board of Medical Specialties, neurosurgery was the last to develop a program of recertification. The American Board of Neurological Surgery is developing a program that ensures the maintenance of basic competency and that engenders a program of lifelong learning. A prototype of this process will be an examination taken every 10 years on modules such spine, vascular, and pediatrics specialties.

In 1920, Cushing (44) likened the growth of medical knowledge to a banyan tree, which in time puts out many roots from the major branches. Some of the branches reach the ground, become attached, and drawing up their own nourishment have in some cases enlarged and become permanent and necessary supports to the parent branches." Cushing warned that the temptation to climb these branches, "mistaking them for the main stem" can lead to "short cuts to specialization without thorough preparation in the fundamentals," ultimately leading to "incompetent if not dangerous practitioners." The massive evolution in spinal surgery today may one day result in it becoming its own subspecialty; however, we need to be cognizant of its origins and respectful of the fact that it is still a vital component of its neurosurgical progenitor.

INFORMATION DISSEMINATION IN SPINAL SURGERY

A voluminous amount of information concerning the treatment of spinal disorders is available from many sources, such as the Internet, printed journals, and television. Information once confined to a consultation with a neurosurgeon or other spine specialist is now available with a few keystrokes on the Internet. The coverage of spinal disorders in the literature has been explosive. In the late 1800s and early 1900s, discoveries of note were published in journals of general interest, such as the *New England Journal of Medicine* and the *Journal of the American Medical Association*. One of the first specialized journals was the *Journal of Bone and Joint Surgery*, which began as a periodical for the American Orthopedic Association in 1922. The first neurosurgical specialty journal, the *Journal of Neurosurgery*, began as a bimonthly publication in January 1944. This format was followed for 18 years, until it became a monthly publication in 1962. Observing the importance of spinal issues and the sharp increase in manuscripts devoted to spinal issues, the *Journal of Neurosurgery* began to publish *Journal of Neurosurgery: Spine* on a quarterly basis in July 1999. Other innovations came with the journal *Spine* and the *Journal of Spinal Disorders*, both of which are dedicated entirely to the spine. The journal *Neurosurgery* was first published about 25 years ago under the auspices of the CNS. It covers broad neurosurgical topic areas, but approximately 25% of its August 2002 issue was devoted to topics related to the spine. At least seven monthly journals covering spine-related topics are available in the United States (Table 1). *The Spine Journal*, the newest addition to the group, is the official journal of the North American Spine Society (NASS).

When one considers that many other international journals deal with spinal disorders, it is clear that the amount of spinal information published each year is dumbfounding. This abundance is underlined by the fact that most other medical and surgical specialties have only one or two journals each. Is there such a thing as too much information? No one can keep up with the information published in all the journals relating to the spine. Readers must be selective and choose journals that provide them with the information they need to care for their particular population of patients.

TABLE 8.1
U.S. Journals that Cover Spinal Topics

Journal of Neurosurgery: Spine	*Journal of Spinal Disorders*
Neurosurgery	*The Spine Journal*
Spine	*Journal of Spinal Cord Medicine*
Journal of Bone and Joint Surgery	

In addition to printed material on spinal disorders, organizations and meetings dealing with spinal disorders have proliferated. Although the AANS and CNS have always dealt with issues concerning spinal disorders, the AANS/CNS Section on Disorders of the Spine and Peripheral Nerves was not formed until 1978. What began as a small and loosely organized group has become the largest specialty section of the two primary neurosurgical organizations. The NASS, which was formed in 1984, portrays itself as "a multidisciplinary medical organization that advances quality spine care through education, research and advocacy." It boasts membership from orthopedic surgeons, neurosurgeons, chiropractors, pain specialists, physiatrists, psychologists, and researchers. Its annual meeting attracts more than 3,000 registrants, and participation has grown with each annual meeting. Other meetings, such as World Spine II, have an international flavor and are a testament to the importance of spinal disorders globally.

The plethora of educational courses sponsored by the Joint Section, NASS, CNS, AANS, and others offer wide opportunities for practicing spinal surgeons to learn state-of-the-art techniques. Keeping education within the domain of our specialty organizations is one way to ensure that spinal surgeons lead the future of their specialty into the third millennium. The best approach to leading the subspecialty into the future is an open and honest assessment of the educational needs of spinal surgeons and an unbiased approach to providing them this information.

Perhaps the major event affecting medical information has been the Internet. The Internet is the most comprehensive source of information on spinal disorders. Each of the seven U.S. journals dealing with spinal disorders has a website that permits subscribers to peruse and download journal topics. Other major sources of information include websites such as PubMed, a service of the National Library of Medicine. PubMed provides access to more than 12 million MEDLINE citations back to the mid-1960s and additional life-science journals. PubMed includes links to many sites that provide full text articles and other related resources. Within seconds, a physician can search for articles related to a topic in spinal surgery, review major therapies, and even locate a specialty center where more information can be obtained.

Unfortunately, the lack of content regulation on the website leaves patients vulnerable to misinformation (170). Websites such as WebMD and Dr. Koop offer comprehensive medical information with links to websites such as those administered by the AANS and the American Academy of Orthopedic Surgeons. Other websites, such as SpineUniverse, deal with specific spinal disorders, offer patient education materials, provide interviews with spinal surgeons, and offer operative videos of various spinal procedures. The content of these websites is regulated and verified to a certain extent. Most information available on the Internet, however, is not.

Entering "spine surgery" as the query on the search engine Google (http://www.google.com), for example, reveals 277,000 "hits" or sites dealing with the topic. The first two listings are "sponsored links" and hold the first two positions because they have paid a fee for the listing. The first three nonsponsored links are for the University of Kentucky, New York University, and Massachusetts General Hospital. Redoing the search several minutes later changes the top three contenders to different links, but the paid links remain the same. Without delving into the specifics of how search engines work, suffice it to say that the amount of information about the spine on the Internet is almost limitless. Given the ubiquity of back pain in our society, it is not surprising that "back pain" has the highest number of hits (Table 2) among a variety of common medical problems.

How are patients to be protected from incorrect information? The nature of the Internet makes it impossible to ensure the veracity of every entry on spinal disorders. Part of leading the future of spinal surgery will be to ensure that patients are directed to websites with content that has been verified. The commercial aspects of the Internet are extremely powerful motivators, but spinal surgeons must strive to ensure the correctness and appropriateness of the information that

TABLE 8.2
Number of Links for Various Disorders on a Typical Search Engine (e.g., Google)

Key Words	No. of Links
Back pain	3,340,000
Heart disease	2,340,000
Menopause	1,060,000
Liver disease	930,000
Kidney disease	822,000
Spine disease	266,000
Disc disease	175,000
Pancreas disease	155,000
Erectile dysfunction	153,000

is provided. Ensuring that patients are well educated means that they have a clear understanding of their disease process, the available treatment options, and the potential risks and benefits of each. The Internet can never supplant the physician-patient relationship. If properly employed, however, it can enhance the information-gathering process and make patients as well informed as they can be.

STATE OF THE ART AND FUTURE DIRECTIONS IN SPINAL SURGERY

Given the progress of the past 100 years, it is hard to imagine that the pace of growth can continue; however, that is exactly what is happening. In April 2000, we published a review entitled "Spinal surgery: The past century and the next." Since then, more dramatic advances within medicine in general and spinal surgery in particular have been made. Spinal surgeons are poised on the brink of an explosion in genetic, biomolecular, and nanotechnological advances that will change the practice of spinal surgery. Being aware of the technologies and progress made in other disciplines makes us realize that all of medicine will benefit from these discoveries. Neurosurgeons have always prided themselves on "thinking outside the box"—in realizing that other areas of medicine may have benefits to offer our patients.

Aristotle saw the interconnected relationship between science and medicine when he expressed the relationship between physicists and physicians as follows:

> [W]e may say of most physical inquirers, and of those physicians who study their art philosophically, that while the former complete their works with a disquisition on medicine, the latter usually base their medical theories on principles derived from Physics (14).

Continuing to search for new applications to the latest innovations in medicine and becoming partners with the scientists will confirm our role as leaders in the future of spinal surgery.

Imaging

Spinal surgery of the future will take advantage of the refinements in both MR imaging and CT technology that will allow these modalities to be used in the operating room on a routine basis. Although these modalities are being used in this setting in clinical trials and in a limited fashion, the technology is still cumbersome (25, 69, 72, 120, 165, 169). Refinements in frameless stereotaxy or image-guided surgery have made the intraoperative use of CT and MR imaging common in spinal surgery. Image justification between fluoroscopy and CT/MR imaging is now available. It obviates intraoperative anatomic registration and significantly decreases or eliminates the need for continuous fluoroscopy during spinal instrumentation surgery. These systems are being refined almost daily, thus helping to improve their accuracy and ease of use.

Future imaging technology will most likely take advantage of global positioning satellites or similar electronic technology to provide real-time information about the exact location of the patient's spine in space. The gold standard of intraoperative imaging will be real-time anatomic localization with continuously updated views of the region of interest to enhance the ease and safety with which complex spinal disorders can be treated surgically.

Intervertebral Disc Disease

During the past 60 years, spinal surgeons have become facile with increasingly minimally invasive strategies for treating lumbar and cervical degenerative disc disease. As technical prowess has increased, the number of segmental arthrodeses has also increased, and the indications for these procedures have become less clear. For example, there is little doubt that fusion is indicated for patients with dynamic instability related to progressive spondylolisthesis. The case for degenerative disc disease, however, is much less well established.

Another problem with fusion surgery is rooted in the debate about Cloward's technique for anterior cervical disc herniation. During the spirited debate that followed his 1958 presentation, Dr. William B. Scoville asked, "May not fusion of a cervical interspace cause this same stress on adjacent interspaces?" (40). This statement is most likely the first reference to what is now referred to as adjacent segment instability or disease. This entity can be a real problem in patients who undergo spinal fusion surgery (53, 58, 73, 127, 171). Theoretically, it could be prevented (or at least minimized) by preserving the load-sharing ability of the degenerated disc instead of immobilizing the segment.

For the past two decades, millions of dollars have been spent on developing artificial disc arthroplasty. Theoretically, such a device could eliminate sources of inflammation and instability associated with a degenerated disc and restore its natural load-sharing and kinematic properties, thus eliminating adjacent-level disease. Numerous prototypes of both lumbar and cervical disc devices have been developed, but none has been approved by the U.S. Food and Drug Administration (FDA) for commercial use in the United States (189). Current prototypes fall into three broad categories:

1. Total disc replacement,
2. Nucleus replacement, and
3. Annulus replacement or repair.

Total disc replacement has garnered significant attention recently, but widely accepted prototypes associated with good long-term clinical results and low risks have not been established (2, 184). The indication for these devices would be replacement of degenerated discs in patients for whom the disc is an anatomic pain generator. In itself, this topic is controversial. The implantation of total disc replacement devices can be a surgical tour-de-force, requiring extensive exposure for their correct placement. In general, it would seem that patients who are candidates for interbody or segmental fusion would benefit from this type of strategy. Ultimately, any acceptable total disc replacement would have to be tested against interbody or segmental fusion with equivocal or superior clinical results. Long-term data would be needed to determine if the replacement disc can serve as a long-term substitute capable of preventing adjacent-segment pathology.

Nucleus replacement is another area of great interest. Because the nucleus pulposus has a less complex structure than that of the annulus and end-plate interface, such a device has the allure of being technically less demanding to insert than a total replacement disc. A nucleus replacement would reinflate the disc space and restore function to the degenerated disc. Choosing the viscosity and determining a suitable agent to meet these criteria have been difficult. Various hydrogels that could mimic the water-transfer capability of the nucleus under cyclical loading have been tried (8, 20–22, 133, 151, 152). Other prototypes include curable polymers that can be injected through a small annular opening to help reduce the extrusion potential. When discs degenerate, the process also usually involves the annulus. Therefore, choosing appropriate candidates for this intervention may be challenging unless nucleus replacement is considered for all patients who undergo discectomy in an attempt to prevent the disc degeneration and collapse that can follow surgery.

The final strategy has been annulus repair. An incompetent annulus is thought to lead to pain by mechanical compression or chemical irritation. Despite the theoretical appeal, it has been difficult to repair the annulus, perhaps in part because of its poor healing potential (4, 5, 74, 86).

In the near future, artificial disc arthroplasty will most likely play a role in the treatment of disc degeneration. The ultimate modality, however, will involve a biological solution. That congenital abnormalities lead to disc degeneration has always been inferred from the histories of patients with families in whom multiple members have had spinal surgery. In the landmark paper by Annunen et al. (12), however, a possible genetic defect coding for a subtype of collagen was elucidated in individuals with intervertebral disc disease. This finding set the stage for possible genetic intervention in patients predisposed to pathologically accelerated disc degeneration. Potentially, such alterations could be made early enough to avert the pain and suffering that are associated with multilevel degenerative disc disease.

Actual global genetic therapies are still a few years off. Still, there has been significant interest in the regeneration of diseased discs using notochordal stem cells or virally mediated local gene therapy (11, 54, 97, 101, 125, 129, 131, 173, 190). An example of this type of strategy would be to mediate the gene transfer of a growth factor, such as transforming growth factor-β_1, through a viral vector. This process could be performed percutaneously and its effect limited to the diseased discs with little or no systemic effects. Such a strategy will likely obviate most of the surgical techniques used today to treat intervertebral disc disease.

SPINAL FUSION STRATEGIES

Borrowing from William Shakespeare, Keim (98) posed the eternal dilemma facing spinal surgeons: "To fuse or not to fuse, that is the question." We are still asking that question today, but the technologies now available have tilted heavily toward the possibility of favorable outcomes. With the advent of osteoinductive factors such as BMPs, the field of spinal surgery will be forever changed. The treatment of most spinal disorders with the "heavy metal" of the 1980s and 1990s will one day be extinct.

Expanding on the work of Urist (180), scientists have further classified, subdivided, and purified these revolutionary agents. The BMPs are powerful growth hormone-dependent auto- and paracrine hormones that induce mesenchymal stem cells to produce heterotopic bone (180). Numerous studies have proven the efficacy of BMPs in animal models of spinal fusion both with and without the application of instrumentation (28, 83, 95). One study demonstrated successful percutaneous fusion using a recombinant, replication-defective adenovirus with the cytomegalovirus promotor and the *BMP-2* gene (6).

The use of BMPs has now been approved by the U.S. FDA for use with anterior lumbar interbody fusion devices. Elsewhere in the spine, use of BMPs is limited to tightly regulated studies (10, 161, 186). Other recent interests include protein gene therapy and delivery devices for these molecules (7, 84, 168, 181). Once the safety of these molecules has been established, spinal fusion will most likely include percutaneous technologies with bioresorbable instrumentation "coated" with a mixture of osteoinductive and conductive agents to ensure rapid, solid fusion. Other techniques may include genetically engineered bone or growth factors made specifically for each patient using his or her own genetic precursors.

BIOMECHANICS

The field of biomechanics is the silent partner of spinal surgery. In a handful of laboratories across the country, techniques and innovations in materials and in vitro testing have contributed numerous advances in spinal surgery. Like spinal surgery, the field of biomechanics is constantly evolving.

In the 1980s and 1990s, biomechanical testing largely consisted of in vitro modeling using motion and position technologies to assess the various forces at work in the normal and pathologic spine both before and after treatment. During this period, innovative studies included implanting into patients with degenerative instability a telemetrized spinal fixator capable of generating real-time stress information across fused segments (158, 159). The information obtained could alter instrumentation through the design of "adjustable" devices that could be made more or less rigid as needed in a given situation.

The future of biomechanics, however, lies in the field of finite-element analysis. Recent studies have combined normative data about spinal motion and the properties of individual spinal elements with powerful computer programs to enhance our understanding of the mobile spine. Although this approach has been pursued for many years, its utility has been limited by computer technology. Advances in computer-generated mathematical modeling have allowed researchers such as Kong et al. (102) to develop a finite-element model of the thoracolumbar spine, which has been used to predict stresses on the facets and discs in four different lifting scenarios.

Newer studies have used these techniques to study issues as varied as the impact of fractures on spinal stability and the effects of various types of instrumentation on mobility (30, 36, 64, 103, 109, 145, 148). In trauma, for example, understanding the forces that cause a certain injury may lead to strategies to improve the safety of automobiles and the workplace. Eventually, this type of modeling will supplant the need for in vitro and in vivo studies and further enhance our understanding of the mobile spine.

SPINAL CORD INJURY

Spinal cord injury (SCI) continues to remain a devastating problem in the United States. Each year, more than 11,000 Americans sustain a SCI, at a cost of more than $1 million per patient (78, 176). Despite significant research, no undisputed pharmacotherapy is available for the treatment of acute SCI. Hadley et al. (70) recently published their "Guidelines for the management of acute cervical spine and spinal cord injuries." The section on pharmacological therapy after acute SCI concluded that there was "insufficient evidence to support" the use of both corticosteroids and GM-1 ganglioside. The conclusions of even this thoughtful document are highly controversial, and we still have no "magic bullet" therapy for SCI (31). Recent advances in immunology and genetics, however, may one day offer a viable treatment to patients with an acute SCI.

One aspect of acute SCI that has garnered significant attention has been the role of the inflammatory response. Methylprednisolone, for example, is known to prevent lipid peroxidation and oxidative injury (9, 49, 135), perhaps in part because it profoundly inhibits polymorphonuclear granulocytes and macrophage/microglia infiltration (9, 35, 96, 128, 135). Current therapeutic strategies have focused on stimulation rather than suppression of the immune response. The administration of autoimmune T cells, implantation of stimulated homologous macrophages, and even vaccination with myelin self-antigens promote functional recovery after acute SCI (9, 79–81, 93, 100, 149, 164, 188).

Other areas of interest include the role of the complement system in the cellular response that follows acute SCI. The complement system has been implicated in diseases such as Alzheimer's and multiple sclerosis, in which its activation is thought to mediate neurodegeneration and demyelination (9, 57, 126). Its role in acute SCI, however, has not been well established. Apparently, complement activation is involved in central nervous system degradation, but it sometimes might also be beneficial to regeneration and recovery. For example, complement-induced demyelination helps to promote regeneration after lateral hemisection (9, 55), in part because of the role of the complement system in opsonization and in the mediation and stimulation of phagocytosis.

Contradictory mechanisms seem to be at work within both the cellular immune response and the complement systems after acute SCI, with both apparently helping and hampering recovery. Given the complexity of the cellular mechanisms, manipulation of a single point along the cascade is unlikely to affect the overall goal of repair leading to functional recovery after an acute SCI. More likely, a combination of agents and manipulations in a carefully timed "cocktail" will be administered to enhance the body's innate ability to repair itself even after this most devastating of injuries.

Perhaps the most exciting prospects for the near future are in the fields of neural transplantation and regeneration. One area of significant interest has been gene therapy. Broadly speaking, these therapies fall into two categories: ex vivo strategies and in vivo strategies.

Ex vivo technologies are cell-based methodologies. Genes are placed into cell populations in vitro, with the modified cells then transplanted into the affected subject. The modified cells serve as biological minipumps, which can produce and secrete therapeutic proteins. In vivo applications involve the direct implantation of genes into target tissues in situ. Both strategies require introducing genes into target cells.

Ex vivo therapies using fibroblasts and neurotrophin-3, among others, have been associated with encouraging results (67, 88, 112, 147). In vivo therapies using glial cell line-derived neurotrophic factor and brain-derived neurotrophic factor have also shown promise (66, 113, 147, 183). As with the inflammatory response, a genetic combination of several growth factors will be the most likely use of this technology. The future treatment of SCI probably will involve strategies that harness the inflammatory response while providing an atmosphere that enhances the appropriate recovery and growth of injured axons.

ADVANCES IN SURGERY

During the past decade, the mantra of spinal surgery has been that of "minimally invasive" approaches. This interest will be intensified in spinal surgeries of the third millennium. Today, laparoscopic and thoracoscopic techniques for spinal surgery are two shining examples of state-of-the-art spinal surgery. These video-assisted techniques combine high-intensity illuminification with sophisticated cameras to provide unparalleled three-dimensional views of spinal anatomy. Thoracoscopic surgery has become common for sympathectomies, biopsies, disc herniations, tumor resection, and deformity correction (26, 43, 50, 51, 137, 142). Laparoscopic techniques are used to treat disc herniations and, subsequently, to implant interbody fusion devices (120, 121, 153–155, 191). Refining these strategies will further decrease the amount of tissue that must be manipulated to attain the surgical goal.

Future spinal surgery will embrace these minimalized technologies. Already, percutaneous techniques are being used to perform traditional macroscopic operations, such as pedicle screw fixation of the lumbar spine (60, 91, 114, 119). Although these procedures are just entering the mainstream of spinal surgery, they have been well received thus far. Not only are patients embracing the concept of minimal access surgery, physicians are clamoring to provide these services in an ever competitive environment.

Spinal surgery of the future will most likely add another technologically advanced aspect—robotics (17, 34, 39, 47, 48, 52, 82, 123, 175). Surgical robotics have been used in multiple procedures, including cardiac surgery, thoracoscopic surgery, orthopedic and gynecological procedures, and urological surgery. The term *robot* invokes thoughts of R2D2 and C3PO from *Star Wars*; however, a robotic device may be as simple as a voice-activated arm that is used to hold and control a camera for thoracoscopic surgery.

Other, more advanced systems allow cardiothoracic surgeons to use hand controls at a remote site to perform endoscopic coronary artery bypass surgery. Advanced robotic systems can be programmed to compensate for and, potentially, even overcome a surgeon's tremor or surpass the limits of human coordination by translating gross hand motions into microscopic movements. These techniques might be adopted for procedures such as the endoscopic treatment of spinal stenosis or other compressive pathologies.

In spinal surgery, robotics might also be used for remote placement of pedicle screws, interbody fusion devices, or other types of instrumentation. Using a robotic interface coupled with an image-guided system will make the placement of these types of instrumentation rapid, safe, accurate, and minimally invasive (1, 118). Another welcome byproduct of robotic technology will be less reliance on intraoperative image intensification, which is already being realized with the basic image-guided spinal devices that are available today.

Progressively smaller incisions with increasing accuracy will translate into less painful and safer surgery. Undoubtedly, robotics will play a role in the future of spinal surgery, especially considering the dramatic increase in percutaneous procedures now occurring in the United States.

How will spinal surgeons of tomorrow become facile with new and innovative techniques? The answer lies in the field of virtual reality (3, 15, 37, 56, 108, 138, 141). Taking its cue from the era of video games and movie special effects, it is now possible to design virtual patients who will aid in teaching and refining the skills of spinal surgeons. Aviation has long employed sophisticated preflight simulators. So accurate and realistic are these "virtual cockpits" that this type of training is mandatory for all military and civilian pilots. It is logical to employ this strategy when evaluating a pilot who will have control of a $25 million aircraft and the lives of hundreds of passengers, but what about surgeons? Why should surgeons not embrace such training tools to perfect the skill of those who daily hold patients' lives in their hands? The answer is that we must. Few will find challenging virtual reality experiences to be unhelpful—especially when patients are not actually harmed.

The technology now exists to design virtual patients with pathologies as varied as complex aneurysms and spinal tumors and spondylolisthesis to provide both residents and attendings physicians the chance to "practice" a particular exposure or procedure in a controlled environment. Eventually, the marriage of robotics and virtual reality will make telesurgery common (18, 38, 71, 146). Spinal surgeons of the future will be able to provide online consultations, assist fellow surgeons, or even perform the surgery themselves from remote locations via broadband technology that does not yet reliably exist.

PROTEOMICS AND NANOTECHNOLOGY

In 1999, Annunen et al. (12) uncovered a genetic defect in individuals with intervertebral disc disease. This finding ushered in the concept of genetics in degenerative spinal disorders. Advances in medical genetics and its associated therapies will make Mr. Spock's tricorder seem as medically advanced as a toaster. In 1986, Thomas Roderick coined the term *genomics*, referring to a new scientific discipline of mapping, sequencing, and analyzing genomes. The emphasis has shifted to genome function and to the proteins coded for by these sequences. Most human disease is caused by the functional dysregulation of protein interactions. Proteins do not exist in isolation and form actively fluctuating networks in response to a given stimulus. New technologies allow cultured cell lines to be compared to microdissected tissue cells from the same patient. The findings indicated a significant lack of correlation in patterns of protein expression (134). Despite the surprisingness of this finding, it has opened the door to a new paradigm in medicine—and to a new specialty. This new field, *proteomics*, includes the study of cellular protein interactions and applies this knowledge to therapeutic interventions (19, 27, 94, 107, 110, 111, 140, 166).

In simple terms, genetic mutations, duplications, losses, or amplifications cause aberrations in the expression of the proteins that are normally coded by these genes. In turn, the aberrations act to "rewire" the normal cellular protein network and dictate an abnormal biological state (111). These networks are studied through protein microarrays that profile the state of specific signal pathways (139). Undoubtedly, other technologies will follow. The field of oncology will most likely be the first beneficiary of this newly formed specialty, but the treatment of spinal disorders and the era of molecular neurosurgery will not lag far behind (117).

This approach is already being applied to disorders such as Alzheimer's and Parkinson's disease (16, 115, 167). Further advances should include treatments for disorders ranging from rheumatoid arthritis to degenerative disc disease. Using emerging technologies, researchers will be able to perform proteomic pathway profiling that, eventually, will lead to patient-tailored therapies (111). A word of caution, however, is in order. Given the controversial nature of genetics, the "ethical, legal and social implications of these rapid advances in a genetic understanding of our species will continue to deserve attention just as intense as the scientific effort" (41).

During the third millennium, the field of nanotechnology should also bestow benefits on spinal surgery. In nanotechnology, research involves dimensions of less than approximately 1,000 nm. Also referred to as molecular nanotechnology or molecular manufacturing, the key feature is to get every atom in the right place (13, 29, 61, 87, 160). Almost any structure imaginable can be constructed. Imagine tiny programmable and controllable microrobots that allow spinal surgeons to execute curative and reconstructive procedures on the cellular and molecular level. These microrobots can be envisioned as delivery devices for various therapeutics or as tiny "repair trucks" dispatched to the site of pathology to begin their microrepair tasks.

As medicine progresses and therapeutic options become more directed, even the term *minimally invasive* will become passé. In the third millennium, treating spinal disorders will require an open mind and a willingness to embrace all that collaborating specialties and basic science have to offer.

EVIDENCE-BASED SPINAL SURGERY

In April 2002, Groopman wrote an article in *The New Yorker* entitled "A knife in the back" (68). It was a well-written indictment of the field of spinal surgery, criticizing the lack of consensus and class I evidence that pervades our specialty. Most would tend to discount what sounds like a one-man diatribe against spinal surgery, but Groopman made several accurate points. First, we have done a poor job, both in medicine in general and in spinal surgery in particular, of providing solid, reproducible evidence to justify the treatments offered. The SCI guidelines published by Hadley et al. (70) offer a striking example of this problem. Of the 22 chapters included in the analysis, only five "standards" are based on class I evidence. Three of these standards involve the prevention of venous thromboembolism after SCI. In other words, spinal surgeons can defend few of their procedures.

In the handful of well-conducted class I studies involving spinal surgery, the results have not always been expected. In one study, for example, use of pedicle screws to augment a single-level fusion for degenerative spondylolisthesis increased the rate of fusion but did not improve clinical outcomes with respect to the associated pain syndrome

(59). Those authors concluded that the routine use of pedicle screw fixation to augment lumbar fusions may be unnecessary. This finding seems to be counterintuitive, but studies to the contrary may need to be produced to justify continued reimbursement for this procedure.

Leading the future of spinal surgery means that all spinal surgeons must be involved in answering the questions that plague the specialty today. Who are the best candidates for a fusion? Which is the best approach? Only carefully designed studies with appropriate outcome measures and long-term follow-up can resolve these issues. These questions will remain controversial as community standards for the practice of spinal surgery evolve.

In the third millennium, the goal of organized spinal surgery will be to foster an atmosphere of interest in finding answers to the most basic questions concerning our specialty. We must strive to establish large, multicenter, randomized, controlled trials to define the procedures that are—and are not—beneficial to patients. By incorporating these studies into practice, the "art" of spinal surgery assumes a more scientifically accepted mantle and will be poised to continue improving the well being of our patients.

CONCLUSION

About 30 years ago, Bergland wrote a Special Article for the *New England Journal of Medicine* entitled "Neurosurgery may die" (24). In that commentary, Bergland stated the following:

> Neurosurgery has stopped evolving. Although it is unlikely that the specialty will follow the dinosaur's path to extinction, for many it is becoming lifeless and uninteresting. The promise and excitement that once permeated neurosurgery have yielded too often to an easy acceptance of the status quo.

Obviously, the major revolution in spinal surgery had not quite begun, or such a nihilistic statement would not have been made. Since those words were written in 1973, however, spinal surgery has changed radically. Excitement and innovation permeate the specialty, with no apparent end in sight. Fields such as proteomics and nanotechnology will affect the practice of spinal surgery tomorrow just as BMPs have affected its practice today.

The progressively sophisticated advances in technology of the past 50 years will only continue to expand. Major innovations in the fields of molecular biology, genetics, and engineering will help to shape the evolution of spinal surgery. Without advocating change for the sake of change itself, spinal surgeons must maintain a critical eye on new developments to ensure that they improve treatment beyond the current standards of care. To lead the future of spinal surgery in the third millennium, spinal surgeons must embrace and help to cultivate these technologies appropriately to provide patients with the best possible care.

REFERENCES

1. Abdel-Malek K, McGowan DP, Goel VK, et al.: Bone registration method for robot assisted surgery: Pedicle screw insertion. **Proc Inst Mech Eng [H]** 211:221–233, 1997.
2. Adams MA, Hutton WC: Mechanics of the intervertebral disc. In: Ghosh P (ed): *The Biology of the Intervertebral Disc,* vol. 2. Boca Raton, FL: CRC Press, 1988, pp 39–72.
3. Ahlberg G, Heikkinen T, Iselius L, et al.: Does training in a virtual reality simulator improve surgical performance? **Surg Endosc** 16:126–129, 2002.
4. Ahlgren BD, Lui W, Herkowitz HM, et al.: Effect of annular repair on the healing strength of the intervertebral disc: A sheep model. **Spine** 25:2165–2170, 2000.
5. Ahlgren BD, Vasavada A, Brower RS, et al.: Annular incision technique on the strength and multidirectional flexibility of the healing intervetebral disc. **Spine** 19:948–954, 1994.
6. Alden TD, Pittman DD, Beres EJ, et al.: Percutaneous spinal fusion using bone morphogenetic protein-2 gene therapy. **J Neurosurg (Spine 1)** 90:109–114, 1999.
7. Alden TD, Varady P, Kallmes DF, et al.: Bone morphogenetic protein gene therapy. **Spine** 27:S87–S93, 2002.
8. Allen JM, Schoonmaker JE, Ordway NR, et al.: Pre-clinical testing of a poly(vinyl alcohol) hydrogel nucleus in baboons. **15th Annual Meeting of North American Spine Society,** New Orleans, 2000.
9. Anderson AJ: Mechanisms and pathways of inflammatory responses in CNS trauma: Spinal cord injury. **J Spinal Cord Med** 25:70–79, 2002.
10. Anderson DG, Andersson GB, Boden SD, et al.: Summary statement: Clinical BMP programs. **Spine** 27:S49, 2002.
11. Anderson DG, Izzo MW, Hall DJ, et al.: Comparative gene expression profiling of normal and degenerative discs: Analysis of a rabbit annular laceration model. **Spine** 27:1291–1296, 2002.
12. Annunen S, Paassilta P, Lohiniva J, et al.: An allele of COL9A2 associated with intervertebral disc disease. **Science** 285:409–412, 1999.
13. Apuzzo ML, Liu CY: 2001: Things to come. **Neurosurgery** 49:765–778, 2001.
14. Aristotle: *On Sense and the Sensible.* In: *Great Books of the Western World,* vol. 8: Chicago: Encyclopedia Britannica, 1952.
15. Arnold P, Farrell MJ: Can virtual reality be used to measure and train surgical skills? **Ergonomics** 45:362–379, 2002.
16. Athan ES, Williamson J, Ciappa A, et al.: A founder mutation in presenilin 1 causing early-onset Alzheimer disease in unrelated Caribbean Hispanic families. **JAMA** 286:2257–2263, 2001.
17. Awad H, Wolf RK, Gravlee GP: The future of robotic cardiac surgery. **J Cardiothorac Vasc Anesth** 16:395–396, 2002.
18. Ballantyne GH: Robotic surgery, telerobotic surgery, telepresence, and telementoring. **Surg Endosc** 16:1389–1402, 2002.

19. Banks RE, Dunn MJ, Hochstrasser DF, et al.: Proteomics: New perspectives, new biomedical opportunities. **Lancet** 356:1749–1756, 2000.
20. Bao QB, Bagga CS, Higham PA: Swelling pressure of hydrogel: A perceived benefit for a spinal prosthetic nucleus. **Transactions of 10th Annual Meeting of International Intradiscal Therapy Society**, Naples, FL, 1997.
21. Bao QB, Higham PA: Hydrogel intervertebral disc nucleus. **US patent 5,047,055,** September 10, 1991.
22. Bao QB, Higham PA: Hydrogel intervertebral disc nucleus. **US patent 5,192,326,** March 9, 1993.
23. Bascoulergue Y: Percutaneous injection of methyl methacrylate in the vertebral body for the treatment of various diseases. **74th Annual Meeting of the Radiological Society of North America, Chicago,** November, 1988.
24. Bergland RM: Neurosurgery may die. **N Engl J Med** 288:1043–1046, 1973.
25. Black PM, Alexander E III, Martin C, et al.: Craniotomy for tumor treatment in an intraoperative magnetic resonance imaging unit. **Neurosurgery** 45:423–433, 1999.
26. Blackman RG, Luque E: Endoscopic anterior correction of idiopathic scoliosis. In: Dickman CA, Rosenthal DJ, Perin NI (eds): *Thoracoscopic Spine Surgery.* New York: Thieme, 1999, pp 183–211.
27. Blume-Jensen P, Hunter T: Oncogenic kinase signaling. **Nature** 411:355–365, 2001.
28. Boden SD, Martin GJ Jr, Morone MA, et al.: Posterolateral lumbar intertransverse process spine arthrodesis with recombinant human bone morphogenetic protein 2/hydroxyapatite-tricalcium phosphate after laminectomy in the nonhuman primate. **Spine** 24:1179–1185, 1999.
29. Bogunia-Kubik K, Sugisaka M: From molecular biology to nanotechnology and nanomedicine. **Biosystems** 65:123–138, 2002.
30. Bozkus H, Karakas A, Hanci M, et al.: Finite element model of the Jefferson fracture: Comparison with a cadaver model. **Eur Spine J** 10:257–263, 2001.
31. Bracken MB: Comments on guidelines for the management of acute cervical spine and spinal cord injuries. **Neurosurgery** 50:S-xiv–S-xix, 2002.
32. Capener N: The evolution of lateral rhachotomy. **J Bone Joint Surg Br** 36:173–179, 1954.
33. Caspar W: A new surgical procedure for lumbar disc herniation causing less tissue damage through a microsurgical approach. **Adv Neurosurg** 4:74–80, 1977.
34. Chapman WH III, Albrecht RJ, Kim VB, et al.: Computer-assisted laparoscopic splenectomy with the da Vinci trade mark Surgical Robot. **J Laparoendosc Adv Surg Tech A** 12:155–159, 2002.
35. Chen A, Xu XM, Kleitman N, et al.: Methylprednisolone administration improves axonal regeneration into Schwann cell grafts in transected adult rat thoracic spinal cord. **Exp Neurol** 138:261–276, 1996.
36. Chen CS, Cheng CK, Liu CL, et al.: Stress analysis of the disc adjacent to interbody fusion in lumbar spine. **Med Eng Phys** 23:483–491, 2001.
37. Chinnock C: Virtual reality in surgery and medicine. **Hosp Technol Ser** 13:1–48, 1994.
38. Clayman RV: Transatlantic robot-assisted telesurgery. **J Urol** 168:873–874, 2002.
39. Cleary K, Nguyen C: State of the art in surgical robotics: Clinical applications and technology challenges. **Comput Aided Surg** 6:312–328, 2001.
40. Cloward RB: The anterior approach for removal of ruptured cervical disks. **J Neurosurg** 15:602–617, 1958.
41. Collins FS, Guttmacher AE: Genetics moves into the medical mainstream. **JAMA** 286:2322–2324, 2001.

42. Cormack AM: Representation of a function by its line integrals, with some radiological applications. **J Appl Phys** 34:2722–2727, 1963.
43. Crawford AH: Anterior release of spinal deformities. In: Dickman CA, Rosenthal DJ, Perin NI (eds): *Thoracoscopic Spine Surgery.* New York: Thieme, 1999, pp 161–181.
44. Cushing H: The special field of neurological surgery after another interval. **Arch Neurol Psychiatry** 4:603–637, 1920.
45. Cushing H: *Consecratio Medici and Other Papers.* Boston: Little, Brown, and Company, 1928.
46. Dandy WE: Röntgenography of the brain after the injection of air into the spinal canal. **Ann Surg** 70:397–403, 1919.
47. Davies B: A review of robotics in surgery. **Proc Inst Mech Eng [H]** 214:129–140, 2000.
48. Detter C, Boehm D, Reichenspurner H, et al.: Robotically-assisted coronary artery surgery with and without cardiopulmonary bypass—From first clinical use to endoscopic operation. **Med Sci Monit** 8:MT118–MT123, 2002.
49. Diaz-Ruiz A, Rios C, Duarte I, et al.: Lipid peroxidation inhibition in spinal cord injury: Cyclosporin-A vs methylprednisolone. **Neuroreport** 11:1765–1767, 2000.
50. Dickman CA, Apfelbaum RI: Thoracoscopic resection of intrathoracic neurogenic tumors. In: Dickman CA, Rosenthal DJ, Perin NI (eds): *Thoracoscopic Spine Surgery.* New York: Thieme, 1999, pp 245–269.
51. Dickman CA, Rosenthal DJ, Perin NI: Thoracoscopic microsurgical discectomy. In: Dickman CA, Rosenthal DJ, Perin NI (eds). *Thoracoscopic Spine Surgery.* New York: Thieme, 1999, pp 221–244.
52. Diodato LH, Scarborough JE, Domkowski PW, et al.: Robotically assisted versus conventional freehand technique during beating heart anastomoses of left internal thoracic artery to left anterior descending artery. **Ann Thorac Surg** 73:825–829, 2002.
53. Dohler JR, Kahn MR, Hughes SP: Instability of the cervical spine after anterior interbody fusion. A study on its incidence and clinical significance in 21 patients. **Arch Orthop Trauma Surg** 104:247–250, 1985.
54. Doita M, Kanatani T, Ozaki T, et al.: Influence of macrophage infiltration of herniated disc tissue on the production of matrix metalloproteinases leading to disc resorption. **Spine** 26:1522–1527, 2001.
55. Dyer JK, Bourque JA, Steeves JD: Regeneration of brainstem-spinal axons after lesion and immunological disruption of myelin in adult rat. **Exp Neurol** 154:12–22, 1998.
56. Eftekhar B, Ghodsi M, Ketabchi E, et al.: Surgical simulation software for insertion of pedicle screws. **Neurosurgery** 50:222–223, 2002.
57. Eikelenboom P, Veerhuis R: The role of complement and activated microglia in the pathogenesis of Alzheimer's disease. **Neurobiol Aging** 17:673–680, 1996.
58. Etebar S, Cahill DW: Risk factors for adjacent-segment failure following lumbar fixation with rigid instrumentation for degenerative instability. **J Neurosurg** 90:163–169, 1999.
59. Fischgrund JS, Mackay M, Herkowitz HN, et al.: 1997 Volvo Award winner in clinical studies. Degenerative lumbar spondylolisthesis with spinal stenosis: A prospective, randomized study comparing decompressive laminectomy and arthrodesis with and without spinal instrumentation. **Spine** 22:2807–2812, 1997.
60. Foley KT, Gupta SK: Percutaneous pedicle screw fixation of the lumbar spine: Preliminary clinical results. **J Neurosurg** 97:7–12, 2002.
61. Freitas RA Jr: The future of nanofabrication and molecular scale devices in nanomedicine. **Stud Health Technol Inform** 80:45–59, 2002.

62. Garfin SR: Editorial on residencies and fellowships. **Spine** 25:2700–2702, 2000.
63. Gill GG, Manning JG, White HL: Surgical treatment of spondylolisthesis without spine fusion. Excision of loose lamina with decompression of the nerve roots. **J Bone Joint Surg Am** 37:493–520, 1955.
64. Goto K, Tajima N, Chosa E, et al.: Mechanical analysis of the lumbar vertebrae in a three-dimensional finite element method model in which intradiscal pressure in the nucleus pulposus was used to establish the model. **J Orthop Sci** 7:243–246, 2002.
65. Gowers WR, Horsley VA: A case of tumour of the spinal cord: Removal, recovery. **Med Chir Tr (S2)** 53:379–428, 1888.
66. Gravel C, Gotz R, Lorrain A, et al.: Adenoviral gene transfer of ciliary neurotrophic factor and brain-derived neurotrophic factor leads to long-term survival of axotomized motor neurons. **Nat Med** 3:765–770, 1997.
67. Grill R, Murai K, Blesch A, et al.: Cellular delivery of neurotrophin-3 promotes corticospinal axonal growth and partial functional recovery after spinal cord injury. **J Neurosci** 17:5560–5572, 1997.
68. Groopman J: A knife in the back: Is surgery the best approach to chronic back pain? **The New Yorker** April 2002, pp 66–73.
69. Grunert P, Muller-Forell W, Darabi K, et al.: Basic principles and clinical applications of neuronavigation and intraoperative computed tomography. **Comput Aided Surg** 3:166–173, 1998.
70. Hadley MN, Walters BC, Grabb PA, et al.: Guidelines for the management of acute cervical spine and spinal cord injuries. **Neurosurg Suppl** 50:S1–S179, 2002.
71. Hall JC: The internet: From basics to telesurgery. **Aust N Z J Surg** 72:35–39, 2002.
72. Hall WA, Martin AJ, Liu H, et al.: Brain biopsy using high-field strength interventional magnetic resonance imaging. **Neurosurgery** 44:807–814, 1999.
73. Hambly MF, Wiltse LL, Raghavan N, et al.: The transition zone above a lumbosacral fusion. **Spine** 23:1785–1792, 1998.
74. Hampton D, Laros G, McCarron R, et al.: Healing potential of the annulus fibrosus. **Spine** 14:398–401, 1989.
75. Hankinson HL, Wilson CB: Use of the operating microscope in anterior cervical discectomy without fusion. **J Neurosurg** 43:452–456, 1975.
76. Harrington PR: The history and development of Harrington instrumentation. **Clin Orthop** 93:110–112, 1973.
77. Harrington PR, Dickson JH: Spinal instrumentation in the treatment of severe progressive spondylolisthesis. **Clin Orthop** 117:157–163, 1976.
78. Harrison CL, Dijkers M: Spinal cord injury surveillance in the United States: An overview. **Paraplegia** 29:233–246, 1991.
79. Hauben E, Agranov E, Gothilf A, et al.: Posttraumatic therapeutic vaccination with modified myelin self-antigen prevents complete paralysis while avoiding autoimmune disease. **J Clin Invest** 108:591–599, 2001.
80. Hauben E, Butovsky O, Nevo U, et al.: Passive or active immunization with myelin basic protein promotes recovery from spinal cord contusion. **J Neuroscience** 20:6421–6430, 2000.
81. Hauben E, Ibarra A, Mizrahi T, et al.: Vaccination with a Nogo-A-derived peptide after incomplete spinal-cord injury promotes recovery via a T-cell mediated neuroprotective response: Comparison with other myelin antigens. **PNAS** 98:15173–15178, 2001.
82. Health Devices: Surgical robotics. Evaluation of the Computer Motion AESOP 3000 robotic endoscope holder. **Health Devices** 31:256–268, 2002.
83. Hecht BP, Fischgrund JS, Herkowitz HN, et al.: The use of recombinant human

bone morphogenetic protein 2 (rhBMP-2) to promote spinal fusion in a nonhuman primate anterior interbody fusion model. **Spine** 24:629–636, 1999.

84. Helm G, Anderson DG, Andersson GB, et al.: Summary statement: Bone morphogenetic proteins: Basic science. **Spine** 27:S9, 2002.
85. Herkowitz HN, Connolly PJ, Gundry CR, et al.: Resident and fellowship guidelines: Educational guidelines for resident training in spinal surgery. **Spine** 25:2703–2707, 2000.
86. Herron L: Recurrent lumbar disc herniation: Results of repeat laminectomy and discectomy. **J Spinal Disord** 7:161–166, 1999.
87. Herzog A: Of genomics, cyborgs and nanotechnology: A look into the future of medicine. **Conn Med** 66:53–54, 2002.
88. Himes BT, Liu Y, Solowska JM, et al.: Transplant of cells genetically modified to express neurotrophin-3 rescue axotomized Clarke's nucleus neurons after spinal cord hemisection in adult rats. **J Neurosci Res** 65:549–564, 2001.
89. Hinshaw WS, Bottomley PA, Holland GN: Radiographic thin-section of the human wrist by nuclear magnetic resonance. **Nature** 270:722–723, 1977.
90. Hodgson AR, Stock FE: Anterior spinal fusion: A preliminary communication on the radical treatment of Pott's disease and Pott's paraplegia. **Br J Surg** 44:266–275, 1956.
91. Horgan MA, Hsu FP, Frank EH: A novel endoscopic approach to anterior odontoid screw fixation: Technical note. **Minim Invasive Neurosurg** 42:142–145, 1999.
92. Hounsfield GN: Computerized transverse axial scanning (tomography). 1. Description of system. **Br J Radiol** 46:1016–1022, 1973.
93. Huang DW, McKerracher L, Braun PE, et al.: A therapeutic vaccine approach to stimulate axon regeneration in the adult mammalian spinal cord. **Neuron** 24:639–647, 1999.
94. Ideker T, Thorsson V, Ranish JA, et al.: Integrated genomic and proteomic analyses of a systematically perturbed metabolic network. **Science** 292:929–934, 2001.
95. Itoh H, Ebara S, Kamimura M, et al.: Experimental spinal fusion with use of recombinant human bone morphogenetic protein 2. **Spine** 24:1402–1405, 1999.
96. Kanellopoulos GK, Kato H, Wu Y, et al.: Neuronal cell death in the ischemic spinal cord: The effect of methylprednisolone. **Ann Thorac Surg** 64:1279–1286, 1997.
97. Kang JD, Boden SD: Orthopaedic gene therapy. Spine. **Clin Orthop** 379:S256–S259, 2000.
98. Keim HA: Indications for spine fusions and techniques. **Clin Neurosurg** 25:266–275, 1978.
99. Kelly DL Jr: Current spine surgery in North America: Progress or violation? **Neurosurgery** 35:86–91, 1994.
100. Kipnis J, Yoles E, Schori H, et al.: Neuronal survival after CNS insult is determined by a genetically encoded autoimmune response. **J Neurosci** 21:4564–4571, 2001.
101. Kohyama K, Saura R, Doita M, et al.: Intervertebral disc cell apoptosis by nitric oxide: Biological understanding of intervertebral disc degeneration. **Kobe J Med Sci** 46:283–295, 2000.
102. Kong WZ, Goel VK, Gilbertson LG: Prediction of biomechanical parameters in the lumbar spine during static sagittal plane lifting. **J Biomech Eng** 120:273–280, 1998.
103. Langrana NA, Harten RD, Lin DC, et al.: Acute thoracolumbar burst fractures: A new view of loading mechanisms. **Spine** 27:498–508, 2002.
104. Larson SJ: Unstable thoracic fractures: Treatment alternatives and the role of the neurosurgeon. **Clin Neurosurg** 27:624–640, 1980.

105. Larson SJ, Holst RA, Hemmy DC, et al.: Lateral extracavitary approach to traumatic lesions of the thoracic and lumbar spine. **J Neurosurg** 45:628–637, 1976.
106. Lee TT, Klose JL, and other participating members of the Congress of Neurological Surgeons Education Committee: Survey on neurosurgery subspecialty fellowship training. **Surg Neurol** 52:641–645, 1999.
107. Legrain P, Jestin JL, Schachter V: From the analysis of protein complexes to proteome-wide linkage maps. **Curr Opin Biotechnol** 11:402–407, 2000.
108. Leitch RA, Moses GR, Magee H: Simulation and the future of military medicine. **Military Medicine** 167:350–354, 2002.
109. Lim TH, Kim JG, Fujiwara A, et al.: Biomechanical evaluation of diagonal fixation in pedicle screw instrumentation. **Spine** 26:2498–2503, 2001.
110. Liotta LA: Molecular profiling of human cancer. **Nat Rev Genet** 1:48–56, 2000.
111. Liotta LA, Kohn EC, Petricoin EF: Clinical proteomics. Personalized molecular medicine. **JAMA** 286:2211–2214, 2001.
112. Liu Y, Himes BT, Solowska J, et al.: Intraspinal delivery of neurotrophin-3 using neural stem cells genetically modified by recombinant retrovirus. **Exp Neurol** 158:9–26, 1999.
113. Liu Y, Kim D, Himes BT, et al.: Transplants of fibroblasts genetically modified to express BDNF promote regeneration of adult rat rubrospinal axons and recovery of forelimb function. **J Neurosci** 19:4370–4387, 1999.
114. Lowery GL, Kulkarni SS: Posterior percutaneous spine instrumentation. **Eur Spine J** 9:S126–S130, 2000.
115. Martin ER, Scott WK, Nance MA, et al.: Association of single-nucleotide polymorphisms of the tau gene with late-onset Parkinson disease. **JAMA** 286:2245–2250, 2001.
116. Martin J: Recent trends in neurosurgery. **J Neurosurg** 15:674–687, 1958.
117. Martuzza RL: Molecular neurosurgery for glial and neuronal disorders. **Stereotact Funct Neurosurg** 59:92–99, 1992.
118. Masamune K, Fichtinger G, Patriciu A, et al.: System for robotically assisted percutaneous procedures with computed tomography guidance. **Comput Aided Surg** 6:370–383, 2001.
119. Mathews HH: Percutaneous interbody fusions. **Orthop Clin North Am** 29:647–653, 1998.
120. Matula C, Rossler K, Reddy M, et al.: Intraoperative computed tomography guided neuronavigation: Concepts, efficiency, and work flow. **Comput Aided Surg** 3:174–182, 1998.
121. McAfee PC, Regan JJ, Geis WP, et al.: Minimally invasive anterior retroperitoneal approach to the lumbar spine. Emphasis on the lateral BAK. **Spine** 23:1476–1484, 1998.
122. Meagher JN: Presidential address: What a neurosurgeon ought to be. **Clin Neurosurg** 20:21–27, 1973.
123. Melfi FM, Menconi GF, Mariani AM, et al.: Early experience with robotic technology for thoracoscopic surgery. **Eur J Cardiothorac Surg** 21:864–868, 2002.
124. Meyerding HW: Spondylolisthesis. **Surg Gynecol** 54:371–377, 1932.
125. Moon SH, Gilbertson LG, Nishida K, et al.: Human intervertebral disc cells are genetically modifiable by adenovirus-mediated gene transfer: Implications for the clinical management of intervertebral disc disorders. **Spine** 25:2573–2579, 2000.
126. Morgan BP: Physiology and pathophysiology of complement: Progress and trends. **Crit Rev Clin Lab Sci** 32:265–298, 1995.
127. Nakai S, Yoshizawa H, Kobayashi S: Long-term follow-up study of posterior lumbar interbody fusion. **J Spinal Disord** 12:293–299, 1999.

128. Naso WB, Perot PL Jr, Cox RD: The neuroprotective effect of high-dose methylprednisolone in rat spinal cord hemisection. **Neurosci Lett** 189:176–178, 1995.
129. Nishida K, Gilbertson LG, Robbins PD, et al.: Potential applications of gene therapy to the treatment of intervertebral disc disorders. **Clin Orthop** 379:S234–S241, 2000.
130. Ojemann RG: Training the neurosurgeon for the twenty-first century. **Surg Neurol** 37:167–174, 1992.
131. Okuma M, Mochida J, Nishimura K, et al.: Reinsertion of stimulated nucleus pulposus cells retards intervertebral disc degeneration: An in vitro and in vivo experimental study. **J Orthop Res** 18:988–997, 2000.
132. Oldendorf WH: Isolated flying spot detection of radiodensity discontinuities—Displaying the internal structural pattern of a complex object. **Trans BioMed Elect** 8:68–72, 1961.
133. Ordway NR, Zheng YG, McCullen GM: Biomechanical evaluation of the functional spine unit with a hydrogel implant. **Transactions of the 11th Annual Meeting of North American Spine Society** Vancouver, BC, Canada, 1996.
134. Ornstein DK, Gillespie JW, Paweletz CP, et al.: Proteomic analysis of laser capture microdissected human prostate cancer and in vitro prostate cell lines. **Electrophoresis** 21:2235–2242, 2000.
135. Oudega M, Vargas CG, Weber AB, et al.: Long-term effects of methylprednisolone following transection of adult rat spinal cord. **Eur J Neurosci** 11:2453–2464, 1999.
136. Paget S: *Sir Victor Horsley: A Study of His Life and Work.* New York: Harcourt, Brace and Howe, 1920, p 12.
137. Papadopoulos SM, Dickman CA: Thoracoscopic sympathectomy. In: Dickman CA, Rosenthal DJ, Perin NI (eds): *Thoracoscopic Spine Surgery.* New York: Thieme, 1999, pp 143–160.
138. Patterson RH Jr: How many residents should we train? The USA experience. **Acta Neurochir Suppl (Wien)** 69:30–32, 1997.
139. Paweletz CP, Charboneau L, Bichsel VE, et al.: Reverse phase protein microarrays which capture disease progression show activation of pro-survival pathways at the cancer invasion front. **Oncogene** 20:1981–1989, 2001.
140. Pawson T: Protein modules and signaling networks. **Nature** 373:573–580, 1995.
141. Pedowitz RA, Esch J, Snyder S: Evaluation of a virtual reality simulator for arthroscopy skills development. **Arthroscopy** 18:E29, 2002.
142. Perin NI: Biopsy of vertebral lesions. In: Dickman CA, Rosenthal DJ, Perin NI. (eds) *Thoracoscopic Spine Surgery.* New York, Thieme, 1999, pp 213–220.
143. Perot PL, Munro DD: Transthoracic removal of midline thoracic disc protrusions causing spinal cord compression. **J Neurosurg** 31:452–458, 1969.
144. Piepgras DG: Post residency subspecialty training in neurosurgery—The impact of subspecialty training on organized neurosurgery and resident training—Benefits, responsibilities and liabilities. **Acta Neurochir Suppl (Wien)** 69:140–144, 1997.
145. Pitzen TR, Matthis D, Barbier DD, et al.: Initial stability of cervical spine fixation: Predictive value of a finite element model. Technical note. **J Neurosurg** 97:128–134, 2002.
146. Pott P, Schwarz M: Robots, navigation, telesurgery: State of the art and market overview [in German]. **Z Orthop Ihre Grenzgeb** 140:218–231, 2002.
147. Poulsen DJ, Harrop JS, During MJ: Gene therapy for spinal cord injury and disease. **J Spinal Cord Med** 25:2–9, 2002.
148. Puttlitz CM, Goel VK, Traynelis VC, et al.: A finite element investigation of upper cervical instrumentation. **Spine** 26:2449–2455, 2001.

149. Rapalino O, Lazarov-Spiegler O, Agranov E, et al.: Implantation of stimulated homologous macrophages results in partial recovery of paraplegic rats. **Nat Med** 4:814–821, 1998.
150. Ratcheson RA: Presidential address: Meeting the challenges to neurosurgical education. **Clin Neurosurg** 33:3–14, 1986.
151. Ray CD, Dickhudt EA, Ledoux PJ, et al.: Prosthetic spinal disc nucleus. **US patent 5,674,295,** October 7, 1997.
152. Ray CD, Schönmayr R: A prosthetic lumbar nucleus "artificial disc." **12th Annual Meeting of North American Spine Society,** New York, 1997.
153. Regan JJ, Guyer RD: Endoscopic techniques in spinal surgery. **Clin Orthop** 335:122–139, 1997.
154. Regan JJ, McAfee PC, Guyer RD, et al.: Laparoscopic fusion of the lumbar spine in a multicenter series of the first 34 consecutive patients. **Surg Laparosc Endosc** 6:459–468, 1996.
155. Regan JJ, Yuan H, McAfee PC: Laparoscopic fusion of the lumbar spine: Minimally invasive spine surgery. A prospective multicenter study evaluating open and laparoscopic lumbar fusion. **Spine** 24:402–411, 1999.
156. Robertson JT: Anterior removal of cervical disc without fusion. **Clin Neurosurg** 20:259–261, 1973.
157. Robinson RA, Smith GW: Anterolateral cervical disc removal and interbody fusion for cervical disc syndrome. **Bull Johns Hopkins Hosp** 96:223,1955.
158. Rohlmann A, Bergmann G, Graichen F, et al.: Telemeterized load measurement using instrumented spinal internal fixators in a patient with degenerative instability. **Spine** 20:2683–2689, 1995.
159. Rohlmann A, Bergmann G, Graichen F, et al.: Influence of muscle forces on loads in internal spinal fixation devices. **Spine** 23:537–542, 1998.
160. Salzberg AD, Bloom MB, Mourlas NJ, et al.: Microelectrical mechanical systems in surgery and medicine. **J Am Coll Surg** 194:463–476, 2002.
161. Sandhu HS, Anderson DG, Andersson GB, et al.: Summary statement: Safety of bone morphogenetic proteins for spine fusion. **Spine** 27:S39, 2002.
162. Schneider RC, Cherry G, Pantek H: The syndrome of acute central cervical spinal cord injury. With special reference to the mechanisms involved in hyperextension injuries of cervical spine. **J Neurosurg** 11:546–577, 1954.
163. Schwartz HG: Education of the neurosurgical resident and his future. **Clin Neurosurg** 21:1–7, 1974.
164. Schwartz M, Moalem G: Beneficial immune activity after CNS injury: Aspects for vaccination. **J Neuroimmunol** 113:185–192, 2001.
165. Schwartz RB, Hsu L, Wong TZ, et al.: Intraoperative MR imaging guidance for intracranial neurosurgery: Experience with the first 200 cases. **Radiology** 211: 477–488, 1999.
166. Schwikowski B, Uetz P, Fields S: A network of protein-protein interactions in yeast. **Nat Biotechnol** 18:1257–1261, 2000.
167. Scott WK, Nance MA, Watts RL, et al.: Complete genomic screen in Parkinson disease. Evidence for multiple genes. **JAMA** 286:2239–2244, 2001.
168. Seeherman H, Wozney J, Li R: Bone morphogenetic protein delivery systems. **Spine** 27:S16–S23, 2002.
169. Seifert V, Zimmermann M, Trantakis C, et al.: Open MRI-guided neurosurgery. **Acta Neurochir (Wien)** 141:455–464, 1999.
170. Sharan AD, Vaccaro AR, Albert TJ, et al.: Internet resources for spine surgeons. **J Spinal Disord** 13:419–421, 2000.
171. Shono Y, Kaneda K, Abumi K, et al.: Stability of posterior spinal instrumentation

and its effects on adjacent motion segments in the lumbosacral spine. **Spine** 23:1550–1558, 1998.

172. Silcox DH III: Laparoscopic bone dowel fusions of the lumbar spine. **Orthop Clin North Am** 29:655–663, 1998.
173. Sive JI, Baird P, Jeziorsk M, et al.: Expression of chondrocyte markers by cells of normal and degenerate intervertebral discs. **Mol Pathol** 55:91–97, 2002.
174. Sonntag VKH: Neurosurgical spine fellowships: The Phoenix model. **Acta Neurochir** 69:130–134, 1997.
175. Specht LM, Koval KJ: Robotics and computer-assisted orthopaedic surgery. **Bull Hosp Jt Dis** 60:168–172, 2002.
176. Stover SL, Fine PR, Go BK: *Spinal Cord Injury: The Facts and Figures*. Birmingham, AL: University of Alabama, 1986.
177. Taillard W: Le spondylolisthesis chez l'enfant et l'adolescent (etude de 50 cas). **Acta Orthop Scand** 24:115–144, 1954.
178. Theodore N, Sonntag VKH: Spinal surgery from the Eisenhower years to the third millennium. In: Barrow DL, Kondziolka D, Laws ER, Traynelis VC (eds): *Fifty Years of Neurosurgery. Golden Anniversary of the Congress of Neurological Surgeons*. Philadelphia: Lippincott Williams & Wilkins, 2000, pp 281–294.
179. Traynelis VC, Andrews BT, Awad IA, et al.: Resident curriculum guidelines for neurosurgery. Congress of Neurological Surgeons Education Committee. **Clin Neurosurg** 47:589–681, 2000.
180. Urist MR: The first three decades of bone morphogenetic protein research. **Osteologie** 4:207–223, 1995.
181. Vaccaro AR, Anderson DG, Toth CA: Recombinant human osteogenic protein-1 (bone morphogenetic protein-7) as an osteoinductive agent in spinal fusion. **Spine** 27:S59–S65, 2002.
182. Verbiest H: A radicular syndrome from developmental narrowing of the lumbar vertebral canal. **J Bone Joint Surg Br** 36:230–237, 1954.
183. Watabe K, Ohashi T, Sakamoto T, et al.: Rescue of lesioned adult rat spinal motoneurons by adenoviral gene transfer of glial cell line-derived neurotrophic factor. **J Neurosci Res** 60:511–519, 2000.
184. White AA, Panjabi MM: *Clinical Biomechanics of the Spine,* 2nd ed. Philadelphia: Lippincott Williams & Wilkins, 1990, p 3.
185. Woolsey RD: The mechanism of neurological symptoms and signs in spondylolisthesis at the fifth lumbar, first sacral level. **J Neurosurg** 11:67–76, 1954.
186. Wozney JM: Overview of bone morphogenetic proteins. **Spine** 27:S2–S8, 2002.
187. Yasargil MG: Microsurgical operation of herniated lumbar disc. **Adv Neurosurg** 4:81, 1977.
188. Yoles E, Hauben E, Palgi O, et al.: Protective autoimmunity is a physiological response to CNS trauma. **J Neurosci** 21:3740–3748, 2001.
189. Yuan HA, Bao QB: Disc arthroplasty. **SpineLine** 11:6–11, 2001.
190. Yung Lee J, Hall R, Pelinkovic D, et al.: New use of a three-dimensional pellet culture system for human intervertebral disc cells: Initial characterization and potential use for tissue engineering. **Spine** 26:2316–2322, 2001.
191. Zdeblick TA: Laparoscopic spinal fusion. **Orthop Clin North Am** 29:635–645, 1998.

CHAPTER

9

Prosthetics and Biologics: The Wave of the Future

VINCENT C. TRAYNELIS, M.D.

This review will address the next wave of technology as it pertains to the treatment of spinal spondylosis. Spinal surgery currently consists of two basic treatment options: decompression and fusion. These may be performed separately or in a combined fashion. The coming decade will witness the addition of a number of prosthetic alternatives, all of which are focused on the maintenance of motion and stability. Additionally, specific biologic factors will improve the success of arthrodesis when that treatment is necessary. Genetic research has tremendous potential in terms of prevention and treatment of degenerative spinal disorders; however, such therapies probably will not reach the clinical arena for at least 10 years.

SPINAL PROSTHESES

Multiple factors must be addressed to produce an effective prosthetic disc. Maintenance of motion, normal alignment, and stability as well as preservation of intervertebral height and durability constitute the most basic requirements. Natural discs also act as shock absorbers, which may be an important quality to incorporate into the design of a prosthesis, particularly those devices being developed for multilevel lumbar reconstruction. Ease and safety of implantation, minimal imaging distortion, and revisability are also significant issues.

Currently, segmental spinal restoration can be divided into two categories: nucleus replacement and total disc replacement. The addition of these two classes of prosthetic devices will double our treatment options. In the future, simple disc herniations, particularly free fragments, may be treated solely with a decompression. A nucleus replacement may be appropriate for a more marked disturbance, such as a recurrent disc herniation with a significant component of axial pain. Total joint arthroplasty has the capability of restoring intervertebral height and represents a potential option for patients with disease more advanced than that of the previous example. Finally, arthrodesis will still be necessary in patients with overt instability, deformity, or complete absence of segmental motion.

NUCLEUS REPLACEMENTS

Nucleus replacements may be considered in situations with significant nuclear degeneration but a relatively healthy annulus and supporting fibers. Contraindications to nuclear disc arthroplasty include an interspace height of less than 5 mm, spondylolisthesis, and Schmorl's nodes.

The most extensively evaluated nucleus replacement is the Prosthetic Disc Nucleus (PDN; Raymedica, Bloomington, MN), and more than 500 patients have received this implant. The implant closely replicates the physiologic function of the nucleus and can restore some disc space height (1). The PDN device consists of a hydrogel core constrained within a woven polyethylene jacket (*Fig. 9.1*). It has been evaluated with mechanical and in vitro testing. The results have been favorable, and the early clinical results are promising (2–4).

Compression and hydration of the hydrogel core and insertion of platinum-iridium wire markers before implantation minimizes the size of the PDN and allows for radiographic identification of the device.

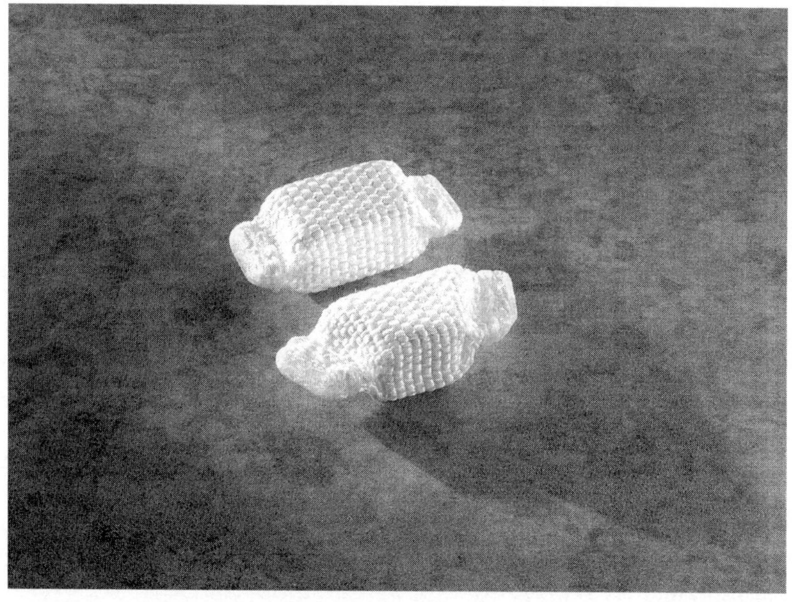

FIG. 9.1 Prosthetic Disc Nucleus.

The permeable, tightly woven, ultrahigh-molecular-weight polyethylene (UHMWPE) jacket is flexible but inelastic. These properties constrain expansion upon hydration yet permit the core to deform and reform in response to compressive forces. Once implanted, the hydrogel immediately begins to absorb fluid, and within 4 to 5 days, maximum expansion is achieved. Currently, the PDN is the only nucleus replacement that can effectively distract the interspace. Because of this distraction capability, it can be implanted into segments as small as 5 mm, whereas the nondistracting nucleus replacements probably will function best in disc spaces that have maintained a height of at least 10 mm.

Several other nucleus replacements are currently under development. No significant volume of clinical data exist concerning the outcomes of patients receiving these implants, making it impossible to present relevant patient outcomes at this time.

Aquarelle (Stryker Howmedica, Rutherford, NJ) is a hydrogel-based nuclear replacement constructed with polyvinyl alcohol (PVA). This viscoelastic material exerts a uniform pressure across the end plates. Biomechanically, the Aquarelle device has performed well in fatigue testing up to 40 million cycles, and extensive cadaveric studies have demonstrated that the device does not extrude. There has been no evidence of local or systemic toxicity to the PVA or its particles in a baboon study (5). Aquarelle is inserted through a 4- to 5-mm, tapered cannula that may access the disc space from either a lateral or posterior avenue.

Newcleus (Sulzer Spine-Tech, Edina, MN) is a spinal nuclear implant constructed with a polycarbonate urethane elastomer (Sulene PCU). Sulene PCU is biocompatible and has been used in multiple cardiovascular applications. The Newcleus device is manufactured in a specific manner that causes it to curl up into a spiral in its natural state. This property enables Newcleus to completely fill the intervertebral space and, potentially, to exert lateral tension on the annulus. Functionally, it probably acts as a spacer with some shock-absorbing capabilities. Newcleus is implanted using the same approach as that for a microdiscectomy, but in the future, it may be possible to introduce the implant percutaneously.

At least two other nuclear replacements are being developed that consist of polymers cured in situ. The ability to insert these implants through a small annular window may be an attractive factor in selected patients, because theoretically, this would allow for implantation via a minimally invasive procedure with minuscule risk of implant migration.

The Prosthetic Intervertebral Nucleus (PIN; Disc Dynamics, Minnetonka, MN) is an in situ curable polyurethane. The PIN is injected into a polyurethane balloon through a catheter and polymerizes in minutes, after which the catheter is removed. BioDisc (Cryolife, Kennesaw, GA) is constructed with a protein hydrogel. This in situ curable protein hydrogel is injected into the disc space and also cures within minutes. Very little additional information is available concerning these implants at this time.

TOTAL DISC REPLACEMENT

Lumbar

The Link SB Charite (Waldemar Link GmbH & Co, Hamburg, Germany), now in its third generation, has been the most widely implanted disc prosthesis, and more than 2,000 patients have received this device (6). The Charité III consists of a biconvex UHMWPE spacer encircled by a radiopaque ring for x-ray localization. This core spacer, which is available in different sizes, interfaces with two casted cobalt-chromium-molybdenum (CrCoMO) alloy end plates. The end plates are coated with titanium and hydroxyapatite to promote bone bonding, and they have ventral and dorsal teeth to discourage migration (*Fig. 9.2*). The end plates are available in different sizes and angulations. The unique design of the Charité III allows the implant to provide unconstrained kinematic motion across the treated spinal segment. Although there is great concern regarding wear debris from hip prostheses in which UHMWPE articulates with metal, this does not appear to occur in the Charité III (6). A number of studies assessing clinical outcome have been published, some with 5-year follow-up, and the overall results with the Charité implant have been good (7–9).

The Prodisc (Aesculap AG & Co KG., Tuttlingen, Germany) was developed by Dr. Thierry Marnay. It is constructed with two CrCoMO alloy end plates with vertical wings (*Fig. 9.3*) and a monoconvex polyethylene core inserted into the caudal end plate. The polyethylene core is firmly anchored to the caudal end plate, which results in a kinematic behavior that is best described as "semiconstrained." Good to excellent results have been reported in the majority of patients receiving this implant (10, 11).

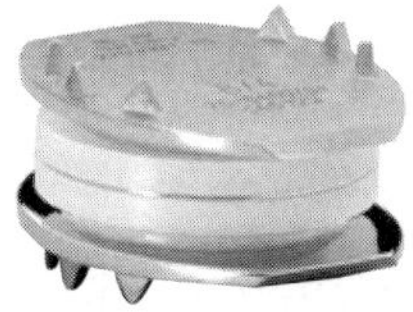

FIG. 9.2 Link SB Charité Disc.

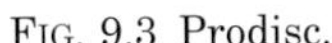

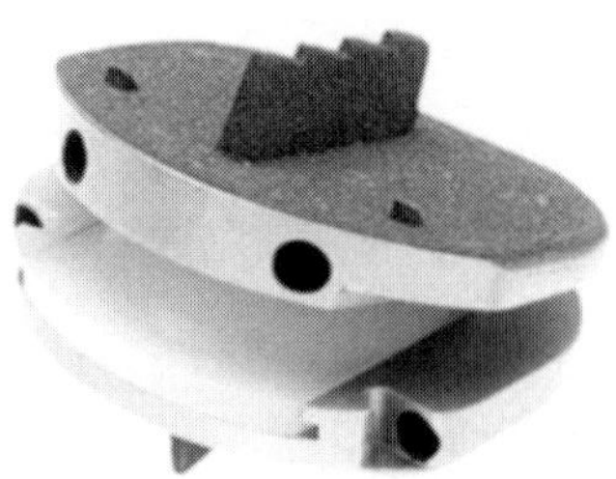

FIG. 9.3 Prodisc.

Cervical

At first glance, it may seem a little more difficult to justify arthroplasty in the cervical spine as opposed to the lumbar region. Evidence is mounting, however, that arthrodesis increases stress and, therefore, the rate of disc degeneration in the cervical spine (12–18).

The Bristol cervical disc has the longest follow-up compared to any other current prosthesis, and the clinical outcomes have been good (19). The Bristol disc is the second generation of the Cummins disc. It is a ball-and-trough-type device constructed of stainless steel, which is secured to the vertebral bodies with screws (*Fig. 9.4*). The Bristol disc allows unconstrained motion across the segment (*Fig. 9.5*).

Wigfield et al. (20, 21) have recently reported that the Bristol artificial disc decreases adjacent level motion as compared to an arthrode-

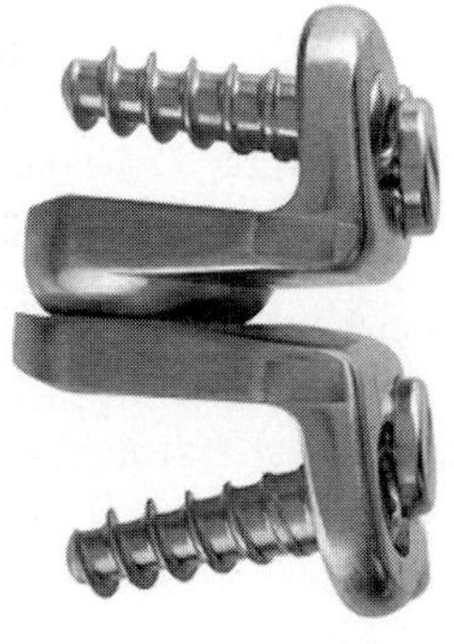

A

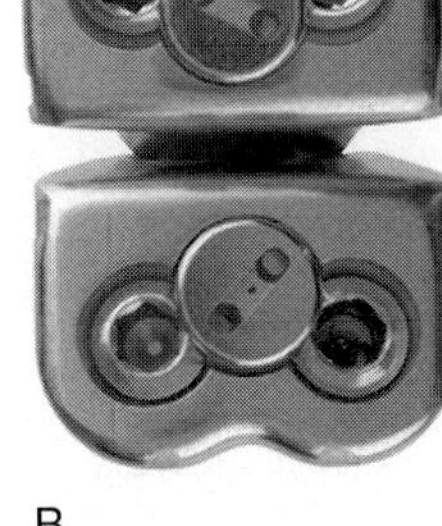

B

FIG. 9.4 The Bristol disc. (*A*) Lateral view. (*B*) Anterior view.

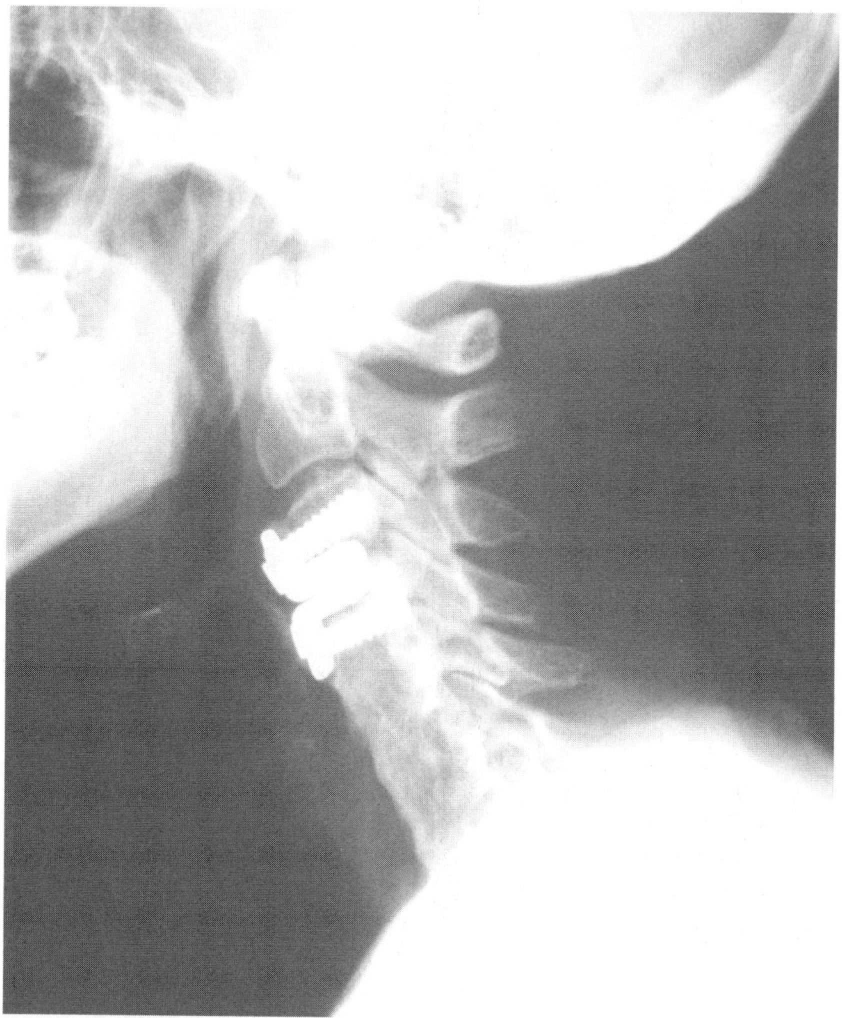

FIG. 9.5 The Bristol disc. (*A*) Lateral cervical radiograph in extension.

sis. Theoretically, this will decrease the incidence of adjacent segment disease. Robertson et al. (22) have reviewed the preliminary data for a prospective, randomized trial comparing the Bristol disc to an instrumented arthrodesis for single-level primary cervical disc disease. The 1-year data demonstrate that the arthroplasty patients had a greater improvement than those in the arthrodesis cohort in the Neck Disability Index, visual analog pain scale scores, and the mental and physical component scores of the SF-36. Segmental cervical motion was maintained across the operated segments in all patients.

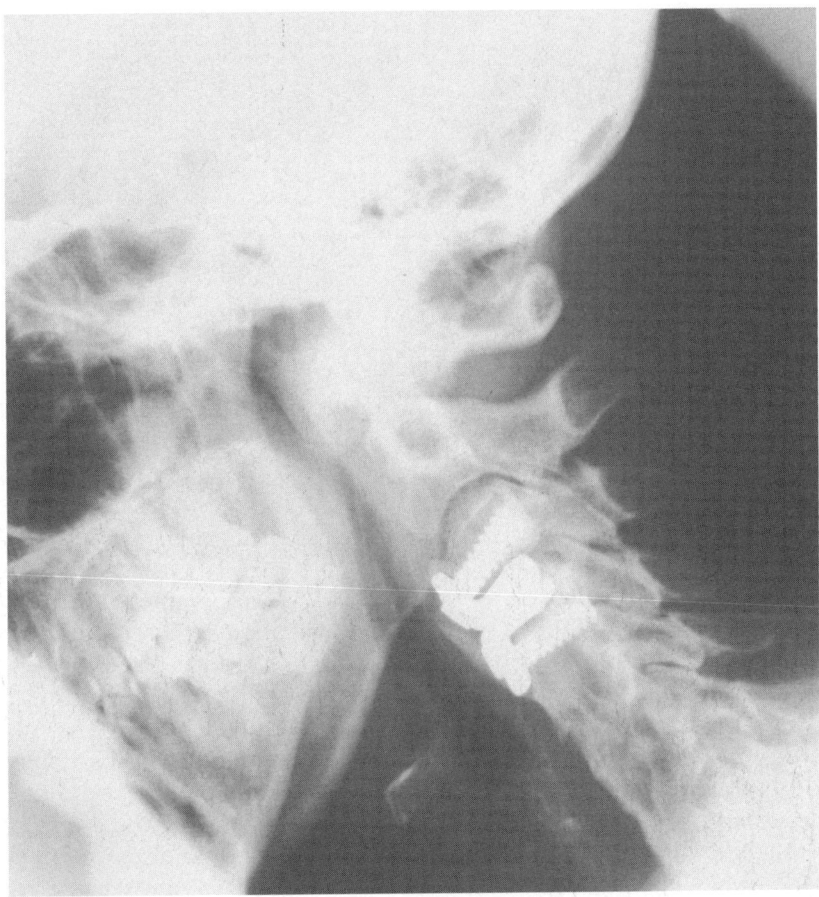

FIG. 9.5 The Bristol disc. (*B*) Lateral cervical radiograph in flexion.

The Bryan Cervical Disc System (Spinal Dynamics Corporation, Seattle, WA) consists of a polyurethane nucleus that is situated between and articulates with two titanium plates (shells) that are fitted to the vertebral body end plates (*Fig. 9.6*). A pliable polyurethane membrane surrounds the nucleus and is secured to the end plates with a titanium wire. The closed environment deters wear-debris migration and also inhibits the intrusion of connective tissue. The implant allows for unconstrained normal range of motion in flexion/extension, lateral bending, axial rotation, and translation. It also provides some cushioning for axial loads.

The initial clinical experience with the Bryan Total Cervical Disc Prosthesis has been promising. Goffin et al. (23) have reported the results of 60 patients receiving the Bryan disc. Although the follow-up

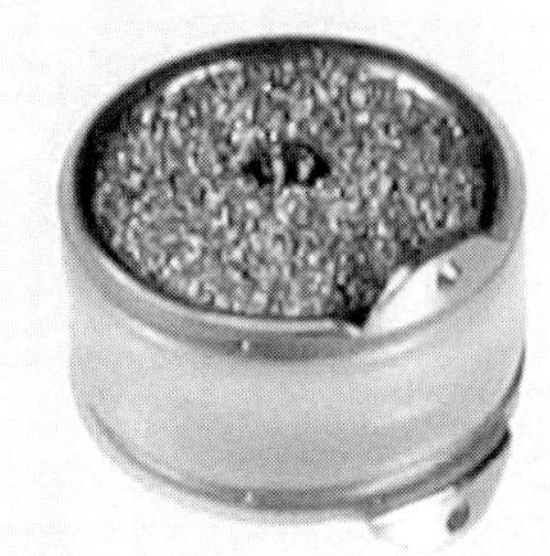

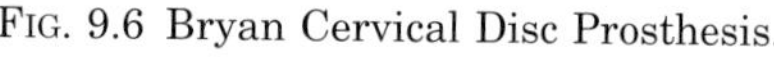
FIG. 9.6 Bryan Cervical Disc Prosthesis.

has only been 1 year, no device failures and no subsidence were found, and motion was maintained at each implanted level. The patient-derived outcomes were excellent.

BONE MORPHOGENETIC PROTEIN

Those patients who require an arthrodesis will benefit from advances in biologic enhancement of the bony healing process. More than 35 years ago, Marshall Urist (24), an orthopedic surgeon, discovered that demineralized bone could induce a cellular response resulting in new bone formation. He later demonstrated that this activity was caused by a protein (or group of proteins) that he named bone morphogenetic protein (BMP) (25, 26). Progress in biochemical techniques and advances in genetic research technology have led to the discovery and purification of numerous specific BMPs. At least a dozen separate BMPs have been detected. The genes or cDNA encoding each of these proteins has been cloned. Analysis of the clones has revealed that the individual proteins are related, and the family of compounds have been named bone morphogenetic proteins. The family consists of dimeric molecules that constitute the largest subgroup of the transforming growth factor-β (TGFβ) superfamily (27).

Bone morphogenetic proteins are local-acting, soluble proteins that bind to specific receptors on the cell surface. These receptors transduce their signal via a group of proteins called Smads, which result in the activation of certain genes. The BMPs act primarily as differentiation factors converting responsive mesenchymal cells into cartilage- and bone-forming cells. The activity of BMPs is controlled at many levels. In the extracellular space, inhibitory proteins may bind BMPs, thereby making them unavailable to the cell-surface receptors; in fact, BMPs may upregulate the activity of these inhibitors, creating a negative-feedback loop. In the intracellular space, BMPs can upregulate the expression of inhibitory Smad proteins. Additionally, a number of negative intranuclear BMP regulators are known. The bone induction process is tightly controlled by each of these processes. The end result of these processes is that bone induction is observed only locally at the site of BMP and matrix implantation. The amount of bone formation is determined by the volume of matrix implanted and the time that the BMP is present (28).

It is relatively easy to promote bone formation both in vitro and in rodent models. Likewise, in lower vertebrates such as rabbits and dogs, bone heals more readily than in humans. Physiologic BMP concentrations are adequate for fracture healing and arthrodesis in ideal conditions, but supraphysiologic concentrations are necessary to produce a significant positive effect in the human condition. The presence of powerful inhibitors of BMP is a major reason for this variation (29, 30).

It is imperative that an adequate concentration of BMPs be delivered to and maintained at the appropriate site to be effective. This is accomplished by loading a carrier material with BMPs. The major role for carrier-based delivery systems is to preserve the concentration of osteogenic factors at the fracture site long enough to allow the migration of mesenchymal cells to the area of injury to proliferate and differentiate. The carrier must accomplish these goals without interfering with the healing process. Ideally, the carrier would be porous and rapidly biodegradable to allow for cellular and vascular ingrowth yet, at the same time, produce a minimal inflammatory response. Spinal fusion requires that the carrier serve as an osteoconductive matrix for bone-forming cells while maintaining a three-dimensional space where bone formation can occur. This is particularly important to prevent soft tissues from entering the site and inhibiting the fusion process. Four major categories of carriers have been utilized for the delivery of osteogenic factors: inorganic materials, natural polymers, synthetic polymers, and composites. Each has specific advantages and disadvantages, and the ideal carrier has yet to be identified (30).

Currently, four BMPs show promise for clinical application in the arena of spinal fusion. These include recombinant human BMP (rhBMP)-2; rhBMP-7, which is also known as osteogenic protein (OP)-1; bovine bone-derived BMP extract; and growth and differentiation factor-5.

Recombinant human bone morphogenetic protein-2 has been evaluated in several human studies of lumbar fusion (31). The most important was one in which rhBMP-2 was compared to autograft in an open anterior lumbar interbody fusion study using titanium cages (INFUSE, LT Cage; Medtronic Sofamor Danek, Memphis, TN). The carrier for the rhBMP-2 was a collagen sponge. This study enrolled 279 patients, and more than 90% completed their 2-year follow-up. Demographically, the two groups were similar. The operative time and blood loss were significantly less in the investigational group (rhBMP-2). In the autograft group, 32% of the patients had some degree of donor site pain at 2 years following surgery. The two groups did not differ in terms of back pain and Oswestry scores. The successful fusion rates at 2 years were 94.5% and 88.7% for the rhBMP-2 and autograft groups, respectively. The U.S. Food and Drug Administration granted permission for an additional arm to be added to the above study in which rhBMP-2-filled cages were inserted laparoscopically. Although only 12-mo data are available from this study, the results are encouraging. Currently, rhBMP-2 is approved for the performance of lumbar fusions with the LT Cage.

Recombinant human OP-1 (rhOP-1; Stryker Biotech, Hopkinton, MA) has demonstrated efficacy in promoting spinal fusion in animal models, and human trials are currently ongoing (32). The early clinical results show an improved outcome with the use of rhOP-1, although statistical significance has yet to be achieved. These trials have not demonstrated any adverse effects related to the use of rhOP-1. Currently, a trial is ongoing in which patients with lumbar spinal stenosis and degenerative spondylolisthesis are treated with decompression followed by an uninstrumented posterolateral fusion using either iliac crest autograft or rhOP-1 putty. The 6-mo results for 36 patients are notable for a 32% higher clinical success rate in the rhOP-1 group.

While the recombinant forms of BMPs, rhBMP-2 and rhOP-1, are single factors manufactured using cell culture techniques, bovine BMP extract (bBMPx) is a highly purified protein extract from bovine bone. This extract contains BMP-2, BMP-3, BMP-4, BMP-6, BMP-7, TGFβ_1, TGFβ_2, TGFβ_3, fibroblast growth factor 1, and other noncollagenous proteins. The bBMPx product is composed of bBMPx and type I collagen (Ne-Osteo; Sulzer Biologics, Austin, TX) (33). The bBMPx has been demonstrated to be safe and efficacious in a rabbit posterolateral transverse process fusion model and was twice as successful as autograft in producing arthrodesis in a primate study. At this time, a human study of a posterolateral lumbar transverse process fusion is ongoing; one side receives autograft and the other bBMPx so that each patient serves as his or her own control. The results have not been formally published.

A number of viral and nonviral techniques are being employed to transduce cells with a BMP gene so that significant quantities of BMP will be produced. Both direct and ex vivo BMP gene therapy have been effective in animal models. Although BMP gene therapy may possess advantages over direct BMP applications, this field is in its infancy, and no specific vector or treatment technique has been developed enough to consider for evaluation in clinical trials.

LIGAMENTOUS RESTORATION

Finally, at least two spinal implant systems are designed to restore ligamentous function. Although these are distinctly different than disc replacements, they have the same goal: maintenance of motion. Disc cell death has been shown to be a function of the magnitude and duration of applied loads (34). This has led to the hypothesis that degeneration of the posterior supporting structures may predispose an individual to accelerated disc degeneration (35).

The Dynesys device (Sulzer Orthopedics, Ltd., Baar) is a dynamic neutralization system that consists of polyester cords and modular polycarbonate-urethane spacers attached to the lumbar spine with pedicle screws (36). The rigidity of the cord and spacer is comparable to that of the posterior ligaments of the lumbar spine. The cord allows for stabilization in flexion, while the spacer stabilizes extension motion. The cords and spacers are attached to the spine with pedicle screws. Cadaveric studies have demonstrated that the Dynesys device restores normal stiffness to the lumbar spine following destabilization. Additionally, Dynesys neutralizes posterior nuclear and annular pressure variations. The device does not appear to affect pressures in the anterior portion of the disc/annulus complex. Dynesys has been shown to reverse Modic's end plate changes. The clinical results have been good. The major problem with this technique appears to be related to screw loosening. Clinical and radiographic findings consistent with screw loosening have been reported in 9.6% of patients receiving Dynesys; however, this has only been confirmed by reoperation in 1.9% of the implants placed.

The spinal degenerative process leads to an increase in the neutral zone during sagittal plane rotation. The Wallis System (Spine Next, Bordeaux, France), designed by Prof. Senegas, eliminates not only this increase but other spondylotic perturbations in spinal mechanics (37). The Wallis system consists of a plastic interspinous block and woven polyethylene ligaments. The Wallis device unloads the adjacent disc in both extension and flexion. Indeed, the interspinous portion of the implant decreases disc loading by 50% in extension alone. A prospective study was performed using the first generation of the Wallis device from 1988 through 1993. Two groups of patients were studied: those undergoing excision of a recurrent disc (group A) and those undergoing recurrent disc excision and Wallis implantation (group B).

The improvement in visual pain and Oswestry scores was higher in group B, but the differences did not achieve statistical significance. Perhaps the most fascinating aspect of the Wallis System has been the observation that not only do Modic's changes reverse after implantation of the device but that some patients also develop MR imaging-documented rehydration of their discs.

This is an exciting time to be involved in the management of degenerative spinal disease. Radical new treatments are on the immediate horizon, and these will not only improve patient outcomes but expand our knowledge of degenerative spondylosis.

REFERENCES

1. Bao Q-B, Yuan HA. New technologies in spine. Nucleus replacement. **Spine** 27:1245–1247, 2002.
2. Ray CD, Schönmayr R, Kavanagh SA, et al.: Prosthetic disc nucleus implants. **Riv Neuroradiol** 12(suppl 1):157–162, 1999.
3. Schönmayr R, Busch C, Lotz C, et al.: Prosthetic disc nucleus implants: the Wiesbaden feasibility study. 2 years follow-up in ten patients. **Riv Neuroradiol** 12(suppl 1):163–170, 1999.
4. Wilke H-J, Kavanagh S, Neller S, Haid C, Claes LE. Effect of a prosthetic disc nucleus on the mobility and disc height of the L4-5 intervertebral disc postnucleotomy. **J Neurosurg** 95:208–214, 2001.
5. Yuan H, et al.: *Preclinical Safety of Aquarelle Hydrogel Disc Nucleus.* North American Spine Society, October 2000.
6. Link HD. LINK SB Charité III intervertebral dynamic disc spacer. **Rachis Revue de Pathologie Vertebrale** 11, 1999.
7. David TH. Lumbar disc prosthesis: a study of 85 patients reviewed after a minimum follow-up period of five years. **Rachis Revue de Pathologie Vertebrale** 11(4–5), 1999.
8. Griffith SL, Shelokov AP, Büttner-Janz K, LeMaire J-P, Zeegers WS. A multicenter retrospective study of the clinical results of the LINK SB Charité intervertebral prosthesis. The initial European experience. **Spine** 19:1842–1849, 1994.
9. Lemaire JP, Skalli W, Lavaste F, et al.: Intervertebral disc prosthesis. Results and prospects for the year 2000. **Clin Orthop** 337:64–76, 1997.
10. Marnay T. L'arthroplastie intervertébrale lombaire. **Med Orthop** 25:48–55, 1991.
11. Marnay T. *Prodisc: 10 Years Experience.* Montpelier, France: Society for Spinal Arthroplasty, 2002.
12. Baba H, Furusawa N, Imura S, Kawahara N, Tsuchiya H, Tomita K. Late radiographic findings after anterior cervical fusion for spondylotic myeloradiculopathy. **Spine** 18:2167–2173, 1993.
13. Cherubino P, Benazzo F, Borromeo U, Perle S. Degenerative arthritis of the adjacent spinal joints following anterior cervical spinal fusion: clinicoradiologic and statistical correlations. **Ital J Orthop Traumatol** 16:533–543, 1990.
14. Clements DH, O'Leary PF. Anterior cervical discectomy and fusion. **Spine** 15:1023–1025, 1990.
15. Döhler JR, Kahn MR, Hughes SP. Instability of the cervical spine after anterior interbody fusion. A study on its incidence and clinical significance in 21 patients. **Arch Orthop Trauma Surg** 104:247–250, 1985.

16. Goffin J, van Loon J, Van Calenbergh F, Plets C. Long-term results after anterior cervical fusion and osteosynthetic stabilization for fractures and/or dislocations of the cervical spine. **J Spinal Disord** 8:500–508, 1995.
17. Hilibrand AS, Carlson GD, Palumbo MA, Jones PK, Bohlman HH. Radiculopathy and myelopathy at segments adjacent to the site of a previous anterior cervical arthrodesis. **J Bone Joint Surg Am** 81:519–528, 1999.
18. Pospiech J, Stolke D, Wilke HJ, Claes LE. Intradiscal pressure recordings in the cervical spine. **Neurosurgery** 44:379–385, 1999.
19. Cummins BH, Robertson JT, Gill SG. Surgical experience with an implanted artificial cervical joint. **J Neurosurg** 88:943–948, 1998.
20. Wigfield C, Gill S, Nelson R, Langdon I, Metcalf N, Robertson J. Influence of an artificial cervical joint compared with fusion on adjacent-level motion in the treatment of degenerative cervical disc disease. **J Neurosurg** 96:17–21, 2002.
21. Wigfield CC, Robertson J, Metcalf N, Langdon I. The influence of an artificial cervical joint versus fusion on adjacent level motion in the treatment of cervical disc disease. **Neurosurgery** 47:516, 2000.
22. Robertson J, Porchet F, Brotchi J, et al.: *A Multicenter Trial of an Artificial Cervical Joint for Primary Disc Surgery.* Montreaux, Switzerland: Society for Spinal Arthroplasty, 2002.
23. Goffin J, Casey A, Kehr P, et al.: Preliminary clinical experience with the Bryan Cervical Disc Prosthesis. **Neurosurgery** 51:840–847, 2002.
24. Urist MR. Bone: formation by autoinduction. **Science** 150:893–890, 1965.
25. Urist MR, Iwata H, Ceccotti PL, et al.: Bone morphogenesis in implants of insoluble bone gelatin. **Proc Natl Acad Sci U S A** 70:3511–3515, 1973.
26. Urist MR, Mikulski A, Lietze A. Solubilized and insolubilized bone morphogenetic protein. **Proc Natl Acad Sci U S A** 76:1828–1832, 1979.
27. Wozney JM. Overview of bone morphogenetic proteins. **Spine** 27:S2–S6, 2002.
28. Ebara S, Nakayama K. Mechanism for the action of bone morphogenetic proteins and regulation of their activities. **Spine** 27:S10–S15, 2002.
29. Martin GJ Jr, Boden SD, Morone MA, Moskovitz PA. Posterolateral intertransverse process spinal arthrodesis with rhBMP-2 in a nonhuman primate: Important lessons learned regarding dose, carrier, and safety. **J Spinal Disord** 12:179–186, 1999.
30. Seeherman H, Wozney J, Li R. Bone morphogenetic delivery systems. **Spine** 27:S16–S23, 2002.
31. McKay B, Sandhu HS. Use of recombinant human bone morphogenetic protein-2 in spinal fusion applications. **Spine** 27:S66–S85, 2002.
32. Vaccaro AR, Anderson G, Toth CA. Recombinant human osteogenic protein-1 (bone morphogenetic protein-7) as an osteoinductive agent in spinal fusion. **Spine** 27:S59–S65, 2002.
33. Damien CJ, Grob D, Boden S, Benedict JJ. Purified bovine BMP extract and collagen for spine arthrodesis. **Spine** 27:S50–S58, 2002.
34. Lotz JC, Chin JR, Urban JP. Intervertebral disc cell death is dependent on the magnitude of duration of spinal loading. **Spine** 25:1477–1483, 2000.
35. Senegas J, Etchevers JP, Vital JM, Baulny D, Grenier F. Le recalibrage du canal lombaire, alternative à la laminectomie dans le traitement des sténoses du canal lombaire. **Revue de Chirurgie Orthopédique** 74:15–22, 1988.
36. Dubois G, DeGermay B, Schwarzenbach O, et al.: *The Different Stages of Dystability of the Lumbar Column and Their Treatments.* Second Global Symposium on Intervertebral Disc Replacement and Nonfusion, Montpelier, France, May 2002.
37. Senegas J. *Mechanical Supplementation by Non-Rigid Fixation (MSN) in Degenerative Intervertebral Lumbar Segments.* Second Global Symposium on Intervertebral Disc Replacement and Nonfusion. Montpellier, France, May 2002.

CHAPTER

10

Minimalism: Is Less More?

RICHARD G. FESSLER, M.D., Ph.D., AND FAHEEM A. SANDHU, M.D.

INTRODUCTION

Enabled by technological advances in imaging and surgical instrumentation, surgeons have labored to accomplish operative goals by less invasive means. Clinical factors such as decreased surgical morbidity, improved functional outcome, and cosmesis are obvious driving forces toward minimalistic surgical procedures. Couple this with financial pressures from an overly burdened medical system to contain costs and reduce resource utilization, and surgical minimalism would seem to be the obvious choice for patients, surgeons, and hospital administrators.

For "less to be more" in a surgical procedure, certain goals must be met.

1. The procedure should result in less blood loss, reduced intensive care needs, less postoperative pain, and decreased length of hospitalization.
2. The technique should be reasonable to master without an exhaustive training period.
3. Operative times should be comparable to those of traditional surgical procedures.
4. The technique should be applicable to many different clinical scenarios.
5. The cost of less invasive procedures should be reasonable.
6. The final objective of the surgery must be accomplished (i.e., "get the job done").
7. The complication rate should not increase.

If all these goals are met, then less can be more.

Minimalism is no stranger to spinal surgery. A number of techniques have been used in the past several decades to address spinal pathologies in a minimally invasive manner. The advent of minimal-access spinal techniques began with chemonucleolysis of herniated discs and progressed to include automated percutaneous discectomy, laser discectomy, arthroscopic discectomy, intradiscal electrothermy, and tubular retractor approaches. All of these approaches have attempted to do more through doing less, but according to the above-outlined goals, success has been variable. We will discuss each of these techniques and determine their effectiveness as minimally invasive procedures.

CHEMONUCLEOLYSIS

Injection of chymopapain into the intervertebral disc was introduced as a minimally invasive spinal procedure more than 30 years ago. Initial results with chemonucleolysis were quite favorable, especially when it was used in specific subsets of patients with lumbar disc disease. Comparing chemonucleolysis and open discectomy, Watts et al. (26) found similar responses to treatment in subdivisions of lumbar disc disease that included degenerative, complex, and previous surgery; however, in the subdivision of simple disc, 89% of patients responded successfully to open discectomy, compared to 60% treated with chymopapain injection. Almost identical results, favoring open discectomy over chemonucleolysis, were reported by Zieger (27) a decade later. Other studies found similar responses to either discectomy or chemonucleolysis but a higher incidence of treatment failures in the chemonucleolysis groups requiring surgical intervention (2). In a prospective, randomized study comparing open discectomy and chemonucleolysis, good outcomes were achieved in 85% of open discectomy cases, compared with 63% of chemonucleolysis cases (25). Of note, 22% of patients treated with chemonucleolysis had increased radicular pain immediately following the procedure; none of the patients in the open discectomy group suffered increased radicular pain following surgery. Also, at 1-year follow-up, 25% of patients failed chemonucleolysis therapy and needed open discectomy, whereas only 3% of discectomy patients required a second operation.

Complications of chemonucleolysis are, in general, significantly less than those associated with open discectomy (3.7% vs. 26%) (4). A small risk of anaphylactic or allergic reaction to chymopapain exists following chemonucleolysis. Failure to successfully treat underlying pathology occurs more commonly following chemonucleolysis; this may result in the need for open surgery or in the presence of persistent neurological deficits (2, 5, 25).

Does chemonucleolysis satisfy the goals of a procedure in which less is more? It certainly is minimally invasive, being performed through a single needle-puncture site. It is technically easy, and it can be done quickly. The costs are reasonable, and complications are lower than with open surgical procedures. It is not applicable to many spinal pathologies, however, and it is limited to the treatment of disc herniations largely of the lumbar spine. Most important, is not effective in treating the underlying pathology. Failures of chemonucleolysis require open discectomy and have poorer outcomes than those treated initially by surgery (25).

AUTOMATED PERCUTANEOUS DISCECTOMY

Automated percutaneous discectomy (APD) was introduced as a minimally invasive means of removing herniated disc material still contained by the annulus. A 2-mm probe is introduced percutaneously into the disc space; disc material is then aspirated. Initial reports using APD demonstrated symptomatic improvement in 64% to 85% of patients (7, 9, 18, 20); however, a large number of patients in these studies, ranging from 13% to 29%, required a second surgery.

Various subsets of patients may derive more benefit from APD compared with other patients. Bonaldi et al. (3) found symptomatic improvement in 86% of patients that had only back pain as their primary complaint, compared to an overall success rate of 75% in their patient group. In another study, by dividing patients in groups according to the shape of their disc protrusion on CT discography, a significant difference in response to surgery was noted, with 80% showing improvement if a broad dye base was present but only 53% showing improvement with a narrow dye base (6).

When APD was compared to chemonucleolysis in a prospective, randomized trial, the results were not favorable (22). Only 37% of patients undergoing APD reported improvement at 1 year. Forty-four percent had significant back pain, and 33% required open surgery. Kahanovitz et al. (14) had similarly poor result in their experience with 38 patients treated with APD. Only 55% of their patients showed improvement, and 31% required another surgery. Complication rates following APD are very low. There have been no reported mortalities, dural tears, or root injury (13). The most common complications are discitis, psoas hematoma, and reoperation.

Does APD satisfy the goals of a procedure in which less is more? Like chemonucleolysis, it is minimally destructive to soft tissue and can be done rapidly on an outpatient basis with few complications. The procedure is, however, very restrictive in its application (i.e., a subset of patients with lumbar disc disease). Additionally, APD is not very effective at definitively treating the disease.

LASER DISCECTOMY

The addition of lasers to the percutaneous method of discectomy was an attempt to more reliably remove disc material from the interspace. A predictable size defect in a predetermined location was possible with the use of a laser. Clinical results were equally encouraging, showing between 85% and 87% improvement 18 mo after surgery (8, 24). The need for another surgery did occur, but at lower frequency than with APD.

Laser discectomy would seem to satisfy many of our goals for a procedure in which less is more, but again, it has limited application and is associated with a significant failure rate. Additionally, the price of the laser necessary to perform this procedure makes its overall cost unreasonable.

ARTHROSCOPIC DISCECTOMY

Arthroscopic or percutaneous endoscopic discectomy were the next evolution in minimally invasive spinal surgeries. In this procedure, a posterolateral approach is used to access the disc space, and an endoscope with a 70° angle helps the surgeon to visualize the procedure on a television monitor. Special suction-cutters and shavers aid in the removal of contained and subligamentous disc fragments.

Results with this technique have been favorable. Kambin (15) reported excellent to good outcome in 88% of his group of 100 patients treated by arthroscopic discectomy. Mayer and Brock (19), in a prospective, randomized study comparing percutaneous endoscopic discectomy and open discectomy, found greater improvements in patients receiving the percutaneous endoscopic discectomy. Two years following endoscopic surgery, 80% of patients had resolution of sciatic pain, compared with 69% of open surgery patients. Additionally, almost twice as many patients had no back pain after endoscopic surgery compared with the open group (47% vs. 25%).

Although arthroscopic discectomy satisfies some of our goals for an effective procedure in which less is more, several other goals remain unfulfilled. Technically, arthroscopic discectomy is a challenging procedure. Additionally, its application is limited to lumbar disc herniations that are contained or small subligamentous fragments. Finally, it is difficult to effectively remove the offending pathology by this technique.

INTRADISCAL ELECTROTHERMY

During an intradiscal electrothermy (IDET) procedure, a slender probe is introduced percutaneously into the disc space, and discogenic pain is reduced by electrothermy of nociceptive receptors within the disc. The procedure has been beneficial to a select group of patients, namely those with discogenic back pain and radiographic evidence of internal disc disruption. In their cohort of 63 patients, Saal and Saal (23) found significantly less pain following IDET as measured by visual analog scale and SF-36 pain scales. Overall, they observed improvement in 71% of patients with a mean follow-up of 16 months. When comparing IDET therapy to physical rehabilitation therapy, Karasek and Bogduk (16) found at 3 mo that only 6% of patients in the physical therapy group had significant reduction in back pain, compared with 66% of those receiving IDET. The effect was sustained for 6 and 12 mo to varying degrees.

Is less more following IDET? It may help to avoid, or at least delay, the need for a spinal fusion procedure, but IDET really is only partially effective in a very select group of patients. It does little to address underlying pathology, and the natural history of degenerative conditions may necessitate future surgery despite the success of an earlier IDET procedure. Long-term outcomes following IDET are not known.

TUBULAR RETRACTORS

Tubular retractors, which are inserted by a muscle-splitting technique over serial dilators, were designed to preserve ligamentous and muscular attachments to the spine while providing an adequate surgical corridor (11). The tubular retractors are amenable to endoscopic or more traditional microscopic techniques. Moreover, they are applicable to any region of the spine.

Tubular retractors have been successfully utilized in a number of surgical procedures. Cervical foraminotomy or discectomy can be effectively accomplished by a microendoscopic technique (MED) that combines a tubular retractor and a magnifying endoscope (1, 10). The MED is also very effective in treating lumbar spine pathologies, and disc herniations, foraminal stenosis, and lumbar stenosis are all treatable by MED (11, 12, 17, 21). Clinical outcomes of pain reduction and improvement of neurological function are comparable to those achieved with open surgery. With MED procedures, however, blood loss, length of hospitalization, and need for postoperative narcotic pain medications are all reduced when compared to open techniques. The rate of complications is not significantly higher with MED techniques. It will be of interest to see if the rate of iatrogenic instability and the need for fusion is reduced among patients who have undergone MED procedures.

Do tubular retractors satisfy the goals that we outlined for less to be more? The procedures are minimally invasive: Incisions are generally 1.5 to 2.0 cm in length; muscle is split, not cut, while ligamentous attachments to the spine are preserved; and blood loss, postoperative pain, and hospitalization are all reduced. Technically, the surgeries are not difficult to perform. A surgeon's existing skill sets can be readily adapted to working through a tubular retractor. Surgery can be performed in the same or a shorter time as traditional open procedures. The techniques can be applied to the entire spinal axis and for the treatment of multiple pathologies. The cost of performing the surgery is not significantly more than that of open surgery, and if one factors in the savings from the reduced need for hospitalization, it may even be less. The complication rate is similar to that of open techniques. Finally, a surgeon can "get the job done" using tubular retractors. Of all the procedures discussed, tubular retractor–based approaches are the only ones that satisfy all our criteria for being truly effective minimally invasive procedures (*Table 10.1*).

CONCLUSIONS

As time evolves, it is becoming increasingly clear that more can be done through less of an incision than was ever imagined to be possible. When is less more in spine surgery? For the surgeon, it means initially investing more time to learn and master the techniques necessary for performing spinal surgery through lesser incisions. Some surgeons have reduced their learning curve by using the operating microscope and tubular retractors instead of the endoscope. The 30° an-

TABLE 10.1
Comparison of the Various Minimally Invasive Spinal Procedures with the Criteria for "Doing More with Less"

	CHMN	APD	LD	ARD	IDET	MED
Minimally invasive	X	X	X	X	X	X
Technique	X	X	X		X	X
Operative time	X	X	X	X	X	X
Diversity						X
Cost	X	X		X	X	X
"Get job done"						X
Complications	X	X	X	X	X	X

X = yes, CHMN = chemonucleolysis, APD = automated percutaneous discectomy, LD = laser discectomy, IDET = intradiscal electrothermy, MED = microendoscopic discectomy.

gle on the endoscope and its proximity to the operative site, however, offer distinct advantages over the microscope, which, in our opinion, allows the surgeon to do more in less space. For the patient, less tissue destruction, less intraoperative blood loss, less time spent in the hospital, and less postoperative pain translate into more rapid recovery and more time spent at work or other regular activities. Finally, less disruption of spinal support structures means more normal spinal function and, ultimately, more time with a healthy, well-balanced spine despite having had spinal surgery.

REFERENCES

1. Adamson TE: Microendoscopic posterior cervical laminoforaminotomy for unilateral radiculopathy: results of a new technique in 100 cases. **J Neurosurg** 95:51–57, 2001.
2. Alexander AH, Burkus JK, Mitchell JB, Ayers WV: Chymopapain chemonucleolysis versus surgical discectomy in a military population. **Clin Orthop** 244:158–165, 1989.
3. Bonaldi G, Belloni G, Prosetti D, Moschini L: Percutaneous discectomy using Onik's method: 3 years' experience. **Neuroradiology** 33:516–519, 1991.
4. Bouillet R: Treatment of sciatica. A comparative survey of complications of surgical treatment and nucleolysis with chymopapain. **Clin Orthop** 251:144–152, 1990.
5. Brown MD, Tompkins JS: Pain response post-chemonucleolysis or disc excision. **Spine** 14:321–326, 1989.
6. Castro WH, Jerosch J, Hepp R, Schulitz KP: Restriction of indication for automated percutaneous lumbar discectomy based on computed tomographic discography. **Spine** 17:1239–1243, 1992.
7. Davis GW, Onik G, Helms C: Automated percutaneous discectomy. **Spine** 16:359–363, 1991.
8. Davis JK: Early experience with laser disc decompression. A percutaneous method. **J Fla Med Assoc** 79:37–39, 1992.
9. Faubert C, Caspar W: Lumbar percutaneous discectomy. Initial experience in 28 cases. **Neuroradiology** 33:407–410, 1991.
10. Fessler RG, Khoo LT: Minimally invasive cervical microendoscopic foraminotomy: An initial clinical experience. **Neurosurgery** 51:37–45, 2002.
11. Foley K, Smith M: Microendoscopic discectomy. **Tech Neurosurg** 3:301–307, 1997.
12. Guiot BH, Khoo LT, Fessler RG: A minimally invasive technique for decompression of the lumbar spine. **Spine** 27:432–438, 2002.
13. Hoffman RM, Wheeler KJ, Deyo RA: Surgery for herniated lumbar discs: A literature synthesis. **J Gen Intern Med** 8:487–496, 1993.
14. Kahanovitz N, Viola K, Goldstein T, Dawson E: A multicenter analysis of percutaneous discectomy. **Spine** 15:713–715, 1990.
15. Kambin P: Arthroscopic microdiscectomy. **Arthroscopy** 8:287–295, 1992.
16. Karasek M, Bogduk N: Twelve-month follow-up of a controlled trial of intradiscal thermal anuloplasty for back pain due to internal disc disruption. **Spine** 25:2601–2607, 2000.
17. Khoo LT, Fessler RG: Microendoscopic decompressive laminotomy for the treatment of lumbar stenosis. **Neurosurgery** 51:146–154, 2002.
18. Maroon JC, Onik G, Vidovich DV: Percutaneous discectomy for lumbar disc herniation. **Neurosurg Clin N Am** 4:125–134, 1993.

19. Mayer HM, Brock M: Percutaneous endoscopic discectomy: surgical technique and preliminary results compared to microsurgical discectomy. **J Neurosurg** 78:216–225, 1993.
20. Onik G, Mooney V, Maroon JC, et al.: Automated percutaneous discectomy: A prospective multi-institutional study. **Neurosurgery** 26:228–223, 1990.
21. Perez-Cruet MJ, Foley KT, Isaacs RE, et al.: Microendoscopic lumbar discectomy: Technical note. **Neurosurgery** 51:129–136, 2002.
22. Revel M, Payan C, Vallee C, et al.: Automated percutaneous lumbar discectomy versus chemonucleolysis in the treatment of sciatica. A randomized multicenter trial. **Spine** 18:1–7, 1993.
23. Saal JA, Saal JS: Intradiscal electrothermal treatment for chronic discogenic low back pain: A prospective outcome study with minimum 1-year follow-up. **Spine** 25:2622–2627, 2000.
24. Sherk HH, Black J, Rhodes A, Lane G, Prodoehl J: Laser discectomy. **Clin Sports Med** 12:569–577, 1993.
25. Van Alphen HA, Braakman R, Bezemer PD, Broere G, Berfelo MW: Chemonucleolysis versus discectomy: A randomized multicenter trial. **J Neurosurg** 70:869–875, 1989.
26. Watts C, Hutchison G, Stern J, Clark K: Comparison of intervertebral disc disease treatment by chymopapain injection and open surgery. **J Neurosurg** 42:397–400, 1975.
27. Zeiger HE Jr: Comparison of chemonucleolysis and microsurgical discectomy for the treatment of herniated lumbar disc. **Spine** 12:796–799, 1987.

CHAPTER

11

Spinal Deformity: The Role of the Neurosurgeon

STEPHEN L. ONDRA, M.D.

INTRODUCTION

The spine is the most complex biomechanical structure in the body. It is unique in its intimate relationships between neurological structures and mobile bony anatomy. Despite this elegant complexity, for decades neurosurgery looked at the spine as a simple bony case for the spinal cord and nerve roots. Little attention was paid to the relationship of the bony and soft-tissue structures or to how they related to function, disease, and pain.

The relationship of spine anatomy to axial pain and global mechanical function was largely left to other specialties to investigate. The major breakthroughs during the last half of the twentieth century in spine bony and soft-tissue research occurred primarily in the realm of orthopedics. Neurosurgery focused its attention on problems of neural element injury and disease.

This artificial division completely ignored the reality that disease and treatment of one component of the spine always has an impact on both. Optimum treatment requires a clear understanding of the spine's entire anatomic and biomechanical composition and relationships. This includes both the axial and appendicular skeletal functional and biomechanical relationships.

This division also left neurosurgery in the precarious position of not being a leader in the revolution that occurred during the 1970s and 1980s regarding spine biomechanics and reconstruction. This fundamental transformation in the treatment of spine disease threatened to leave our field in its wake. Because spine disease composes 60% to 70% of our field, the consequences could have been catastrophic.

During this time, visionary leaders recognized the gap. Through their efforts, neurosurgery began to participate in the latest thought and development regarding spine surgery and disease. They kept our specialty meaningful in the debate by making contributions to the field.

This effort held the door open for our specialty to participate in the full spectrum of spine disease, its treatment, and research.

Spine disease is a spectrum of problems. As a spectrum, it is not easy—or often appropriate—to put boundaries on treatment. When one thinks of spinal deformity, the disease that invariably comes to mind is adolescent idiopathic scoliosis. This is an important component of spinal deformity, but it is also a small portion of a spectrum of diseases that result in alteration of the normal relationships and alignment of the spine in the coronal, axial, and sagittal planes. The heart of spinal deformity research and treatment lies in the understanding of spinal balance and how deformation of that balance is compensated. This discipline examines how normal compensation places stress on spine anatomy, compensating skeletal structures and associated neurological structures. The field of spinal deformity studies reconstruction of the spine and it's effect on balance and function. Lastly, there are groups of diseases, ranging from neurological conditions to primary bone diseases, that create spinal deformity and affect its treatment.

Any surgeon treating patients with spine disease will have a more full understanding of the patient's condition and treatment implications if that surgeon also has a full appreciation of the concepts and issues regarding spinal balance. Because spinal deformity is at the cutting edge of this study, it is essential that our specialty be educated in these principles and participate in their study.

SAGITTAL BALANCE AND THE TREATMENT OF DISEASE

Spine diseases that results in problems of sagittal balance are the most common group of problems encountered by the spine surgeon. Sagittal balance can be thought of in local, regional, spinal, or global terms (2, 3). It is simply the relationship of the spine along a plumb line dropped from the first cervical vertebra. This line should pass through each normal curve of the spine at its inflection to another curve (C1, T1, L1, and S1). Additionally, there are known normative relationships within a curve. When a local or regional curve becomes diseased, it may lose its normal curvature (8), which will result in a loss of sagittal balance. A line falling anterior to the sacrum is considered to be a positive sagittal balance; a line falling posterior is considered to be a negative sagittal balance. Both are pathologic.

When the normal sagittal relationship is lost, the plumb line will shift in front of or in back of the pelvic axis. This results in a functional disorder in which standing posture and gait are disturbed. This relationship of the spine to the pelvis defines the concept of global spinal balance. To correct imbalance, a variety of compensatory mechanisms are available. With a loss of lordosis in the cervical or lumbar spine, the first compensatory mechanism is simply to extend adjacent segments in the region. This will bring the plumb line back in line over the posterior superior edge of the S1 end plate. It will also result in closing of the formaninal and spinal canal cross-section. This can be a potential problem in an already stenotic spine. It also adds strain to the facets, their capsules, and associated ligaments (6, 9). Extensor muscle strain is also created by the need for an actively maintained sustained posture. This ligamentous strain can result in back pain.

When regional correction will not fully compensate, global mechanisms can be employed. Other regional curves can be altered, and the appendicular skeleton will change posture. These latter mechanisms become increasingly common in the aging rigid spine. Hip and knee flexion are two of the most common. This requires immense effort and energy consumption. It also profoundly affects gait and function and can result in excessive wear and disease in the hips, knees, and ankles.

It should be apparent how important the issues of sagittal balance are in understanding a patient's disease and treatment, but the question that is often brought up is whether these issues are relevant to most neurosurgical practices. The answer can be found by looking at some of our most common problems and their treatment.

The lumbar disc asymmetry creates 80% of the lumbar lordosis (2, 3). Two thirds of that lordosis exists between L4 and S1, the location of most diseases treated by neurosurgeons. Most diseases will then have some effect on sagittal balance. At what point, however, does degenerative disc disease change from a simple problem of local pain to a regional problem of loss of lordosis or flat back? When does this become a global problem of a sagitally decompensated spine (*Figs. 11.1 through 11.5 and 11.7*).

A laminectomy results in a loss of 20% of the spine's tension band resistance to flexion (1, 6, 11). If the patient already has a strain created on the tension band by a positive sagittal balance, the result can be further decompensation and pain. A worse situation is to fuse that patient in a decompensated position or flat back. This can occur from poor positioning that did not preserve lordosis. It can also result from implants that eliminate the discs' normal contour. The placement of nonlordotic interbody devices must be carefully weighed against what they will do in terms of the sagittal contour of the spine. Appreciation of the importance of such a contour can result in better implant choice to maintain or improve lordosis and sagittal contour. The most un-

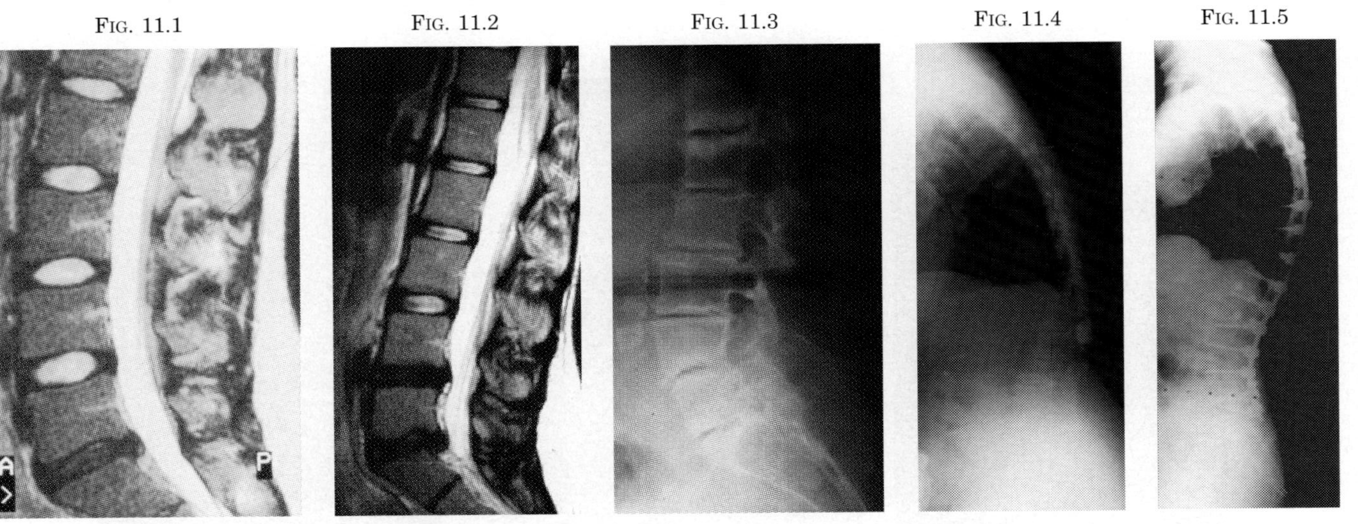

FIG. 11.1 FIG. 11.2 FIG. 11.3 FIG. 11.4 FIG. 11.5

FIGS. 11.1–11.5 *Figure 11.1* demonstrates a degenerative lumbar disc at L5-S1. Note the subtle but clear loss of segmental lordosis. *Figure 11.2* is a patient with two-segment disease associated with a more profound loss of sagittal contour. *Figure 11.3* is a multisegment disc degeneration with a complete loss of lumbar lordosis. *Figure 11.4* has a complete sagittal decompensation with severe back pain and a profound loss of functional ability. *Figure 11.5* demonstrates the patient's reconstruction with profound improvement in both back pain and function.

FIG. 11.6 FIG. 11.7 FIG. 11.8

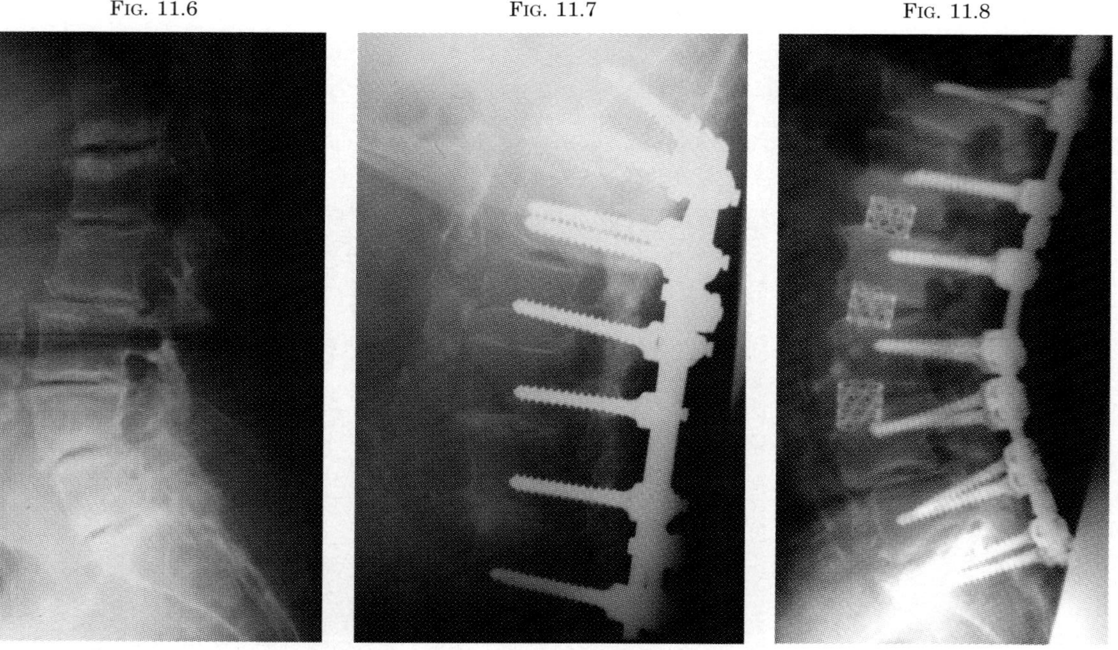

FIGS. 11.6–11.8 *Figure 11.6* is a patient with a complete loss of lumbar lordosis because of degenerative disease and a loss of sagittal balance. His original surgery, seen in *Figure 11.7*, resulted in a fusion but no sagittal correction. This left him fully decompensated and painful. Sagittal correction, shown in *Figure 11.8*, resulted in decreased pain and improved functional ambulation.

fortunate of circumstance arises from poor design. Long-segment constructs that reduce lordosis also limit sagittal balance and the ability to compensate. Attempts to compensate at the rigid spine create large cantilever forces that strain soft tissues and the spinal pelvic junctions (4, 9).

This iatrogenic flat back results in the need for skeletal compensation, postural imbalance, and gait dysfunction—as well as a profoundly unhappy patient. Correction of this is possible but demanding on both the patient and the surgeon (*Figs. 11.6 through 11.8*).

Patients with degenerative progression invariably have a loss of lumbar lordosis or a thoracolumbar junction kyphosis. Fusion in these patients must account for this kyphotic deformity, or they will invariably develop an iatrogenic, debilitating flat back.

TENSION BAND RESISTANCE AND SAGITTAL BALANCE

Equally dramatic examples exist in the cervical spine. Laminectomy in children results in a kyphosis rate of 38% to 90% depending of the level of tension band loss, patient age, and neurological function (1, 11). In adults, the cervical kyphosis rate is quoted at 11% to 17% (1, 11). Such a kyphosis results in pain, skeletal imbalance, and spinal cord stretch over the kyphotic segments. If kyphosis exists before treatment or is predictable as a result of treatment, correction should be considered. Patients who develop profound spinal deformity can undergo successful treatment, correction, and stabilization. Prevention of the occurrence of a predictable kyphosis is always preferable.

An example of how cervical and cervical thoracic junction deformity can affect global balance and function is seen in this patient with kyphosis that results in a positive sagittal balance (*Figs. 11.9 through 11.11*). This patient compensated by hyperlordosing her already degenerative lumbar spine, resulting in back pain. Recognition of the sagittal deformity and its correction not only prevented further kyphosis but eliminated the compensatory hyperlordosis and associated back pain. Not recognizing this could have resulted in inappropriate low back surgery and possible worsening of symptoms.

When kyphosis has been untreated and continues to progress, it can result in severe skeletal and neurological deterioration. Although correction of this is daunting, it is possible with acceptable results. We have treated 15 patients with profound (up to 90°) kyphosis with reduction to the neutral or lordotic position. In that group, we have had no paralysis as a result of surgical intervention, though one patient did have a paralysis as a result of equipment malfunction in the head-holding device. One patient had C5 unilateral motor loss. All have

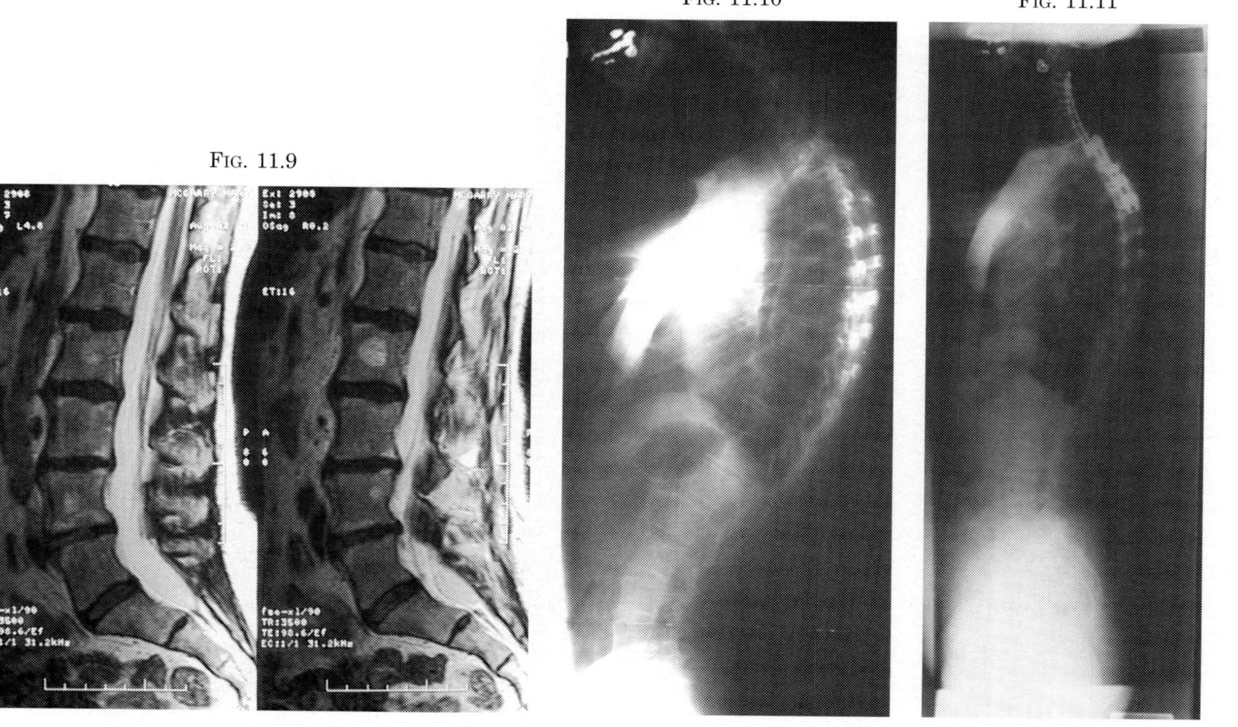

FIG. 11.9

FIG. 11.10

FIG. 11.11

FIGS. 11.9–11.11 This patient presented with low back pain, intermittent radiculopathy, and the MR image seen in *Figure 11.9*. *Figure 11.10* demonstrates the importance of scoliosis films to fully understand the global spine. It shows a cervical thoracic junctional kyphosis and lumbar hyperlordosis to compensate. This led to the correction of the cervical thoracic kyphosis. Elimination of the painful compensatory behavior, seen in *Figure 11.11*, also eliminated the back and leg pain.

maintained correction, and as of this writing, there has been no late neurological deterioration.

CORONAL IMBALANCE AND SPINE DISEASE TREATMENT

Coronal imbalance is the classic association with spinal deformity and scoliosis. Again, there is a spectrum of disease, from a patient with degenerative scoliosis to an infant or adolescent with idiopathic, congenital, or neuromuscular scoliosis.

Pediatric neurosurgeons often encounter scoliosis as a result of congenital abnormalities, such as tethered cord, myelomeningocele, diastemametamyelia, or neuromuscular diseases (5). It is important for the pediatric neurological surgeon to fully understand the skeletal implications of disease and treatment. A comprehensive treatment plan can then be developed and, when necessary, the skeletal deformity treated. All too often, such children are lost to follow up until they are profoundly deformed and correction an arduous process.

Adult spine surgeons frequently encounter degenerative lumbar spinal deformity. Such deformity has a more powerful effect per degree on coronal balance than most pediatric disease simply because of the more caudal location of the curve. The impact of a degree of coronal deviation doubles for every 10 cm that curve is distant from the C7 plumb line. In children, the structural curve is typically limited to the thoracic spine, allowing for lumbar compensation. As a result, the coronal decompensation is often minimal. In adults, the lumbar curve is typically both structural and the major curve. In this case, coronal decompensation can be profound. This can result in the hips and knees having to compensate and often in asymmetric pressure and wear.

For these reasons, appreciation and, when necessary, correction of coronal deformity in adults is necessary. This can be done even in the elderly spine. We have treated more than 60 patients older than 60 years with advanced adult scoliosis. Independently reviewed 2-year follow-up data are available on 25 of these patients. The average age is 70 years, with a range of 62 to 78 years. All achieved correction of coronal and sagittal imbalance. Good to excellent outcomes were achieved in 80% of patients when scored by an independent observer. Pain scores decreased by 51%, and 40% of patients eliminated all narcotic pain medication. The complication rate was a daunting 110%, but most were self-limited. Surprisingly, no deaths or neurological injury occurred in this group despite the extensive nature of the surgery. These results are comparable with those other series in the literature dealing with adult scoliosis (4, 7, 10). The age distribution is by far

FIG. 11.12 FIG. 11.13 FIG. 11.14 FIG. 11.15

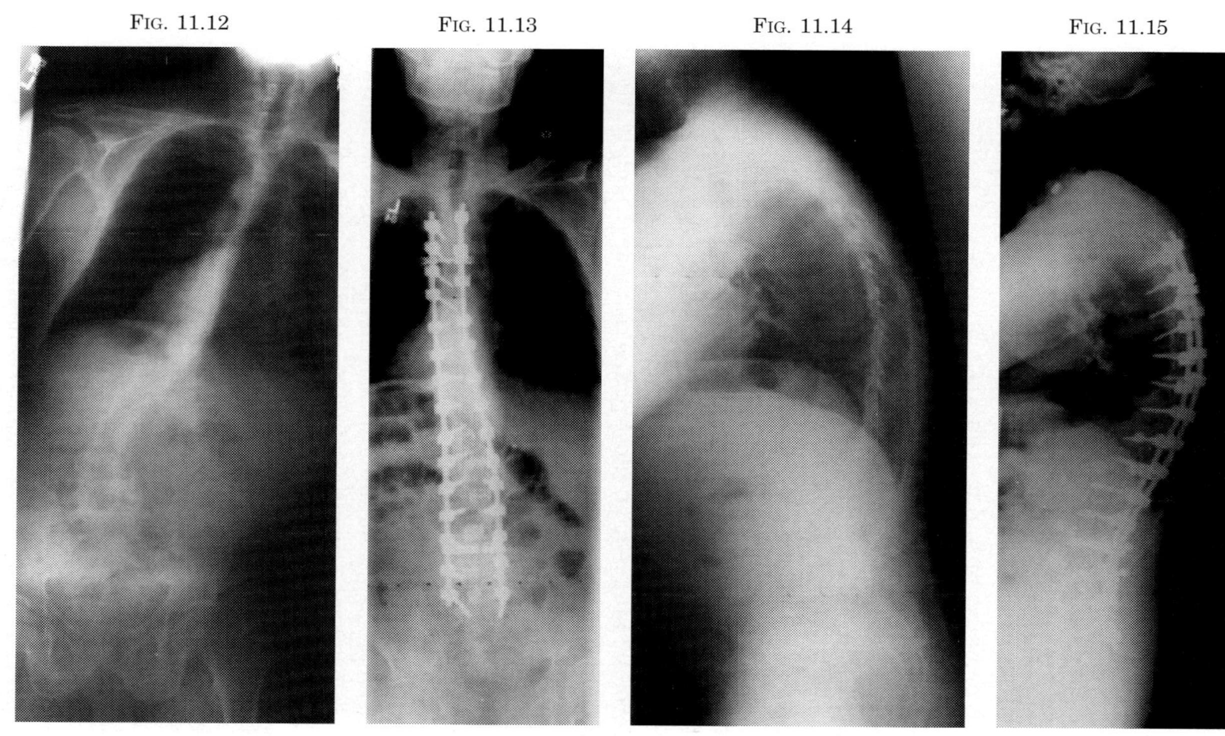

FIGS. 11.12–11.15 *Figures 11.12* and *11.14* demonstrate full coronal and sagittal decompensation because of adult degenerative scoliosis. *Figures 11.13* and *11.15* demonstrate reconstruction in both the coronal and sagittal planes.

the oldest, demonstrating that in a properly selected patient with expected longevity, age is not an absolute barrier. These results are also comparable in terms of success rates for other spine procedures (*Figs.11.12 through 11.15*).

THE NEUROSURGEON AND SPINE SURGERY IN THE FUTURE

What, then, is neurosurgery's role in spinal deformity? As surgeons, it is our responsibility to embrace and understand the principles of spinal deformity to help us better analyze and treat our patients. We also have a responsibility to bring our unique expertise and perspective to the treatment of the full spectrum of deforming spine disease.

Neurosurgeons have a unique understanding and comfort in working with neurological structures. This expertise can translate into better treatment of spinal deformity in the cervical spine. The issues of spinal balance and their correction, however, have received little attention in the cervical spine. Thus, treatment of such conditions as cervical scoliosis remain primitive and limited. The application of principles of correction such as pedicle subtraction have had limited use beyond the lumbar spine.

Adolescent idiopathic scoliosis is generally recognized as an autosomal dominant disease. Its pathophysiology remains obscure, but both the pineal gland and brain stem dysfunction have been implicated as possible mechanisms. Neurosurgeons have a chance to contribute to the fundamental understanding of this group of diseases.

We can add our experience and creativity, ranging from minimal access surgery to the coming revolution of prosthetics and biological modifiers, to change the face of spinal deformity surgery.

Most neurosurgeons will treat tumors and vascular disease of the brain; few will treat the most advanced disease states. This requires specialized training and the dedication of a subspecialist. Despite this, all neurosurgeons learn and improve their level of care by what is discovered in the treatment of these extreme disorders. The same is true of spinal deformity. Not all neurological spine surgeons will choose to treat deformity or other advanced areas of disease and care. All of us, however, will benefit from the body of knowledge that is acquired by the care of such disease and its addition to our specialty's training programs, fellowships, and continuing medical education.

In the end, the neurosurgeon's role in spinal deformity is as a physician, surgeon, and investigator to advance our understanding and to improve the care of all patients with spine disease.

REFERENCES

1. Bell DF, Walker JL, O'Connor G, Tibshironi R: Spinal deformity after multilevel cervical laminectomy in children. **Spine** 19:406, 1994.
2. Bernhardt M, Bridwell KH: Segmental analysis of the sagittal plane alignment of the normal thoracic and lumbar spine and thoracolumbar junction. **Spine** 14:717, 1989.
3. Jackson RP, McManus AC: Radiographic analysis of sagittal plane alignment and balance in standing volunteers and patients with low back pain matched for age, sex, and size: prospective controlled clinical study. **Spine** 14:1611, 1994.
4. Kostuik JP: Treatment of scoliosis in the adult thoracolumbar spine with special reference of fusion to the sacrum. **Orthop Clin North Am** 19:371, 1988.
5. Park TS, Coil WS, Maggio WM, Mithcell DC: Progressive spasticity and scoliosis in children with myelomeningocele. **J Neurosurgery** 62:367, 1985.
6. Shirazi Adl, Drovin G: Load bearing role of facets in a lumbar segment under sagittal loadings. **J Biomech** 20:601, 1987.
7. Swank S, Lonstein JE, Moe J, Bradford DS: Surgical treatment of adult scoliosis. A review of 222 cases. **J Bone Joint Surg** 63:268, 1981.
8. Wambolt A, Spencer DL: A segmental analysis of the distribution of lumbar lordosis in the normal spine. **Orthop Trans** 11:92, 1987.
9. White AA, Panjabi MM: *Clinical Biomechanics of the Spine.* Philadelphia: JB Lippincott, 1978.
10. Van Dam BE, Bradford DS, Lonstein JE, et al.: Adult idiopathic scoliosis treated by posterior spinal fusion. **Spine** 12:32, 1987.
11. Yasuoka S, Peterson HA, MacCarty CS: Incidence of spinal column deformity after multilevel laminectomy in children and adults. **J Neurosurg** 57:441, 1982.

CHAPTER

12

Development of Evidence-Based Guidelines for the Management of Acute Spine and Spinal Cord Injuries

BEVERLY C. WALTERS, M.D., AND MARK N. HADLEY, M.D.

One of the most successful enterprises of organized neurosurgery is the completion and publication of the *Guidelines for the Management of Severe Head Injury*. A joint project of the American Association of Neurological Surgeons (AANS), including the Section on Neurotrauma and Critical Care of the AANS and the Congress of Neurological Surgeons (CNS), and the Brain Trauma Foundation, these evidence-based guidelines were published for the profession in 1995 and then in the peer-reviewed medical literature in 1996 and again in 2000 (1, 2). The success of clinical application of the *Guidelines* in improving the outcomes of patients afflicted with severe nonpenetrating brain injury has been shown in several publications (3–5). Other guidelines in neurotrauma have been published (e.g., penetrating brain injury [6]) or are in the process of publication (e.g., surgical management of brain injury, pediatric brain injury). More recently, a large-scale effort to provide *Guidelines for the Treatment of Acute Cervical Spine and Spinal Cord Injuries* was sponsored by the Section on Disorders of the Spine and Peripheral Nerves of the AANS and the CNS. The various rationales behind the choice of spinal cord injury as a significant topic for guideline development included the facts that this entity represents a significant societal health care burden, that the patients are generally young and at the peak or beginning of their productivity, and that their outcomes are severe in terms of functional disability. In addition, several areas were identified as controversial, with a considerable amount of conflicting literature. It was felt that neurosurgeons were ideally positioned to lead this effort, because the specialty is the one that is most involved with the entire spectrum of acute spinal cord injury care, both operative and nonoperative. The product of this venture was extensively peer-reviewed and presented in *Neurosurgery* as a special supplement, marking the first time that such guidelines have been published in a neurosurgical subspecialty publication (7).

These guidelines followed the same evidence-based principles as extolled in the landmark publication on severe head injury. In this model, evidence from the medical literature is gathered and critically evaluated regarding both type and quality. The concept behind this process is to reflect the strength of the extant scientific evidence with recommendations of varying strength. The best scientific evidence is that derived from well-designed, randomized, controlled trials (exemplifying true human experimentation), with lesser clinical studies, such as case-control studies or nonrandomized comparative studies, resulting in lesser recommendations. The more common case series or observational studies are relegated to the type of recommendation that carries the least weight (in the same category as expert opinion). In a fashion embraced by the American Medical Association and formalized as policy by the parent neurosurgical organizations, evidence is designated as indicated in the summary in *Table 12.1*.

Guideline development in organized neurosurgery follows the recommendations given by the Institute of Medicine, and summarized previously, as indicated below (8):

1. There should be a link between the available evidence and the recommendations.
2. Empirical evidence should take precedence over expert judgment in the development of guidelines.
3. The available scientific literature should be searched using appropriate and comprehensive search terminology.
4. A thorough review of the scientific literature should precede guideline development.
5. The evidence should be evaluated and weighted depending upon the scientific validity of the methodology used to generate the evidence.

TABLE 12.1
Levels of Evidence for Studies of Therapeutic Effectiveness

Evidence Class	Source of Evidence
Class I	Evidence from one or more well-designed, randomized, controlled clinical trials, including overviews of such trials.
Class II	Evidence from one or more well-designed, comparative clinical studies, such as nonrandomized cohort studies, case-control studies, and other comparable studies.
Class III	Evidence from case series, comparative studies with historical controls, case reports, and expert opinion.

6. The strength of the evidence should be reflected in the strength of the recommendations, thus reflecting scientific certainty (or lack thereof).
7. Expert judgment should be used to evaluate the quality of the literature and to formulate guidelines when the evidence is weak or nonexistent.
8. Guideline development should be a multidisciplinary process, involving key groups affected by the recommendations.

Following the conceptual underpinnings of the guidelines process, there is the implementation of the process itself. The first necessary aspect is the commitment of a specialty group to invest the necessary resources—time, money, and energy—in the effort. In this case, the Section on Disorders of the Spine and Peripheral Nerves of the AANS and the CNS provided parental sponsorship and fiscal support. Next comes the choice of the author group, which should include specialists and subspecialists in the topic chosen for review. Then, scheduled meetings of the guideline author group occur, involving intensive work sessions in which the clinical questions are articulated from the general topic to be reviewed. An example of the process from the *Guidelines for the Management of Acute Spine and Spinal Cord Injuries* would be "Should methylprednisolone be given to patients with spinal cord injury to improve patient functional outcome?" Each of the recommendations in the final document began with a clinical question of this nature.

The next step is to search the pertinent medical literature, a task that has been made much more thorough in a shorter period of time by using high-speed Internet connections through personal computers. Searching the National Library of Medicine's MEDLINE database, a large number of potential articles can be located and their abstracts reviewed for relevancy to the topic at hand. In most guideline efforts, studies pertaining to humans alone are cited as justification for the ultimate recommendations, with animal or in vitro studies providing the biological background for the proposed management stratagem. In addition, most recommendations in American medicine come from literature found in English language–only publications. Although this may limit the recommendations, most studies done in other countries and originally published in foreign languages are ultimately found in the English-language literature. When this is not the case, these studies are usually referenced in reviews and other English-language publications. In addition, translation time and expense usually inhibit full use of the worldwide literature. This may be a weakness of the process as instigated in American efforts, but a decision was made in this instance to limit searches to the English-language literature in the interests of both time and fiscal restraints.

Once the search has been completed, the abstracts are reviewed for appropriateness to the clinical question at hand. Each paper that has passed through the "abstract filter" is obtained and examined carefully by the author group regarding type of study (e.g., diagnosis, clinical assessment, or therapeutic effectiveness), and its quality is assessed using standard, stringent clinical epidemiologic criteria. In addition to the levels of evidence assigned for the literature on therapeutic effectiveness indicated in *Table 12.1*, additional criteria were established for the task of creating the *Guidelines for the Management of Acute Spine and Spinal Cord Injuries*, including diagnostic tests (e.g., clearance of the cervical spine in trauma) and clinical assessment (i.e., initial and ultimate condition of the patient with spine injury).

The criteria for diagnostic tests are based upon the studies examined having included enough patients with possible injury (i.e., patients in trauma consistent with the production of spinal injury) and without injury and having been conducted and compared to a "gold standard" reference test indicating the presence or absence of the suspected injury. These criteria have been formalized previously and are illustrated in *Tables 12.2 and 12.3* and *Figure 12.1* (9).

The criteria for classification of evidence on clinical assessment were also devised for the purposes of these guidelines. This was undertaken using the well-established criteria of clinical epidemiologists that revolve around the fact that clinical assessment is carried out by humans interpreting their observations and that different observers may interpret their observations differently. It is essential to have reliability of the assessment both from observer to observer and from observation to observation by the same observer on different occasions. Clearly, some agreement will occur between observers and observations by chance alone. Therefore, reliability must be measured *beyond chance*. This is accomplished through a statistical technique called the "kappa (κ) statistic." This statistic takes into account what agreement you would expect to find versus the observed agreement (10). To understand the calculation for κ, the Bayesian 2×2 table can once again be employed. This is illustrated in *Figures 12.2 and 12.3.*

A value relationship for the κ scores has been proposed and was used in the *Guidelines* document. The strength of agreement for a κ of 0.81 to 1.00 has been considered to be "almost perfect," of 0.61 to 0.80 to be "substantial," and of 0.41 to 0.60 to be "moderate" agreement. Agreement below 0.41 is graded from fair to poor. Therefore, the classification of evidence on clinical assessment into the class I,

TABLE 12.2
Formulae for Calculating Accuracy of Diagnostic Tests

Test Feature	Formula[a]	Clinical Question
Sensitivity	$a/a + c$	If a patient has a positive radiograph, how likely is the patient to have a C-spine injury?
Specificity	$d/b + d$	If a patient has a negative radiograph, how likely is the patient to not have a C-spine injury?
Positive predictive value	$a/a + b$	If a patient has a C-spine injury, how likely is the patient to have a positive test?
Negative predictive value	$d/c + d$	If a patient does not have a C-spine injury, how likely is the patient to have a negative test?
Accuracy	$a + d/a + b + c + d$	What is the overall accuracy of the test?

[a]Variables are as defined in *Figure 12.1.*

II, and III paradigm was carried out using the criteria outlined in *Table 12.4* in an attempt to relate reliability performance to strength of recommendations.

Once the levels of evidence were determined, depending upon the type of study reviewed (i.e., therapy, diagnosis, or clinical assessment), each paper was classified into class I, II, and III. These were placed

		GOLD STANDARD		
		Patient has injury	Patient has no injury	
TEST RESULT:	Positive: Appears to have injury	TRUE POSITIVE (a)	FALSE POSITIVE (b)	(a) + (b)
C-SPINE FILM	Negative: Appears to have no injury	FALSE NEGATIVE (c)	TRUE NEGATIVE (d)	(c) + (d)
		(a) + (c)	(b) + (d)	(a) + (b) + (c) + (d)

FIG. 12.1 Bayesian table for calculating the attributes of diagnostic test literature.

TABLE 12.3
Levels of Evidence for Studies of Diagnostic Test Accuracy

Evidence Class	Source of Evidence
Class I	Evidence provided by one or more well-designed, clinical studies of a diverse population using a "gold standard" reference test in a blinded evaluation appropriate for the diagnostic applications and enabling assessment of sensitivity, specificity, positive predictive value, negative predictive value, and when appropriate, likelihood ratio.
Class II	Evidence provided by one or more well-designed, clinical studies of a restricted population using a "gold standard" reference test in a blinded evaluation appropriate for the diagnostic applications and enabling assessment of sensitivity, specificity, positive predictive value, negative predictive value, and when appropriate, likelihood ratio.
Class III	Evidence provided by expert opinion or studies that do not meet the criteria for the delineation of sensitivity, specificity, positive predictive value, negative predictive value, and when appropriate, likelihood ratio.

		Observer #1		
		YES	NO	
Observer #2	YES	AGREE (a)	DISAGREE (b)	(a) + (b) = f_1
	NO	DISAGREE (c)	AGREE (d)	(c) + (d) = f_2
		(a) + (c) = n_1	(b) + (d) = n_2	(a) + (b) + (c) + (d) = N

FIG. 12.2 Bayesian table for calculating κ.

$$\kappa = \frac{N(a + d) - (n_1 f_1 + n_2 f_2)}{N^2 - (n_1 f_1 + n_2 f_2)} \quad \text{or} \quad \kappa = \frac{2(ad - bc)}{(n_1 f_1 + n_2 f_2)}$$

FIG. 12.3 Formula for calculating κ from the Bayesian table. Variables are as defined in *Figure 12.2*.

TABLE 12.4
Levels of Evidence for Studies of Clinical Assessment

Evidence Class	Source of Evidence
Class I	Evidence provided by one or more well-designed, clinical studies in which interobserver and intraobserver reliability are represented by a κ statistic of 0.60 or greater
Class II	Evidence provided by one or more well-designed, clinical studies in which interobserver and intraobserver reliability are represented by a κ statistic of 0.40 or greater
Class III	Evidence provided by one or more well-designed, clinical studies in which interobserver and intraobserver reliability are represented by a κ statistic of less than 0.40

in evidentiary tables that showed the main thrust of the paper and its relative strength. These papers were then used to generate recommendations at a standard, guideline, or option level based upon the presence of class I, II, or III studies.

The topics covered included general issues, such as immobilization before hospital admission; transport recommendations; clinical assessment of the patient with spinal cord injury, both initially and ultimately at last time of follow up; radiographic assessment; closed reduction of fracture-dislocation injuries; and intensive care unit management, including blood pressure management, pharmacologic therapy, deep-vein thrombosis prophylaxis and treatment, and nutritional support. Detailed recommendations for individual types of injuries were painstakingly generated, including treatment of spinal cord injury without radiographic abnormality (SCIWORA), atlanto-occipital dislocation injuries, occipital condyle fractures, isolated fractures of the atlas in adults, isolated fractures of the axis in adults, combination fractures of the atlas and asic in adults, os odontoideum, subaxial cervical spinal injuries, central cord syndrome, and vertebral artery injuries. Pediatric cervical spine and spinal cord injuries were treated separately.

This comprehensive coverage of the topic of acute spine and spinal cord injuries involved the review of more than 845 publications and yielded 85 recommendations in 22 topics. The literature was not distinguished by many class I or II studies; therefore, only six practice standards and seven guidelines were generated. The remaining 72 recommendations were at a practice-option level derived from class III studies. The six practice standards included the following:

1. Radiographic assessment of the cervical spine is not recommended in trauma patients who are awake, alert, and not intoxicated; who are without neck pain or tenderness; and who do not have significant associated injuries that detract from their general evaluation.

2. A three-view cervical spine series (anteroposterior, lateral, and odontoid views) is recommended for radiographic evaluation of the cervical spine in patients who are symptomatic after traumatic injury.
3. Three-view cervical spine films should be supplemented with CT scans to further define areas that are suspicious or not well visualized on the plain cervical radiographs.
4. Prophylactic treatment of thromboembolism in patients with severe motor deficits because of spinal cord injury is recommended.
5. Use of low-molecular-weight heparins, rotating beds, adjusted-dose heparin, or a combination of modalities is recommended as a prophylactic treatment strategy.
6. Low-dose heparin in combination with pneumatic compression stockings or electrical stimulation is recommended as a prophylactic treatment strategy.

The guidelines, based upon class II evidence, included the following:

1. The Functional Independence Measure (FIM) is recommended as the functional outcome assessment tool for clinicians involved in the assessment and care of patients with acute spinal cord injuries.
2. Low-dose heparin therapy alone is not recommended as a prophylactic treatment strategy for deep-vein thrombosis.
3. Oral anticoagulation alone is not recommended as a prophylactic treatment strategy for deep-vein thrombosis.
4. In children who have experienced trauma and are alert; conversant; have no neurological deficit, no midline cervical tenderness, and no painful distracting injury; and are not intoxicated, cervical spine radiographs are not necessary to exclude cervical spine injury and are not recommended.
5. In children who have experienced trauma and who are not alert or nonconversant or have neurological deficit, midline cervical tenderness, or painful distracting injury or are intoxicated, it is recommended that anteroposterior and lateral cervical spine radiographs be obtained.
6. CT scanning is recommended for establishing the diagnosis of occipital condyle fractures. Clinical suspicion should be raised by the presence of one or more of the following criteria: patients with blunt trauma sustaining high-energy craniocervical injuries, altered consciousness, occipital pain or tenderness, impaired cervical motion, lower cranial nerve paresis, or retropharyngeal soft-tissue swelling.
7. Type II odontoid fractures in patients 50 years and older should be considered for surgical stabilization and fusion.

Of interest, no standard—and only one guideline—was generated regarding the operative care of acute spine and spinal cord injury, namely that of dealing with type II odontoid fractures. All other operative recommendations were made at the level of practice options, indicating the dearth of high-quality scientific literature regarding direct surgical care of these patients.

Not surprisingly, the most controversial aspect of the *Guidelines* has been the recommendations regarding pharmacologic therapy, particularly methylprednisolone in acute spinal cord injury. This is clear in the proliferation of comments published in the *Neurosurgery* volume containing the *Guidelines*. These comments represent an additional level of published peer-review aside from the extensive review provided by the guideline development process, which included review by both the Board of Directors of the AANS and the Executive Committee of the CNS, the Executive Committees of the Spine Section and Trauma Section, and the Committee of the Assessment of Quality before submission for publication. In the chapter evaluating the literature, detailed examination of the literature showed that although several randomized, controlled trials demonstrated the efficacy of methylprednisolone, considerable flaws in those studies decreased their value as supportive evidence for use. Typically, a randomized, controlled trial is considered to be a class I study, and supportive of a practice standard. However, when significant flaws are detected, such as outcome measures that are imprecise and unreliable or unrelated to long-term function (an important issue in spinal cord injury), then the "downgrading" of the trials legitimately takes place. The criticism that can be made of this process is that consensus to reduce the stature of the trial interjects a process that is a modification of the evidence-based medicine paradigm. However, from the beginning of the guideline development process, the concept of evaluation and weighting has been present and recommended by the Institute of Medicine (8). That disagreement exists in this process is inevitable, especially where vested interests are involved and firmly held beliefs are challenged.

In summary, an extensive literature review was undertaken to generate practice recommendations for neurosurgeons and others who are intimately involved in the acute care of spine and spinal cord injuries. Using evidence-based medicine concepts, this literature was evaluated for its quality and then classified accordingly. This classification process led to the development of practice recommendations meant to help clinicians treating acute spine and spinal cord injury and to improve the ultimate outcome of patients afflicted with this potentially devastating condition. Whether these recommendations will be widely adopted or useful in improving patient outcome remains to be seen.

However, before publication of the *Guidelines*, a group developed a critical pathway for the treatment of patients with spinal cord injury and found that they could improve outcome, reduce complications, and decrease costs, similar to the findings in patients with severe head injury (11). It may well be that the *Guidelines* can contribute to the frontiers of medicine in the same way.

REFERENCES

1. Bullock R, Chesnut RM, Clifton GL, et al.: Guidelines for the management of severe head injury. **J Neurotrauma** 13(2):639–734, 1996.
2. Bullock R, Chesnut RM, Clifton GL, et al.: Guidelines for the management of severe head injury. **J Neurotrauma** 17, 2000.
3. Spain DA, McIlvoy LH, Fix SE, et al.: Effect of a clinical pathway for severe traumatic brain injury on resource utilization. **J Trauma** 45(1):101–104, 1998.
4. McIlvoy L, Spain DA, Raque GH, Vitaz TW, Boaz P, Meyer K: Successful incorporation of the Severe Head Injury Guidelines into a phased-outcome clinical pathway. **J Neurosci Nurs** 33(2):72–78, 2001.
5. Vukic M, Negovetic L, Kovac D, Ghajar J, Glavic Z, Gopcevic A: The effect of implementation of guidelines for the management of severe head injury on patient treatment and outcome. **Acta Neurochir (Wien)** 141(11):1203–1208, 1999.
6. Aarabi B, Alden TD, Chesnut RM, et al.: Guidelines for the management of penetrating brain injury. **Neurosurgery** 5(suppl 2):S1–S85, 2001.
7. Hadley MN, Walters BC, Grabb PA, et al.: Guidelines for the management of acute cervical spine and spinal cord injuries. **Neurosurgery** 3(50):S1–S199, 2002.
8. Committee to Advise the Public Health Service on Clinical Practice Guidelines IoM: *Clinical Practice Guidelines: Directions for a New Program.* Washington, DC: National Academy Press, 1990.
9. Walters BC: Clinical practice parameter development in neurosurgery. In: Bean JR (ed): *Neurosurgery in Transition: The Socioeconomic Transformation of Neurological Surgery.* Baltimore: Williams & Wilkins, 1998, pp 99–111.
10. Cohen J: A coefficient of agreement for nominal scales. **Educ Psychol Meas** 20:37–46, 1960.
11. Vitaz TW, McIlvoy L, Raque GH, Spain D, Shields CB: Development and implementation of a clinical pathway for spinal cord injuries. **J Spinal Disord** 14(3):271–276, 2001.

III

General Scientific Session III Freedom to Expand the Neurosurgeon's Domain

CHAPTER

13

Freedom to Expand the Neurosurgeon's Domain: The Modern Neurovascular Team

CAMERON G. McDOUGALL, M.D.

Thank you for the honor of speaking this morning. I have been asked to discuss the modern neurovascular team within the context of this morning's theme, "Expanding the Neurosurgeon's Domain." It should become apparent from my discussion that I do not interpret the modern neurovascular team as an expansion of our domain but rather as the natural evolution of our specialty.

For those of you not yet fully awake this morning, I am going to make this very simple. It will be simple because you already know my key message. The key message is that the future of neurovascular surgery belongs to those who are willing to lead—willing to lead the way in providing uncompromising, high-quality, cost-effective patient care.

When I first began thinking about this presentation, I was hiking in the Grand Canyon. Each spring, a group of people associated with our institution spend a day hiking across the Canyon. The hike is 24 miles long. Traveling from the South Rim to the North Rim, the last 7 miles requires a vertical climb of 6,000 feet. Members of our group travel at their own pace: Some take their time and enjoy the breathtaking scenery, while others challenge themselves to cross the Canyon as quickly as they are able. This past spring, I went on the hike as I usually do. Ten or 12 miles into crossing the Canyon, it happened that I was keeping pace with three colleagues. In front was Dr. Spetzler, who is, as some of you may know, a neurovascular surgeon with a reputation for being competitive. I was immediately behind Dr. Spetzler, and close behind me was a bright young medical student. The fourth and last in our group was an acquaintance who just happens to be a cardiologist.

The Canyon is spectacularly beautiful, but traveling as I was behind Dr. Spetzler, my view was somewhat less inspiring than it might have been, and so my mind began to wander. I found myself thinking about this morning's topic. I asked myself what constitutes a neurovascular team—or any team for that matter. As we continued to run through the Canyon, I thought about the four of us and wondered "Are we a team working together with a common goal, or are we simply competitors?"

It seemed to me that the four of us were analogous with the modern neurovascular team. Currently, the classic microneurovascular surgeon leads the pack. Coming along behind are the recently created endovascular therapists, hoping to create a paradigm shift in the way neurovascular disease is managed—hoping, if you will, to see a change in the landscape. However, what is avant-garde today will be passé tomorrow. So, hot on the heels of today's revolution will come the next generation, with new ideas and technologies that are as-of-yet unimagined. And always, not far off in the background, are the other specialties. They are the dark horses in this race, coming up unexpectedly from behind. Coincidentally, they include, as in this analogy, cardiologists, who like some other colleagues we may not view as traditional participants in managing neurovascular disease but who, in some settings, see an opportunity to expand *their* domain.

Back to the neurovascular team. Who are the current players? For our purposes, which are intended to be illustrative and not comprehensive, they can be divided into the *micro* and the *macro*. Clearly, many individuals and support staff are essential to the smooth functioning of the neurovascular team. The microplayers are those who are likely to coexist within the walls of one institution. They may include neurosurgeons, neurologists, endovascular therapists, intensive care specialists, diagnostic neuroradiologists, and cardiologists.

The macroplayers include organizations large enough to affect the practice of neurovascular surgery on a scale larger than a single institution and who affect the practice of medicine as a whole (industry, payers, government).

That neurosurgeons have a preeminent role in the neurovascular team is not seriously questioned by those of us here today. The crux of our discussion is as follows: How do neurosurgeons relate to the other members of the team, and how will this team evolve in the future? The impetus for this discussion is the increasing role being played by endovascular therapists. As in most situations where major changes are occurring, there is bound to be stress, conflict, and anxiety about changes not unanimously perceived as positive. Who are the endovascular therapists? Most endovascular therapists now in practice are interventional neuroradiologists: diagnostic radiologists who have received variable amounts of fellowship training in diagnostic neuroradiology and interventional neuroradiology.

Recently, the Accreditation Council for Graduate Medical Education (ACGME) approved two fellowship pathways for training in what is to be called endovascular surgical neuroradiology (ENS). The current pathways for an individual to become certified in ENS are through neuroradiology or through neurosurgery. The potential exists for a third pathway to be developed to allow neurologists to receive training in this field. Neurosurgeons require 2 years of training, one of which may be enfolded into a neurosurgical residency. The fellowship training period for radiologists is 3 years: 1 year of diagnostic neuroradiology followed by 2 years of interventional neuroradiology. To my knowledge, no program has yet received accreditation status, although several are in the process of obtaining accreditation. My estimate is that about 50 neurosurgeons have training similar to that required by the ACGME. Although this number is small, it has increased 5- to 10-fold in the past 7 years. By comparison, the American Society of Interventional and Therapeutic Neuroradiology (ASITN) boasts more than 400 members.

Given the diverse backgrounds of the neurovascular team members, institutions are often challenged to create effective, smoothly functioning teams. There is no single "best way" to structure a neurovascular team. Accordingly, in an effort to minimize interdepartmental conflicts, different centers have structured their teams differently. Given that most endovascular therapists are neuroradiologists, one of the more common ways to draw the specialties together is to arrange joint appointments in radiology and neurosurgery departments. At some institutions, the neurosurgery department simply hires interventional neuroradiologists exclusively into their department. Increasingly, of course, neurosurgeons are participating directly in endovascular therapy.

Across this country and around the world, there are many variations in the division of labor. However, the key to assembling a successful team is a leader who fosters diverse expertise while maintaining effective communication and cooperation. There must be free and open cooperation among providers so that patients are treated according to the *best clinical practice* and not treated in any given manner simply because of the vagaries of referral patterns. Strengths and weaknesses of comprehensive centers invariably differ from institution to institution. Therefore, it is appropriate that similar patients be managed differently at different centers. But, it is inappropriate for patients to be locked into one treatment modality simply because the consulted physician chooses to function in isolation and is unable to offer an alternative treatment when appropriate and, simultaneously, is unwilling to refer a patient to a colleague who could provide the most appropriate alternative treatment.

It is natural for both neurosurgeons and interventional neuroradiologists to perceive each other as encroaching on one another's territory. When individuals from different clans meet in disputed territory, a certain amount of suspicion, acrimony, and *schadenfreude* can be expected to ensue. It also may be natural to react in nonproductive ways. Neurosurgeons may react by saying they control the flow of patients. Neuroradiologists may react by exerting control over angiography suites. Both may respond by selectively using literature to further their own agendas.

Let us be clear. Our obligation is to serve the needs of our patients, not to advance one specialty over another. Imagine yourself as the patient. Would you not be outraged to learn that a group of individuals feels that it has a right to further its agenda by exerting control over your health care? Would you not be outraged to learn that a group of individuals might control access to technology to advance their needs over the interests of those they are charged to serve? Even if such an attitude were not morally objectionable, it ultimately is futile to think that one "controls" patients or "owns" a procedure.

Neurosurgeons can rest on their considerable laurels in neurovascular surgery. They can criticize with legitimate validity the weaknesses of new technologies, and they can assert that as the clinicians, they "control" the patients. But, in this age of instant information transfer, imagine how long such control will last if a new treatment is developed that is equivalently effective but is also any combination of safer, less invasive, or more economical.

This situation is not new to neurosurgery. Twenty years ago, neurosurgeons were confronted with a changing world in which their continued preeminence as the experts in management of diseases of the spine and spinal cord was in question. For a time, neurosurgeons felt embattled—outnumbered and outflanked by the changes occurring in orthopedics as these aggressive competitors began to move into spinal instrumentation in large numbers. Neurosurgeons could have clung to a claim of superiority based on some sort of traditional basis. Thanks, however, to leaders such as Dr. Sonntag and others of his generation, neurosurgery instead rose to the challenge. These leaders mobilized neurosurgery with renewed major commitments to research, teaching, and the provision of exemplary patient care. Through the efforts of these leaders, neurosurgeons, despite their relatively few numbers, regained preeminence in the treatment of diseases of the spine and spinal cord. This success was achieved not through controlling patients, not through controlling technology, and not through political maneuvering but through leadership directed at improving the lives of the patients we serve.

Today, the field of neurovascular surgery is changing. Some of these changes are from outside traditional neurosurgery. I do not suggest that we embrace these changes blindly. However, we owe it to our patients to seek and deliver the best treatments—wherever we find them.

To do this will require working cooperatively with colleagues from other disciplines. We must have the confidence to be willing to draw from other disciplines into the service of our patients. These partnerships will require creativity, ingenuity, and tolerance to flourish. On the macro scale, we must collaborate with industry and other organizations, such as the ASITN, to advance our common goals. We are too few, and the forces affecting us and our patients are too great, to dilute our efforts by balkanization or duplication of political organizations.

Techniques will evolve, but principles of caring for patients remain unchanged. We must have the strength and courage needed to adapt positive changes and to reject developments that do not improve patient care. Our patients will be best served if we lead by example. We must set and maintain uncompromised standards. We must evaluate new developments fairly. We must dedicate the energy and resources needed to lead the development and dissemination of even more innovative treatments.

Our Canyon hike ended with the four of us finishing individually, with the classic microneurovascular surgeon in front. But, spurred on by one another, we all achieved personal bests, and we all were better for the shared experience. This time, the cardiologist finished last in the group. I now consider him a good friend, and I know that he is training hard so that next year the order may be different. There is no time for any of us to stand still. The future of neurovascular surgery belongs, as it always has, to those who will lead.

CHAPTER

14

Shunt Technology: Contemporary Concepts and Prospects

R. MICHAEL SCOTT, M.D., AND JOSEPH R. MADSEN, M.D.

What is really new in shunt technology? We have divided this brief talk into four sections:

1. What is new (or rediscovered) in the treatment and pathophysiology of hydrocephalus?
2. What are the new (or rediscovered) technical approaches to the avoidance of permanent shunts?
3. How does one use the new valve devices that have been recently marketed, including the adjustable valves and the antisiphoning devices?
4. What can technology and tissue engineering offer to us in the future to control hydrocephalus in our patients?

WHAT IS NEW IN THE PATHOPHYSIOLOGY AND TREATMENT OF HYDROCEPHALUS?

The traditional pathophysiology of cerebrospinal fluid (CSF) absorption and production holds that CSF is produced in the ventricles, passes through the brain, and is absorbed over the surfaces of the brain at a steady state, which can be determined by perfusion experiments. This can be called the "direct current" model of CSF flow.

In the past year, Michael Egnor and colleagues from Stony Brook published a series of articles in *Pediatric Neurosurgery* discussing a model of pulsatile flow in communicating hydrocephalus that many of us have found to be both instructive and thought-provoking (3, 4). Egnor et al. point out that blockage of absorption of CSF does not explain the pattern of ventricular enlargement that one observes in the typical case of communicating hydrocephalus. They feel that disturbances of the pulsatile flow of CSF lead to the ventricular dilatation that we see in patients with hydrocephalus.

It had been demonstrated by Dandy, Bering, and DiRocco, both in the laboratory and the operating room, that increased intraventricular pulsations cause ventriculomegaly, as cited by Egnor (4). In our own patients, we note that ventricles shrink in the absence of pulsations, and our patients with shunts placed in one lateral ventricle typically have a smaller ventricle on the side of the ventricular catheter, probably because of reduced pulsations in the shunted ventricular system.

Egnor et al. feel that in some patients with difficult-to-understand shunt syndromes, disturbances in normal CSF pulsatility are major factors both in the perpetuation of their syndrome and in why standard shunting system may not necessarily function well. They have proposed that novel shunting systems could reestablish normal pulsatility in CSF by, for example, connecting shunts from the cervical subarachnoid space and the ventricle above a valve mechanism. Mathematical models of shunt flow suggest that with a variable heart rate, sporadic and, perhaps, chaotic patterns of valve opening over time would be expected (10) (*Fig. 14.1*). The analysis of the computational models can get complex, but those interested in learning more should review the publications of Egnor et al.

New (or Rediscovered) Technical Approaches to the Avoidance of Permanent Shunts

Several innovative treatments of hydrocephalus are worthwhile mentioning in this context, including ventriculosubgaleal shunts in premature infants with intraventricular hemorrhage, the third ventriculostomy, and the in utero repair of myelomeningocele.

Ventriculosubgaleal shunts represent another rebirth of an old technique. They have attracted interest recently because of advantages over traditional tapping reservoirs to manage the posthemorrhagic hydrocephalus of prematurity (5, 13, 16). Of note in this discussion, their long survival allows the small subset of patients who are initially dependent on CSF drainage but then "outgrow" it to get by without a permanent shunt. There is no quantitative way to determine how much fluid is actually absorbed by the subgaleal space, but in this discussion, it is interesting that intraventricular pulsations could be dampened by blind shunting into the subcutaneous space, which for proponents of the pulsatile theory of hydrocephalus would be a possible mechanism of action of subgaleal shunting.

The third ventriculostomy, again a resurrection of an old technique, has become a cornerstone in the treatment of hydrocephalus second-

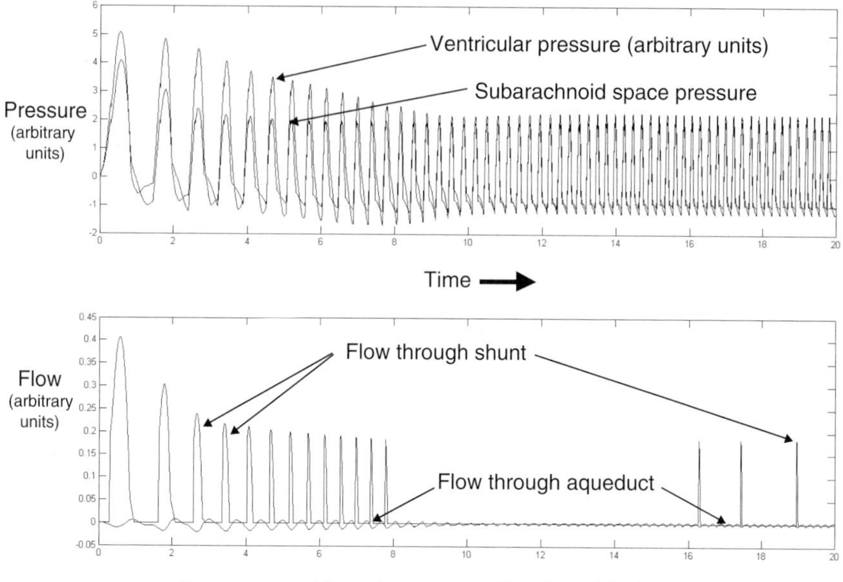

FIG. 14.1 Pulsatile flow models predict unexpected shunt behavior. This computer-generated set of data demonstrates ventricular pressure, subarachnoid pressure, flow through the shunt, and flow through the aqueduct as a function of time using a modified version of the circuit model proposed by Egnor et al. (4, 10). With a model of mixed communicating and obstructive hydrocephalus, and a varying heart rate, the ventricular and subarachnoid space pressures rapidly approximate each other, but the flow through the shunt has a sporadic, intermittent nature, not opening with each heart beat.

ary to obstruction of the aqueduct, particularly in patients beyond the second year of life.

One of the unexpected dividends from in utero closure of myelomeningoceles has been the concomitant reduction of symptomatic hydrocephalus in the operated patients. Early data suggest that these children have a reduced incidence of Chiari II malformation, and many have not required shunt placement (11, 14, 15). A prospective, randomized trial has been sponsored by the National Institutes of Health and is scheduled to begin within the next year. If confirmed, this happy result appears to occur because early closure of the back stops decompression of CSF through the myelomeningocele site, and the resulting normalized circulation of CSF restores the pressure gradients in the posterior fossa, which are necessary in the embryo to allow normal development of the fourth ventricle and cerebellum to proceed. The finding of reduced incidence of hydrocephalus in the in utero–operated patient with myelomeningocele was truly an unexpected dividend from this technology, which many of us thought would have limited utility.

HOW DOES ONE USE THE NEW VALVE DEVICES THAT HAVE BEEN RECENTLY MARKETING, INCLUDING THE ADJUSTABLE VALVES AND THE ANTISIPHONING DEVICES?

There have been a huge number of shunt designs since the first models of Holter and others. After analyzing 2,400 shunt papers and looking at all the available shunt product information from 1974 through 1997, Aschoff et al. (1) concluded that there had been at least 177 different valves produced during this period of time, with approximately 450 pressure ranges and at least 1,200 different types of prefixed assemblies. The sheer number and variety of shunt valves, catheters, reservoirs, connectors, etc., is overwhelming, and it is difficult to know how best to employ the devices that are currently available.

The typical shunt valve has a reservoir of some type and a valve apparatus set to open and close over a specific pressure range. New valves with adjustable pressure settings have come onto the market during the past decade and are, perhaps, among the more interesting of the new shunt valve technologies. The Codman-Medos Programmable valve is the prototype of these systems, but the Strata adjustable valve is also currently available. No doubt, others will soon be on the market as well. Scanning electron photomicrographs of these devices depict ingenious mechanisms that allow percutaneous adjustment of the valve pressure. In the case of the Codman-Medos system (*Fig. 14.2*) a ruby ball is held in place by a spring valve that is set to open at a given pressure. A spiral cam (*Fig. 14.3*) adjusts the tension on the spring holding a ball valve in place; the ball valve is fitted on its undersurface with alternating north/south magnets, permitting a percutaneous magnetic device to change the pressure settings in the valve without operative intervention. The cam rotation progressively elevates the counterbalance on the spring, increasing the pressure on the ball valve and elevating the opening pressure of the valve. In the Strata system (*Fig. 14.4*), which has an integral antisiphon device, a percutaneously regulated magnetic device elevates and turns the valve seat in which the ball and spring sit, altering the amount of tension on the ball valve within its seat as it rotates.

Other relatively recently designed devices include redesigned antisiphon and flow-control devices. The antisiphon device that is part of the Delta system (*Fig. 14.5)* has a flexible diaphragm that closes off distal flow when excessive negative pressure occurs from below.

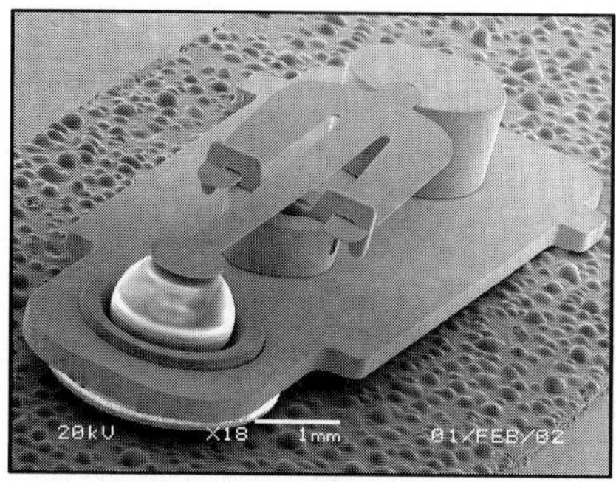

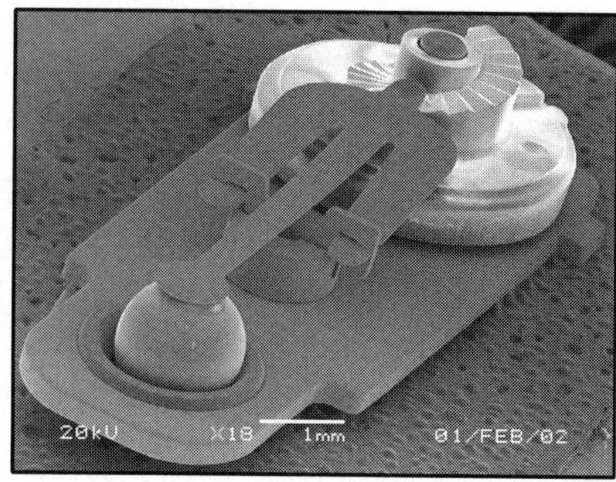

FIG. 14.2 Scanning electron micrographs of Codman Hakim valves. On the left, a ruby ball is held in place with a metal spring; on the right, the tension on the spring is adjusted by rotation of a rotor. [Courtesy Codman; used with permission.]

A ball valve–type antisiphon device, manufactured by Codman, consists of a ball and spring valve surrounded by concentric baffles (*Fig. 14.6*). When excessive negative force or siphoning occurs, the midposition spring ball valve moves distally, occluding the normal path of CSF flow and diverting CSF through baffles on the outside of the system to create increased resistance to distal drainage.

Who are the patients who might benefit from this new technology?

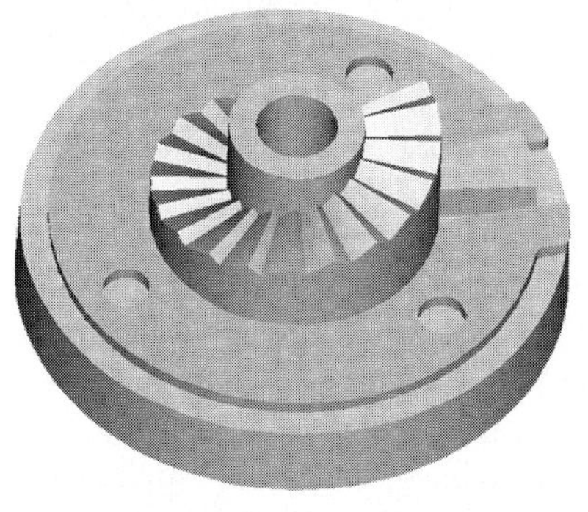

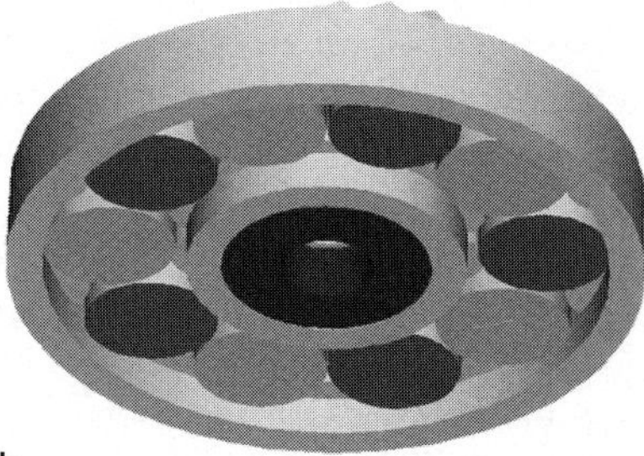

FIG. 14.3 The magnetic mechanism of the Hakim adjustable valve involves 10 small magnets, which result in externally adjusted setting over a range of pressures. [Courtesy Codman; used with permission.]

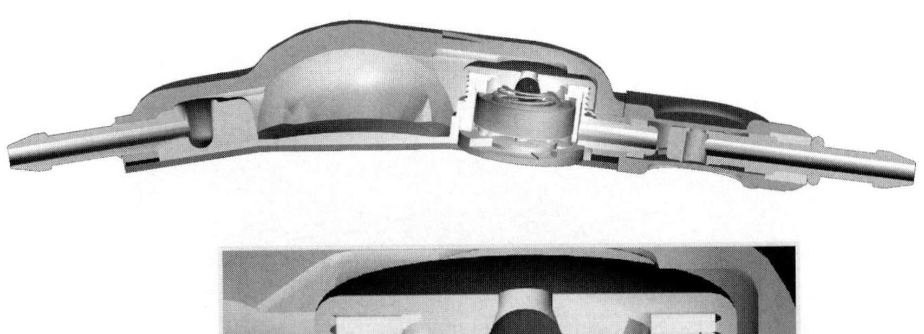

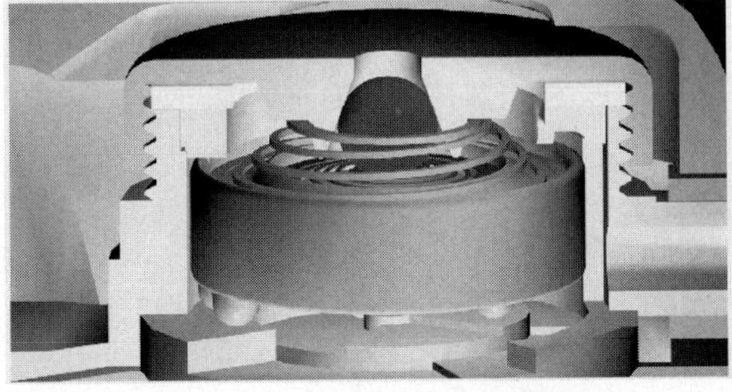

FIG. 14.4 The Strata valve. A screw-mounted chamber changes tension on the spring, which varies pressure of a ruby ball in a cone. This device has a magnetic moment, so that a compass-like device can read the setting after it is changed with a handheld magnet. [Courtesy Medtronic Neurosurgery; used with permission.]

We would mention four particular pediatric patient groups in this context:

1. Infants,
2. Shunted patients with symptoms despite the presence of small ventricles,

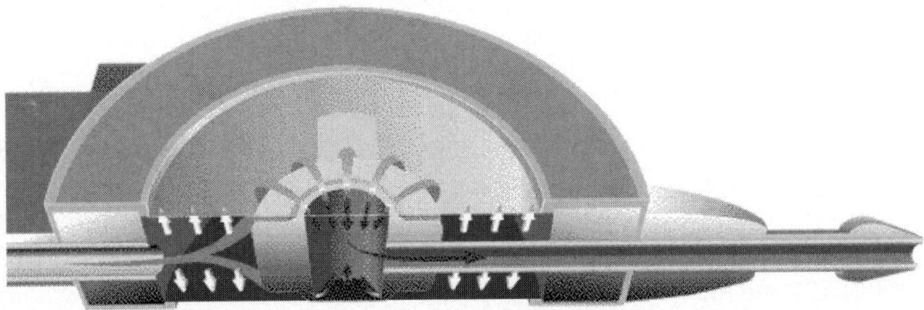

FIG. 14.5 The Delta chamber, one of the available designs of an antisiphon device. Significant negative pressure downstream from the chamber pulls the diaphragm closed and stops flow; this can be overcome with further elevation of pressure upstream. [Courtesy Medtronic Neurosurgery; used with permission.]

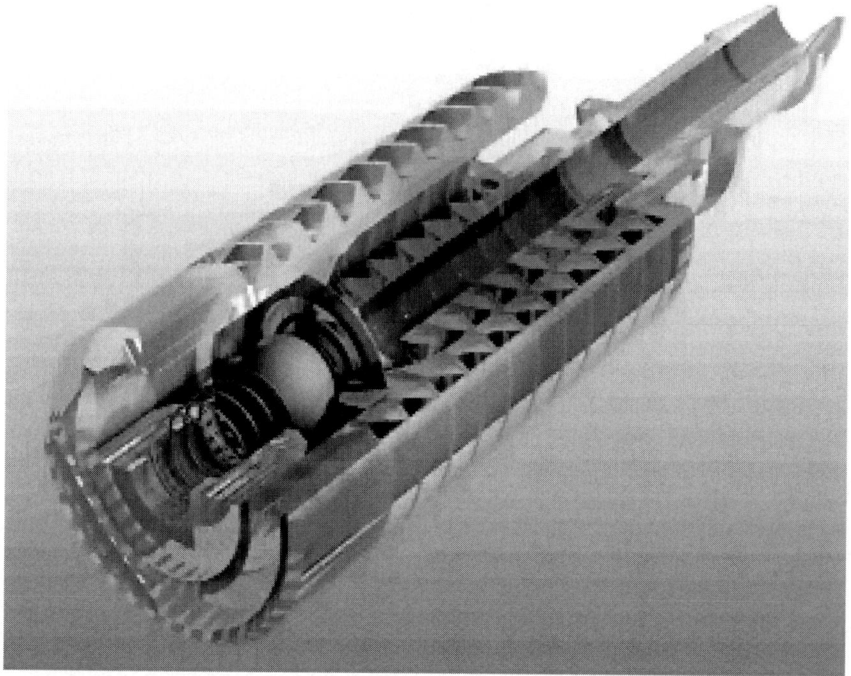

FIG. 14.6 The Codman SiphonGuard device gives flow-rate control by imposing a higher-resistance fluid path when significant negative pressure is exerted on the outflow. Unlike the Delta chamber style of device, this one is insensitive to atmospheric pressure in the management of its flow. Courtesy of Codman; used with permission.

3. Shunted third ventriculostomy candidates, and
4. Patients of all ages with massive ventriculomegaly at the time of shunt placement.

The normal-pressure hydrocephalus population, at the other end of the age spectrum, would be an additional group.

In infants, the rationale for use of adjustable valve technology has been that intracranial pressure changes physiologically with age and that it might be difficult to choose a valve setting that remains appropriate over periods of continued growth and postural change. An adjustable valve might be placed at the time of the first shunt, allowing the surgeon to utilize periodic ultrasound to monitor the ventricular size, thus adjusting the valve pressure as necessary. The end point here, of course, would be the maintenance of a satisfactory ventricular size along with a decompressed fontanelle. One potential problem with this treatment philosophy is that the valves are bulky and may cause skin erosion in very small children.

In the symptomatic patient who is shunted with small ventricles, the rationale for using adjustable valve technology has been to reduce drainage through the shunt and, hopefully, the patient's symptoms by gradually dialing up the opening pressure of the valve to find an ideal pressure setting. An alternative treatment involved the placement of an antisiphon device. The end point here would be reduction in symptoms and, potentially, fewer shunt revisions.

In the shunt-dependent third ventriculostomy candidate, an adjustable valve could be used to gradually increase ventricular size over time to make the ventriculostomy a safer procedure; after the third ventriculostomy is performed, the adjustable valve can still be used to gradually increase the pressure and wean the patient off the previously place shunt. Many neurosurgeons would probably opt to use an external drain to accomplish this task, but in certain patients, ventricular expansion is difficult to achieve.

In the patient with massive ventriculomegaly or, typically, an adult with normal-pressure hydrocephalus, the rationale for use of this technology has been that standard shunting may decompress the ventricles too rapidly. In these patients, the solution has been to place an adjustable valve, beginning the decompression of the ventricles with a high valve pressure. Gradually, the pressure can be reduced, and the patient can be observed to determine their clinical response. It is hoped here that the end point will be not only effective treatment of the symptoms but also a reduced incidence of subdural hygromas and hematomas.

Clinical trials may now be in order to determine the best strategy for setting the shunt valve pressure and other characteristics in the above group of patients. Controlled trials that examine one strategy of valve reprogramming over another may be very useful in determining the optimal use of these devices. In a sense, the clever designs of these products have provided us with excellent hardware, and we, as clinicians, have to determine the inputs that are optimal for these devices—in other words, their "software." Absent informed instructions on the best approach for setting the devices, a global assessment of their utility remains a matter of opinion and experience.

As a practical matter, I (RMS) have been reluctant to employ these new valves except in very specific circumstances. I believe that a neurosurgeon should stick with a familiar shunt system, which should have components that are easy to take apart and to assess in the operating room when malfunction occurs. I personally place medium-pressure valves in most neonates—in fact, all of my patients—to avoid overdrainage syndromes. I avoid changing valve pressures empirically, although in the patients in my practice with very large ventricles secondary to tumors or other long-standing hydrocephalus problems, I tend to use high-pressure valves to avoid the development of subdural hygromas. I do not believe that small changes in valve pressures can make a defined difference in most of our patients. If one considers the pressure changes that occurs in the head when one moves from the recumbent position to the sitting position and then to the standing position, it is very hard to understand how alteration in a valve pressure over even a 200-mm-of-water range can make any difference at all in the typical patient, except if that patient stays recumbent. Finally, our major problem with shunts continues to be the blocked ventricular catheter, and none of these technologies have effectively dealt with that problem.

My coauthor (JRM) would disagree with many of the statements in the above paragraph. He would argue that the flexibility permitted by having a valve that can be noninvasively changed must be a strong benefit to some patients, and if such flexibility allows avoidance of even a fraction of shunt revisions, it would be worth the cost to society of using the more expensive and sophisticated valves. We would certainly both agree, however, that more data are needed to resolve this question.

FUTURE TECHNOLOGIES

Future technologies in the evolution of shunts will certainly involve the more refined use of microelectronic systems or, possibly, tissue engineering solutions.

Microelectromechanical systems (MEMS) (*Fig. 14.7*) are currently in commercial use in a variety of situations where intermittent pressure-sensing is required (6, 9, 12). Ink-jet printers or air bags in automobiles are examples in which this technology is currently employed. It seems to me that there is no reason why the current devices that we use for pressure measurement in the brain cannot be miniaturized to use feedback from the brain parenchyma itself to alter the functioning of valves placed in the subcutaneous tissues. The application of this technology to neurosurgery certainly will come in the not-too-distant future.

Tissue engineering is another very exciting technology that has already been employed in experimental animals to treat a variety of conditions, to manufacture heart valves, and to manufacture shunts (2,

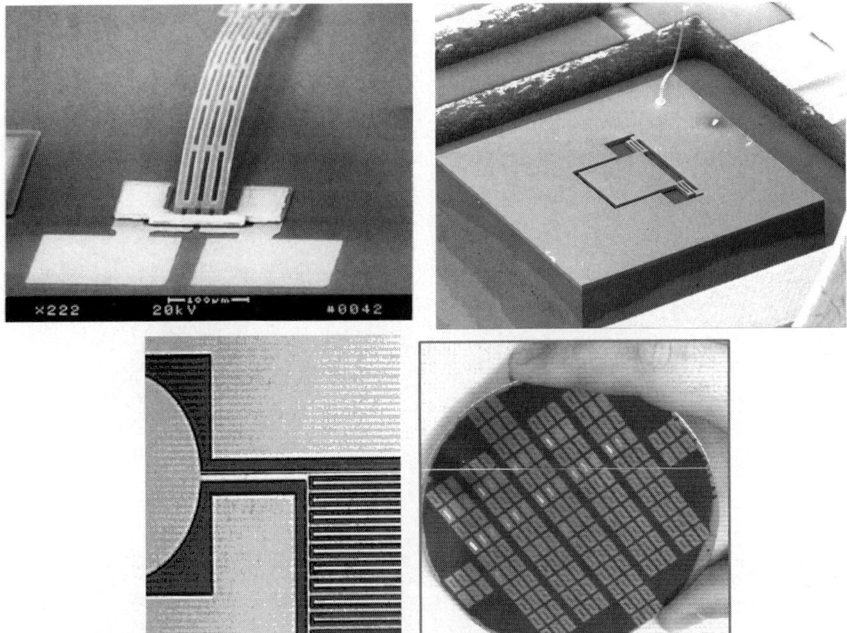

FIG. 14.7 Three examples of typical microelectrical mechanical systems (MEMS). These devices are made using a photoengraving technique very similar to that which produces microcircuit chips, with many such devices "printed" onto a silica wafer (*lower right*). They can thus be mass produced and will have many applications in medicine in the future, probably including shunts. The photomicrographs are more than a 10-fold higher magnification compared to the pictures in *Figure 14.2*. [Photographs courtesy Drs. Dentcho Ivanov and Gordon Thomas, New Jersey Institute of Technology.]

7). This technology utilizes a culture of the patient's own cells to create a living device on a matrix.

A tube can be constructed of cultured cartilage cells that when implanted can convey fluids within the body and become lined by endothelial or ependymal cells (8) (*Fig. 14.8*).

It is apparent that these shunts comprised of living and, eventually, autologous cells can survive and conduct CSF as well as adapt to the animal within which they are implanted. It is also apparent to us that these shunts can malfunction, and obviously, they will not solve all of the problems that the clinician has with current shunt systems.

How should the neurosurgeon deal with these new technologies? The neurosurgeon must stay current and pay attention to the literature.

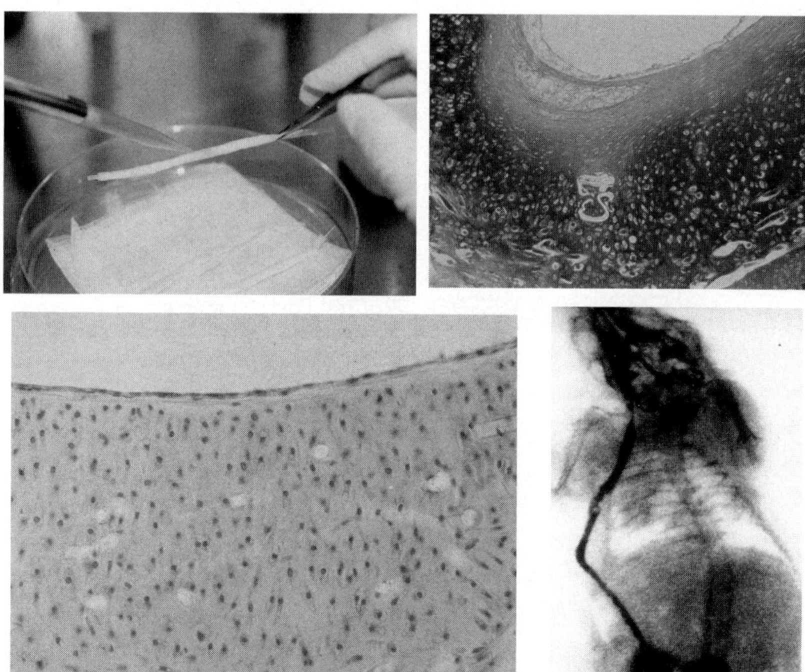

FIG. 14.8 Tissue engineering as an approach to hydrocephalus. By culturing isolated chondrocytes on a bioreservable scaffold, it is possible to produce a shunt tube that is living and could be made from autologous cells. These tubes seem to develop an epithelium and can be shown to be patent with radiographic studies when allowed to grow in hydrocephalic rats. [Modified from Lee et al (8); with permission.]

Look for well-controlled studies that evaluate these shunt systems for specific end points. Note that to our knowledge, there has been no study as yet that has demonstrated the benefit of one shunt design over another. The thinking neurosurgeon should not jump on any new technology bandwagon without thoroughly understanding the mechanics of the new system and how it will specifically benefit his or her patient with hydrocephalus. Nevertheless, it is the neurosurgeon's responsibility and opportunity to perfect the use of existing technology and to play an active role in the creation of tomorrow's technology.

REFERENCES

1. Aschoff A, Kremer P, Hashemi B, Kunze S: The scientific history of hydrocephalus and its treatment. **Neurosurg Rev** 22(2–3):67–93, 1999.
2. Atala A, Lanza RP (eds): *Methods of Tissue Engineering*. San Diego: Academic Press, 2001.

3. Egnor M, Rosiello A, Zheng L: A model of intracranial pulsations. **Pediatr Neurosurg** 35(6):284–298, 2001.
4. Egnor M, Zheng L, Rosiello A, Gutman F, Davis R: A model of pulsations in communicating hydrocephalus. **Pediatr Neurosurg** 36(6):281–303, 2002.
5. Fulmer BB, Grabb PA, Oakes WJ, Mapstone TB: Neonatal ventriculosubgaleal shunts. **Neurosurgery** 47(1):80–83, 2000.
6. Gad-El-Hak M (ed): *The MEMS Handbook*. New York: CRC Press, 2001.
7. Lanza RP, Langer R, Vacanti JP (eds): *Principles of Tissue Engineering*, 2nd ed. San Diego: Academic Press, 2000.
8. Lee IW, Vacanti JP, Taylor GA, Madsen JR: The living shunt: a tissue engineering approach in the treatment of hydrocephalus. **Neurol Res** 22(1):105–110, 2000.
9. Madou MJ: *Fundamentals of Microfabrication: The Science of Miniaturization,* 2nd ed. New York: CRC Press: 2002.
10. Madsen JR, Egnor M: Pulsatile dynamics of intracranial pressure and response to shunting: A computational mechanical model using Simulink. Program No. 106.9. 2002 Abstract Viewer and Itinerary Planner. Washington, DC: Society for Neuroscience, 2002. On CD-ROM.
11. Paek BW, Farmer DL, Wilkinson CC, et al.: Hindbrain herniation develops in surgically created myelomeningocele but is absent after repair in fetal lambs. **Am J Obstet Gynecol** 183(5):1119–1123, 2000.
12. Senturia SD: *Microsystem Design.* New York: Kluwer Academic Publishers, 2001.
13. Soul JS, Madsen JR: Neonatal hydrocephalus. In: Hansen AR, Puder M (eds): *Neonatal Surgical Intensive Care*. Hamilton, ON, Canada: BC Decker Inc., 2003, pp 386–394.
14. Sutton LN, Adzick NS, Bilaniuk LT, Johnson MP, Crombleholme TM, Flake AW: Improvement in hindbrain herniation demonstrated by serial fetal magnetic resonance imaging following fetal surgery for myelomeningocele. **J Am Med Assoc** 282(19):1826–1831, 1999.
15. Tulipan N, Hernanz-Schulman M, Lowe LH, Bruner JP: Intrauterine myelomeningocele repair reverses preexisting hindbrain herniation. **Pediatr Neurosurg** 31(3): 137–142, 1999.
16. Tubbs RS, Smyth MD, Wellons JC III, Blount JP, Grabb PA, Oakes WJ: Life expectancy of ventriculosubgaleal shunt revisions. **Pediatr Neurosurg** 38(5):244–246, 2003.

CHAPTER

15

Modern Paradigms of Pain Management

KIM J. BURCHIEL, M.D., F.A.C.S.

INTRODUCTION

New *technology* for the surgical management of pain has increased our capabilities for achieving satisfactory pain control in the majority of patients with chronic pain. The trend toward minimally invasive pain surgery *procedures* has diminished morbidity and costs. Novel *pain care delivery systems* are needed to exploit these changes and innovations in ways that maximize benefit to patients and appropriate utilization of neurosurgical expertise. The future of *pain medicine* lies in the development of primary practitioners in the field and integration with specialists, such as neurosurgeons. This brief overview will highlight advances in the treatment of chronic pain, which will set the direction of the field for the next generation of neurosurgeons.

TECHNOLOGY

Pain surgery technology is now on a par with many of the "high-tech" specialties of neurosurgery, including endovascular neurosurgery, spinal surgery, functional and stereotactic neurosurgery, and radiosurgery. Technology for neurostimulation now includes multi-contact electrodes for peripheral nerve, spinal cord, and brain stimulation. Electrode arrays now offer an unprecedented degree of control for selective stimulation. Multichannel generators for stimulation can be either self-contained or radiofrequency-coupled. Patient-oriented systems can assist with mapping of stimulation paresthesias and with spinal cord stimulation, decreasing the need for physician time, increasing specificity, prolonging battery life, and increasing patient satisfaction (2). Drug-delivery pumps for intrathecal therapy are programmable to a degree that often exceeds our clinical needs. Intrathecal catheter design and implant protocols promise increased success and longevity of the system (1).

PROCEDURES

Pain surgeons have a full armamentarium of procedures to relieve chronic pain and cancer pain. Neuromodulation procedures, which are fundamentally testable and reversible, include *neurostimulation* and *intrathecal drug delivery*. Neurostimulation can be used to improve pain control at virtually any level of the nervous system, including the motor cortex. Intrathecal opioids and adjuvant agents continue to be a mainstay of surgical pain therapy.

Ablative lesions, while less common than neuromodulation, still play a role in surgery for pain. Procedures that can be considered for specific indications include dorsal root entry zone (DREZ) and the so-called Caudalis-DREZ lesions, anterolateral cordotomy, dorsal root ganglionectomy, sympathectomy, midline myelotomy, cingulotomy/pulvinotomy, and medial thalamotomy (3).

We now have an unprecedented array of surgical techniques to alleviate pain. Now more than ever, the delivery of neurosurgical pain care is dependent on the means by which patients access care and the organization of the delivery system for pain care. Third-party payers have fundamentally changed the delivery of pain care from intensive, inpatient programs to almost exclusively outpatient settings. The intensity of pain services available to patients has, on the average, also diminished. Patients and physicians must simply make do with less. Managed care continues to seek opportunities to limit services and diminish short-term costs. *Neurosurgeons interested in the field of pain medicine need to appreciate both the threats and the opportunities of this new marketplace.*

Large, multidisciplinary pain clinics have virtually disappeared. Payers have questioned these clinics as being too expensive and too cumbersome, with dubiously cost-effective outcomes. As opposed to the salad days of pain clinics during the 1970s and 1980s, virtually no inpatient services remain for pain rehabilitation. The outpatient "pain center" is now the dominant model for the provision of pain care. Unfortunately, many of these surviving centers have been reduced to little more than venues for procedure-based practices. Clearly, pain medicine is a multispecialty specialty, but anesthesiologists continue to dominate the field both in numbers and national leadership.

The mega-multidisciplinary "pain clinic" will continue to be replaced by smaller, more mutable teams comprised of neurosurgeons, anesthesiologists, neurologists, psychologists, physiatrists, and nurse specialists. Distributed "clinics without walls," which need to subspecialize, communicate, and collaborate, should thrive; this should be particularly true of those that master the art of networking. Thus, the future of pain care will look more like a matrix than a single repository of expertise.

What is not news are the principles of pain medicine that endure despite the changes in the delivery of care. These principles can be distilled to five key points: First, although a cliché, pain is a "biopsychosocial" phenomenon. Monolithic approaches to treatment are doomed to failure, specifically when the biological aspect is emphasized to the exclusion of the psychological or social aspects of a given condition. Second, application of our most accurate overall knowledge is crucial to established an accurate diagnosis and, thus, to provide effective treatment. Third, most pain treatments will be nonsurgical. Neurosurgeons treat a tiny fraction of pain cases, which generally are refractory to all other modalities. Fourth, rehabilitation is the optimal approach. Often, the best that we can hope for from our surgical procedures is a relatively pain-free interval during which the patient can be remobilized. With rare exceptions, passive pain treatment with surgery alone is unlikely to provide lasting benefit. Fifth, adherence to the tenets of pharmacological means of pain care is critical. Drugs must be used with current pharmacological knowledge, incorporating an understanding of their mechanisms of action and addiction medicine.

PAIN SURGERY

The surgical management of pain has a special role in the comprehensive delivery of pain care. In general, this surgery should be performed by neurosurgeons; however, few neurosurgeons have been trained in the full spectrum of pain-relieving surgeries. Many other disciplines, including anesthesiology, physiatry, and neurology, look to the field of interventional pain management as a way to broaden their respective field and scope of practice.

My hope is that this turf war of the future will give way to a field that, while populated largely by nonneurosurgeons, will preserve a unique role for neurosurgeons who are interested in pain care. Neurosurgeons, after all, have special training that gives them the capability of analyzing a patient's condition from many perspectives (e.g., spinal care and spine surgery in a patient with low back pain). Cross-training in pain medicine could give the neurosurgeon additional expertise to bring to bear on the most complex pain problems. On the other hand, I am skeptical that many neurosurgeons would willingly put themselves in the "first position" with regard to a large population of patients with chronic pain. What neurosurgeons need is a colleague and collaborator. The cross-disciplinary pain medicine specialist of the future will be the "hub" for pain care, with the knowledgeable neurosurgeon located on one of the "spokes" of the health care wheel.

THE PAIN MEDICINE SPECIALIST

Will the pain medicine specialist of the future be a neurosurgeon? We have only recently begun to train the pain Medicine "generalists" of the future, so this is a difficult question at present. Currently, board-certified anesthesiologists, neurologists, psychiatrists, and physiatrists can participate in a 1-year pain medicine fellowship under the auspices of the American Board of Anesthesiologists (ABA). At the completion of the fellowship, a certifying exam must be passed, after which a Certificate of Added Qualifications (CAQ) is given in pain medicine by the fellowship graduate's primary Board. This CAQ has the quality imprimatur of the American Board of Medical Specialties (ABMS), which is currently the quality standard against which other boards are compared in the United States. An alternative route, open to board-certified neurosurgeons and other ABMS-certificate holders (as well as to almost anyone qualified to sit for the ABA certifying exam in pain medicine), is the certificate offered by the American Board of Pain Medicine (ABPM). The ABPM is a multispecialty board that qualifies individuals to sit for a 2-day, psychometrically validated, comprehensive examination based on training, experience, and in some cases, formal pain fellowships offered in conjunction with a sister organization, the American Academy of Pain Medicine.

In all likelihood, the pain medicine practitioner of the future will be a "primary care" doctor for patients with chronic pain. It seems unlikely that proceduralists, neurosurgeons included, will commonly take on this role. These "pain docs" will be our close ally, however similar to the roles that intensivists now play in intensive care units and that physiatrists now facilitate in postoperative or postinjury rehabilitation. The three C's of "Consultation, Communication, and Collaboration" will be the hallmark of the successful pain specialist.

THE ROLE OF THE NEUROSURGEON IN PAIN MEDICINE

Much as it us now, our future role in the evaluation of patients with chronic pain will be to consider them first from a neurosurgical perspective. Does the patient have a condition that would benefit from a neurosurgical approach to the primary pathology (e.g., a fusion for spinal instability)? Once all reasonable neurosurgical options have been evaluated and rejected, the neurosurgeon should take the perspective of the pain surgeon. A full consideration of neuromodulation and neuroablative options to alleviate the pain can—and should—be entertained. This ability to render both a neurosurgical opinion and a pain care opinion makes the neurosurgeon an extremely valuable resource to the patient and his or her physician. The model of the cross-trained neurosurgeon has many contemporary parallels, such as the endovascular neurosurgeon and the surgical neurooncologist.

TRAINING THE PAIN SURGEON

Pain training for a neurosurgeon should last from 6 to 12 mo and incorporate experience in approximately 100 procedures, including both neuromodulation and ablation. At least some of the training should take place in a multidisciplinary environment in conjunction with anesthesiologists, psychologists, physiatrists, neurologists, and other pain practitioners. Currently, the Society of Neurological Surgeons is accrediting training programs in the neurosurgical management of pain. This mechanism will bring a large measure of quality assurance to fellowship offerings in the surgical management of pain.

CONCLUSION

The evolution of pain medicine is being driven by societal needs and public awareness of pain as a major health care issue. The new paradigm will see the proliferation of pain medicine generalists working closely with cross-trained pain surgery specialists, including neurosurgeons. Matrix pain clinics will become the dominant practice structure. As they are today, communication and collaboration will be the hallmark of quality care in patients with complex chronic pain conditions.

REFERENCES

1. Follett KA, Burchiel KJ, Deer T, et al.: Prevention of intrathecal drug delivery catheter-related complications. **Neuromodulation** 6:1, 2003.
2. North RB, Calkins SK, Campbell DS, et al.: Automated, patient-interactive, spinal cord stimulator adjustment: A randomized controlled trial. **Neurosurgery** 52(3):572–580, 2003.
3. Steele TR, Burchiel KJ: Ablative neurosurgical techniques in the treatment of chronic pain: Overview. In *Surgical Management of Pain*, K.J. Burchiel (ed.). New York: Thieme, 2002, pp. 636–646.

CHAPTER

16

The Neurosurgeon as an Intensivist

ALEX B. VALADKA, M.D.

To a layperson—and even to many health care workers—the concept of a neurosurgeon acting as an intensivist may seem like an oxymoron. After all, the most highly respected and sought-after neurosurgeons are those with unparalleled technical expertise in the operating room. The mark of a master neurosurgeon is often considered to be excellence in the performance of a technically demanding case, such as clipping a large basilar tip aneurysm, resecting a large acoustic schwannoma, or realigning and instrumenting a complex spinal deformity. From this perspective, details of perioperative management may seem to be inconvenient tasks that are not part of "real" neurosurgery.

Technical superiority, however, is only part of being a neurosurgeon. Surgery is not simply cutting and sewing. It is much more. It is, in fact, an entire approach and philosophy toward dealing with illness and disease.

This brief overview will explore some of the reasons why neurosurgeons may not feel welcome or comfortable in the intensive care unit (ICU), followed by reasons for neurosurgeons to overcome these concerns and to increase their involvement in the ICU. Finally, a few recent advances and possible future developments in critical care will be summarized in the hope they may inspire and motivate neurosurgeons to maintain an active role in all aspects of their patients' care.

WHY DO NEUROSURGEONS AVOID THE ICU?

The typical neurosurgeon is constantly surrounded by a swirl of office visits, surgeries, ever-increasing regulatory and administrative tasks and paperwork, and similar demands on his or her time. Against this backdrop, it is easy to understand why many neurosurgeons may be more than happy to shift some patient care responsibilities to an intensivist. After all, caring for patients who are critically ill often requires that physicians spend a fair amount of time at the bedside, poring over large amounts of complex data. Rounds of this type can be very different than rounds on postoperative patients who will be leaving the hospital after a brief stay. In the latter case, rounds may consist of a brief examination, a review of vital signs, and a wound check, followed by socializing and chatting with the patient and his or her family. For patients in the ICU, however, families may not be readily available during the early morning or late evening hours, when many neurosurgeons make rounds. Thus, in addition to the time spent at the bedside, the neurosurgeon has to spend as much—or even more—time finding the family and answering their many questions. Families of patients who are critically ill often require a great deal of emotional support as well. Finally, carrying out these extended conversations with families may require the neurosurgeon to make several return trips to the ICU or, at least, to spend considerable amounts of time on the telephone.

In addition to the greater amount of time required to care for patients in the ICU, the neurosurgeon must also adapt to the unpredictability of critical care medicine. These patients may require immediate attention at a moment's notice at any time of the day or night. These demands often result in many pages or phone calls to the office—or even to the operating room—for questions about medications, ventilator changes, intravenous fluids, abnormal laboratory results, and similar issues.

Keeping current with advances and new trends in critical care may also be difficult for the neurosurgeon. It is difficult enough for a busy general neurosurgeon to keep abreast of new developments in the many branches of neurosurgery, such as trauma, spine, tumor, cerebrovascular, and other areas. More time is required to keep one's knowledge current in such additional areas as antibiotics, sepsis, nutrition, ventilator management, pressors, treatment of high blood pressure, and other branches of critical care.

Finally, and perhaps of greatest concern, various political forces are coming together to undermine the leadership role of the neurosurgeon in the ICU. In many hospitals, allowing neurosurgeons to manage ventilators, order parenteral nutrition, insert pulmonary artery catheters, and perform similar procedures are things that "just aren't done." Long-standing local custom may suggest that those types of procedures "belong" to pulmonologists, cardiologists, or intensivists. Even neurosurgeons who are quite adept at these procedures because of extensive experience acquired during residency may find that continuing such behavior in their new practice location breeds ill will, animosity, political battles, and even a greater likelihood of such nightmares as inquiries from hospital quality-assurance committees and malpractice attorneys. At the national level, a growing movement is advocating that every ICU in this country be staffed by "credentialed" critical care physicians. This is one of the three "safety measures" identified by the Leapfrog Group, which describes itself as a coalition of more than 100 public and private organizations that provide health care benefits (1). It was founded by the Business Roundtable, which defines itself as "an association of chief executive officers of leading corporations with a combined workforce of more than 10 million employees in the United States and $3.5 trillion in revenues. The chief executives are committed to advocating public policies that foster vigorous economic growth and a dynamic global economy" (2). The Leapfrog Group states that its motivation for taking up the cause of patient safety was a highly publicized 1999 report by the Institute of Medicine (IOM), *To Err Is Human* (3). That report was highly flawed, however, and its methodology was quite weak. In fact, its conclusions and methodology have been challenged by several thoughtful commentators (4, 5), including an author of the two studies from which the annual number of medical errors was extrapolated (6). Like many such "feel good" initiatives, however, the weaknesses of the actual report have been cast aside by the expediencies of political opportunity.

The three initial "leaps" in patient safety advocated by the Leapfrog Group are computerized physician order entry, evidence-based hospital referral (i.e., referring patients who need certain medical procedures to "hospitals with characteristics shown to be associated with better outcomes," which generally means hospitals that perform a greater number of those procedures each year), and staffing ICUs with physicians who are Board-certified (or eligible for Board certification) in critical care medicine. These efforts appear to be intended to reduce employers' health care costs by decreasing the number of medical errors. The members of the Leapfrog Group have considerable purchasing power regarding health care services, and it is expected that they will leverage this purchasing power to reward hospitals that implement their recommended procedures.

As mentioned above, this emphasis on patient safety grew out of the flawed IOM report *To Err Is Human*. The tremendous publicity enjoyed by this report has energized efforts by malpractice attorneys to win large settlements or awards for alleged harm resulting from "medical mistakes." These efforts have fueled a tremendous increase in the cost of professional liability insurance for physicians (7). In some areas, the cost of such insurance has become so prohibitive that communities find themselves without specialists in essential areas like obstetrics and neurosurgery (8). It remains to be seen whether these and other attempts to improve patient safety will have other consequences that effectively deny medical care to large segments of the population.

Another concern of the Leapfrog Group is contained in its assertion that more than 500,000 of the greater than 4 million patients admitted to ICUs in this country die every year (9). An article by Zimmerman et al. (10), in which the mortality rate of 37,668 patients admitted to 285 ICUs was found to be 12.35%, is cited in a manner that implies that such a mortality rate is a problem. The article by Zimmerman et al., however, which evaluated the accuracy of a particular scoring system for predicting hospital mortality, reported that the predicted mortality rate in these patients was 12.27%—a rate that was not significantly different from the observed rate. These statistics suggest that many patients admitted to ICUs are quite ill. In these unfortunate patients, death is frequently expected, but these patients are still admitted to the ICU for aggressive resuscitative efforts in the hope that they may be part of the small minority who make a seemingly miraculous recovery. Furthermore, admitting severely injured neurosurgical patients to an ICU not only gives such patients every opportunity for recovery, but also expedites the process of organ donation in those patients who progress to brain death despite aggressive interventions (11). The implication that death in these patients represents some sort of deficiency in quality of care cannot go unchallenged. This issue is especially of concern to neurosurgeons, because the study by Zimmerman et al. found that head trauma was one of the diagnoses for which predicted and observed mortality rates differed the most. The predicted death rate was 13.0%, but the observed rate was 17.7%. Does this discrepancy mean that the neurosurgeons who treated these patients with head injury provided substandard care? Or does it suggest that the scoring system under evaluation—like other such systems—tends to underweight the prognostic importance of isolated severe brain injury? If the latter is true, then surely reviewers cannot ascribe the greater-than-expected number of deaths to an epidemic of medical errors.

As an aside, it should be noted that the Leapfrog Group refers to the published literature to bolster its recommendation that ICUs be staffed by trained intensivists. Their ICU Physician Staffing Factsheet states, "At least nine studies to date have examined the relationship between ICU staffing and patient outcomes. In every case, intensivist model ICUs were associated with lower mortality rates" (9). The reference cited in support of this claim is an abstract which refers, at different times, to 6, 7, 8, 10, 11, 12, 15, and 16 studies—but never to nine (12). Although an intensivist staffing model was favored by most of the reviewed studies, the phrase "in every case" is not substantiated by the cited abstract. Because such evidence is only class III, it is a poor foundation upon which to build sweeping changes in the delivery of critical care services. At worst, such discrepancies between descriptions of published reports and the actual reports themselves may represent misinterpretation and distortion of published data.

Regardless of the accuracy or validity of its basis, this message from the Leapfrog Group has been taken up the Society of Critical Care Medicine (SCCM). In an e-mail communication to members of the SCCM on July 30, 2002, Maureen A. Harvey, RN, MPH, CCRN, FCCM, the President of the SCCM, declared, "In 80% of U.S. ICUs, patients and families are still suffering needlessly. Patients are dying needlessly." She strongly implied that such needless death and suffering would be avoided if every ICU established an intensivist model (i.e., a model in which an intensivist directs care).

How can neurosurgeons respond to these powerful forces that seem to be intent on keeping them out of the ICU?

REASONS TO STAY INVOLVED

Although the problems enumerated above are formidable indeed, fortunately they are outweighed by the reasons why neurosurgeons should remain heavily involved in the ICU.

In many cases, one of the most fundamental reasons might be the requirements of contracts that neurosurgeons may have with their hospital for the provision of emergency services. If such a contract stipulates that the neurosurgeon will continue to provide critical care services to patients even after they have been stabilized, admitted to the hospital, and taken to surgery (if necessary), then failure of the neurosurgeon to remain involved in the care of such patients could be interpreted as a violation of that contract.

Another basic reason for neurosurgeons to stay involved is rooted in economics. The costs of running a neurosurgery practice continue to rise, but income and collections are generally dropping or, at best, remaining stagnant. In such a climate, it is foolish for neurosurgeons to fail to bill appropriately for any services they provide. Although most postoperative care is bundled into the CPT code for the operative procedure, it may be possible to bill for critical care services if the postoperative patient develops a complication that creates a new diagnosis (e.g., the onset of pneumonia in a patient who has had a trauma craniotomy).

Many patients with nonoperative traumatic or spontaneous intracranial hemorrhage require observation in the ICU for several days. The neurosurgeon continues to round on these patients, speak with their families, deal with paperwork concerning disability and insurance benefits, explain the patient's absence to employers or schools, and perform similar duties—all while facing the ever-present threat of malpractice claims. The neurosurgeon should certainly consider billing for direct patient care–related activities carried out for the benefit of these patients. In addition, time spent counseling patients and families (when appropriate) is also billable as long as such activity is appropriately documented. Fortunately, billing for evaluation and management services likely will become much more streamlined in the future. On May 16, 2002, the Advisory Committee on Regulatory Reform for the Secretary of Health and Human Services voted overwhelmingly to recommend that the Centers for Medicare & Medicaid Services (formerly the Health Care Financing Administration) have no Evaluation and Management Documentation Guidelines. Thus, the current, burdensome requirements to document a large number of specific items for a certain number of organ systems (the numbers of which increase as reimbursement increases) may soon be replaced by a system grounded much more in common sense. Such a change would be welcomed by most surgical specialty societies because it would greatly facilitate the submission of claims by specialists for the time and effort they invest in caring for these patients.

Another important reason for neurosurgeons to maintain a presence in the ICU is continuity of care, especially if the neurosurgeon has performed an emergency operation on a patient. Such continuity may be very reassuring to patients and to their families as they deal with the stress of major—and often unexpected—illness. From the point of view of risk management, such obvious expression of a neurosurgeon's ongoing interest and involvement may prevent or, at least, help to defend against litigious actions that result from a patient's injury and that ensnare the neurosurgeon in their tangled web. (Along these lines, it is worth mentioning that—contrary to popular perception—it is by no means clear whether physicians who provide emergency services have a greater likelihood of becoming targets of professional liability actions than comparable physicians who do not provide emergency care.)

Without question, the most important reason for neurosurgeons to remain involved with patients in the ICU is that no other physicians are as experienced, qualified, or comfortable in dealing with neurologic emergencies. Although the neurosurgeon may feel uncomfortable or intimidated by certain aspects of critical care (e.g., ventilator management or pressor therapy), it is worth remembering that many other specialists are at least as uncomfortable with managing central nervous system disease. This point is emphasized by a review of the contents of two specialty society journals for the calendar year 2001. *The Journal of TRAUMA Injury, Infection, and Critical Care* is sponsored by the American Association for the Surgery of Trauma and is the official journal of the Eastern Association for the Surgery of Trauma, the Trauma Association of Canada, and the Western Trauma Association. *Critical Care Medicine* is the official journal of the Society of Critical Care Medicine. These journals publish supplements, editorials, case reports, current opinion, and letters to the editors. In 2001, only 11% of the material published in *The Journal of TRAUMA* was relevant to the brain, spine, spinal cord, or peripheral nerves. For *Critical Care Medicine*, the corresponding figure is 6.9%. These percentages stand in sharp contrast to such statements as, for example, the head is the most frequently injured part of the body in patients with polytrauma (13), the social impact of disabilities resulting from central nervous system injuries far outweigh those of injuries to any other organ system (14), and, as far back as 1985, the annual financial burden of traumatic brain injury was estimated to be between $75 and $100 billion in the United States alone (15), with some estimates that at least one-third of the cost of trauma is attributable to central nervous system trauma. Considering the sheer magnitude of the effects of central nervous system disease on patients in the ICU, one would think that journals devoted to trauma and critical care would have a greater interest in educating their readers about management of neurologic disease. It appears that most such articles are published in *Neurosurgery*, the *Journal of Neurosurgery*, and similar journals targeted toward a neurosurgical audience.

This apparent dichotomy between managing the brain versus managing the rest of the body is also important, because many of the treatments that currently are or have been recently recommended for patients who are critically ill may have adverse effects on central nervous system metabolism (16). For example, in patients with abdominal injuries, trauma surgeons may prefer that blood pressure be kept rather low to prevent rupture of injured arteries or vascular organs. In managing the adult respiratory distress syndrome, intensivists may often restrict fluid intake and allow permissive hypercapnia. These same maneuvers, however, may be contraindicated in patients with head injury, because they might reduce cerebral blood flow, elevate intracranial pressure, and impair oxygen delivery to the brain. Sorely needed are specialists with the background and experience to appreciate how such therapeutic interventions may affect the nervous system. At the very least, someone must be constantly prepared to serve as an "advocate" for the central nervous system in an ICU environment that often focuses primarily on the heart, lungs, and immune response.

Realistically, it is not possible for most practicing neurosurgeons to spend the bulk of their day in the ICU as they perhaps did during internship or junior residency. Furthermore, it is difficult enough for neurosurgeons to remain current in the many branches of neurosurgery, much less to keep informed about critical care medicine. Outside of academic institutions with a strong resident presence and a dedicated neurosurgical ICU, the most realistic model for delivery of neurotrauma care may be for neurosurgeons to work closely with intensivists, anesthesiologists, trauma surgeons, or whichever specialists "run" the ICU in their hospitals. Such specialists could assume most of the work of managing these patients, including antibiotics, nutrition, ventilator management, etc. Any changes that could affect cerebral pathophysiology directly, however, would have to be approved by the neurosurgeon. For example, ventilator changes that could affect the arterial partial pressure of carbon dioxide in patients with intracranial hypertension would require neurosurgical approval.

It is worth noting that even the Leapfrog Group and the SCCM do not call for exclusion of non–critical care specialists from the ICU. Rather, their recommendations call only for ICUs to be run by intensivists. Both optimization of patient care as well as administrative and political concerns suggest that such intensivists would be wise to cooperate as closely as possible with appropriate specialists. Echoing the same sentiment, many trauma surgeons who were surveyed about the management of patients with head injury at their hospitals expressed a desire to see greater involvement of neurosurgeons in these cases (17). The role of the neurosurgeon in this type of ICU has been summarized by private practice neurosurgeon Jeff Lobosky, who writes, "It is exceedingly important . . . that we, as the primary advocates ensuring optimal neurologic recovery, appreciate both the invaluable skills as well as the potential shortcomings of all members of the treatment team" (18).

It is worth noting that the types of relationships that exist between physicians of different specialties are highly dependent upon the personalities of the individuals involved. Over time, most physicians who move to a new medical community develop referral patterns based upon such factors as friendship and complementary personalities. Similarly, at a given hospital, a physician from any one of several specialties may emerge as the primary provider of ICU care because of interest, training, and/or experience. As long as such care is delivered in an efficient, high-quality, collegial manner, the exact specialty of that physician assumes lesser importance. Legislating mandatory interspecialty cooperation may not be nearly as effective as less rigorous patterns of consultation and, in fact, may be counterproductive.

THE FUTURE OF NEUROSURGICAL CRITICAL CARE

As neurosurgeons, we are sometimes humbled by the fact that our relentless pursuit of technical perfection has not always produced better outcomes for our patients. For example, outcome for patients with glioblastoma remains frustratingly poor despite continued refinements in surgical technique, intraoperative navigation, and adjunctive therapy. Our current debate about clipping versus coiling various types of aneurysms often overlooks the fact that many patients with aneurysmal subarachnoid hemorrhage remain devastated by this disease and its attendant complications (19, 20). This high rate of morbidity and mortality probably will not be appreciably affected by the technique that is used to secure a ruptured aneurysm. In terms of traumatic brain injury, the apparent reduction in mortality during the last few decades has resulted primarily from better prehospital care and ICU management, not from any surgical breakthrough on the part of neurosurgeons (21). As far as treatment of the actual neurologic injury itself, we frequently can do no better than the treatment described at least 37 centuries ago in the Edwin Smith papyrus, which refers to certain particularly severe head injuries as "an ailment not to be treated" (22). Thus, in response to the attitude mentioned earlier that critical care is not "real" neurosurgery, it might, perhaps, be pointed out that although "real" neurosurgery has benefited a great many patients over the years, there remain many areas in the neurosurgical domain that require novel and different approaches if we are to continue to relieve suffering and improve the quality of life for our patients.

Before initiating new strategies to treat traumatic brain injury, one may wish to perform a careful reassessment of the appropriateness with which current therapies are used or, perhaps, misused. Some treatments that confer benefit when used appropriately may not confer benefit—or might actually be harmful—when used prophylactically. Such is the case for prophylactically treating head-injured patients with barbiturates (23), hyperventilation (24), pharmacologic paralysis (25), and induced hypertension (26). On the other hand, recent data suggest that the old standby mannitol, when administered in higher-than-usual doses, may significantly improve outcome in certain types of patients with head injury (27). Newer data indicate that certain commonly used sedative and anesthetic agents may adversely affect neurologic recovery in patients with traumatic brain injury (28).

Decompressive craniectomy is a treatment that "seems" to be effective, but a well-designed study that rigorously evaluates its effectiveness has not been conducted. Such a trial, however, is (at the time of this writing) in the planning stages and may soon be underway. Finally, although the National Acute Brain Injury Study: Hypothermia did not show benefit in its primary outcome measure (29), a detailed analysis of the results of that study has generated another, more focused hypothermia trial that (at the time of this writing) will soon be accruing patients.

Several large pharmaceutical trials have failed to demonstrate benefit for many drugs that were evaluated as potential treatments for traumatic brain injury or for subarachnoid hemorrhage. Intensive analyses of the methodologies and results of these trials, however, have yielded important lessons about the design and execution of these types of investigations (30). Although they have been expensive, these lessons should greatly improve the planning of future studies.

Greater appreciation for the role of genetic polymorphisms is also beginning to emerge. For example, certain mutations in the gene for endothelial nitric oxide synthase appear to be associated with coronary artery spasm and with myocardial infarction in the absence of organic coronary artery stenosis (31, 32). It is tempting to speculate that similar mutations may predispose affected patients to cerebral ischemia after traumatic brain injury and to vasospasm after aneurysmal subarachnoid hemorrhage. Such investigations, in conjunction with the increasingly frequent application of techniques from genomics and proteomics to the study of trauma (33) and other central nervous system diseases, may soon make it possible to tailor an individual patient's therapy to his or her specific genetic makeup. Currently, investigators can do little more than identify that the presence of the apolipoprotein E-ϵ 4 genotype predicts a poor outcome in survivors of traumatic brain injury (34). In the future, it may be necessary to use different treatments in apparently similar patients who are found to have different isoforms of key genes.

Continued growth of information and imaging technologies will also greatly facilitate the care of patients in the ICU, especially for neurosurgeons and other busy specialists. Through handheld wireless devices like those distributed at the 2002 meeting of the Congress of Neurological Surgeons (CNS), physicians may soon have remote wireless access to patients' vital signs, laboratory values, imaging studies, and even real-time live images of their beds. This immediate availability of information will enable a larger number of critical and time-sensitive decisions to be made immediately, without the need for physicians to delay decision-making while they are en route to a patient's bedside.

Finally, continued evolution of portable bedside CT scanners and MR imagers will make it possible to obtain important information about cerebral blood flow and metabolism without the need to move patients out of the ICU–or even out of their beds (35, 36). Performing such imaging studies at the bedside will obviate transporting patients to a radiology suite in a distant part of the hospital, thereby reducing the exposure of patients to the risks of intrahospital transport (36–38).

This is an exciting era for all of us to be involved in critical care medicine. As Hunt Batjer announced in his CNS Presidential Address several years ago (39), this is truly only the end of the beginning in neurosurgery. We as neurosurgeons have made tremendous advances in our technical sophistication. In the future, as we continue to improve our surgical skills, we will also gain a greater understanding of cerebral metabolism, both during illness and under normal conditions. Patient-specific interventions will be the norm rather than the exception. Transforming these dreams into reality is a striking manifestation of the 2002 Annual Meeting themes of Discovery, Leadership, and Freedom. Through such efforts, the distinction between "neurosurgeon" and "intensivist" will blur, so that our descendants will be able to transition seamlessly between the dual roles of neurosurgeon and intensivist.

REFERENCES

1. About us. **Website of the Leapfrog Group** [http://www.leapfroggroup.org/about.htm], accessed September 6, 2002.
2. BRT Newsroom. **Website of the Business Roundtable** [http://www.brt.org/newsroom.htm], accessed September 6, 2002.
3. Kohn LT, Corrigan JM, Donaldson MS (eds): *To Err is Human. Building a Safer Health System.* A report from the Committee on Quality of Healthcare in America, Institute of Medicine, National Academy of Sciences. Washington, D.C.: National Academy Press, 1999.
4. Anderson RE: How many deaths are due to medical errors? **JAMA** 284:2188, 2000.
5. McDonald CJ, Weiner M, Hui SL: How many deaths are due to medical errors? **JAMA** 284:2187, 2000.
6. Brennan TA: The Institute of Medicine report on medical errors—Could it do harm? **N Engl J Med** 342:1123–1125, 2000.
7. Agovino T: Soaring malpractice insurance squeezes out doctors, clinics. **The Associated Press,** July 18, 2002.
8. Coble YD Jr: West Virginia's trauma patients lost their golden hour—AMA letter to the editor. **Charleston Daily Mail**, Charleston, WV, August 30, 2002.
9. Fact Sheet: ICU Physician Staffing. **Website of the Leapfrog Group** [http://www.leapfroggroup.org/FactSheets/ICU_FactSheet.pdf], accessed September 6, 2002.
10. Zimmerman JE, Wagner DP, Draper EA, Wright L, Alzola C, Knaus WA: Evalua-

tion of acute physiology and chronic health evaluation III predictions of hospital mortality in an independent database. **Crit Care Med** 26:1317–1326, 1998.

11. Dickerson J, Valadka AB, LeVert T, et al.: Organ donation rates in a neurosurgical intensive care unit. **J Neurosurg** 97:811–814, 2002.
12. Pronovost PJ, Young TL, Dorman T, Robinson K, Angus DC: Association between ICU physician staffing and outcomes: a systematic review. **Crit Care Med** 27:A43, 1999.
13. Narayan RK: Emergency room management of the head-injured patient. In: Becker DP, Gudeman SK (eds): *Textbook of Head Injury.* Philadelphia: WB Saunders, 1989, pp. 23–66.
14. Watts C, Eyster EF: National Head and Spinal Cord Injury Prevention Program of the American Association of Neurological Surgeons and the Congress of Neurological Surgeons. **J Neurotrauma** 9:S307–S312, 1992.
15. *Injury in America: A Continuing Public Health Problem.* Washington, DC: National Academy Press, 1985, p 1.
16. Contant CF, Valadka AB, Gopinath SP, Hannay HJ, Robertson CS: Adult respiratory distress syndrome: A complication of induced hypertension after severe head injury. **J Neurosurg** 95:560–568, 2001.
17. Valadka AB, Andrews BT, Bullock MR: How well do neurosurgeons care for trauma patients? A survey of the membership of the American Association for the Surgery of Trauma. **Neurosurgery** 48:17–24, 2001.
18. Lobosky JM: Neurosurgical Critical Care: A perspective from private practice. **Perspect Neurol Surg** 8:111–121, 1997.
19. Hop JW, Rinkel GJ, Algra A, van Gijn J: Case-fatality rates and functional outcome after subarachnoid hemorrhage: A systematic review. **Stroke** 28:660–664, 1997.
20. Hop JW, Rinkel GJ, Algra A, van Gijn J: Quality of life in patients and partners after aneurysmal subarachnoid hemorrhage. **Stroke** 29:798–804, 1998.
21. Marshall LF: Head injury: recent past, present, and future. **Neurosurgery** 47:546–561, 2000.
22. Breasted JH: *The Edwin Smith Surgical Papyrus*, vol. 1–2. Chicago: University of Chicago Press, 1930.
23. Ward JD, Becker DP, Miller JD, et al.: Failure of prophylactic barbiturate coma in the treatment of severe head injury. **J Neurosurg** 62:383–388, 1985.
24. Muizelaar JP, Marmarou A, Ward JD, et al.: Adverse effects of prolonged hyperventilation in patients with severe head injury: a randomized clinical trial. **J Neurosurg** 75:731–739, 1991.
25. Hsiang JK, Chesnut RM, Crisp CB, et al.: Early, routine paralysis for intracranial pressure control in severe head injury: Is it necessary? **Crit Care Med** 22:1471–1476, 1994.
26. Robertson CS, Valadka AB, Hannay HJ, et al.: Prevention of secondary ischemic insults after severe head injury. **Crit Care Med** 27:2086–2095, 1999.
27. Cruz J, Minoja G, Okuchi K: Major clinical and physiological benefits of early high doses of mannitol for intraparenchymal temporal lobe hemorrhages with abnormal pupillary widening: a randomized trial. **Neurosurgery** 51:628–638, 2002.
28. Alexander H, Statler KD, Kochanek PM, et al.: Effects of seven anesthetics on outcome in experimental traumatic brain injury. **J Neurotrauma** 17:972, 2000.
29. Clifton GL, Miller ER, Choi SC, et al.: Lack of effect of induction of hypothermia after acute brain injury. **N Engl J Med** 344:556–563, 2001.
30. Maas AI, Steyerberg EW, Murray GD, et al.: Why have recent trials of neuroprotective agents in head injury failed to show convincing efficacy? A pragmatic analysis and theoretical considerations. **Neurosurgery** 44:1286–1298, 1999.

31. Nakayama M, Yasue H, Yoshimura M, et al.: T^{-786} → C mutation in the 5′-flanking region of the endothelial nitric oxide synthase gene is associated with coronary spasm. **Circulation** 99:2864–2870, 1999.
32. Nakayama M, Yasue H, Yoshimura M, et al. T^{-786} → C mutation in the 5′-flanking region of the endothelial nitric oxide synthase gene is associated with myocardial infarction, especially without coronary organic stenosis. **Am J Cardiol** 86:628–634, 2000.
33. Jenkins LW, Peters GW, Dixon CE, et al.: Conventional and functional proteomics using large format two-dimensional gel electrophoresis 24 hours after controlled cortical impact in postnatal day 17 rats. **J Neurotrauma** 19:715–740, 2002.
34. Friedman G, Froom P, Sazbon L, et al.: Apolipoprotein E-ϵ4 genotype predicts a poor outcome in survivors of traumatic brain injury. **Neurology** 52:244–248, 1999.
35. Butler WE, Piaggio CM, Constantinou C, et al.: A mobile computed tomographic scanner with intraoperative and intensive care unit applications. **Neurosurgery** 42:1304–1310, 1998.
36. Gunnarsson T, Theodorsson A, Karlsson P, et al.: Mobile computerized tomography scanning in the neurosurgery intensive care unit: increase in patient safety and reduction of staff workload. **J Neurosurg** 93:432–436, 2000.
37. Andrews PJ, Piper IR, Dearden NM, Miller JD. Secondary insults during intrahospital transport of head-injured patients. **Lancet** 335:327–330, 1990.
38. Kollef MH, Von Harz B, Prentice D, et al.: Patient transport from intensive care increases the risk of developing ventilator-associated pneumonia. **Chest** 112:765–773, 1997.
39. Batjer HH: Presidential address—The end of the beginning (again!). **Clin Neurosurg** 47:1–18, 2000.

CHAPTER

17

Certification of Neurosurgeons: A Transition from Neurosurgical Certification and Recertification to Maintenance of Certification

Report from the American Board of Neurological Surgeons

DAVID G. PIEPGRAS, M.D.

BACKGROUND

Completion of postgraduate specialty training remains a landmark achievement for the young specialist, one for which he or she both desires and deserves recognition as having achieved a high level of expertise. As early as 1908, the first specialty group, the American Academy of Ophthalmology and Otolaryngology, proposed a process of assessing the specialists in their field "for competency to perform their specialty practice." In 1917, the first nationally recognized medical specialty Board of Ophthalmology (NSBO) was established. Otolaryngology followed in 1924 with their program of required training and certification. Neurosurgery established its specialty board in 1940 with the espoused purpose to encourage the study, to improve the practice, to elevate the standards, to advance the science, and to serve the cause of public health. Eight additional boards have been recognized in the subsequent years.

As specialty and subspecialty medicine has flourished, there has been a need for an umbrella organization to coordinate and facilitate the common purpose and activities of the specialty boards. That role was met first in 1933 by the formation of the Advisory Board for Medical Specialties, which in 1970 was reorganized and incorporated as the American Board of Medical Specialties (ABMS). The ABMS is an organization of its approved medical specialty boards, whose stated mission is to maintain and improve the quality of medical care by assisting the member boards in their efforts to develop professional and educational standards for evaluation and certification of physician specialists. The ABMS mission statement goes on to say that the intent of certification of physicians is to provide assurance to the public that a physician specialist certified by a member board of the ABMS has successfully completed an approved educational program and evaluation process to assess his or her knowledge, skills, and experience required to provide quality patient care in that specialty.

Specifically for neurosurgeons, the process of certification is voluntary and consists of verification of having met the basic training, professional, and practice standards, with affirmation by secure examination of the command of a basic fund of knowledge relative to neuroscience. The initial certification is finalized through passage of an oral examination to affirm the candidate's possession of fundamental clinical knowledge and sound judgment.

RECERTIFICATION

There has been a growing awareness among our profession as well as the public that initial certification is not enough to assure quality care throughout one's career, and during the past several decades, there has been a call for periodic recertification of physician specialists. Importantly, since its inception in 1969, the American Board of Family Practice issued 7-year, time-limited certificates with a requirement for some evaluation of office practice and cognitive knowledge as well as completion of a CME requirement to become recertified. At its outset, recertification was envisioned as an impetus—indeed, a requirement—for physicians to keep up with new knowledge. Other boards followed suit as it became recognized that updating knowledge and other basic skills was essential to maintain high-quality patient care. Recertification became an expectation of the ABMS and was affirmed in policy statements dating back to 1973. By 1998, 20 of the 24 member boards had recertification in place, primarily based on retaking an examination, maintaining licensure, and for the majority of boards, meeting some CME requirement. Neurosurgery was slow to join this movement, however, and had the somewhat ignominious distinction of being the last board to adopt a plan for recertification, instigated not only by the Board's understanding of its virtues but by the expectations of the ABMS as well. The American Board of Neurological Surgeons (ABNS) issued its first time-limited certificates in May 1999, with a 10-year life span.

Meanwhile, however, expectations have been changing, and recognition is growing that a test of factual knowledge every 10 years is inadequate to assure a continuum of a high level of knowledge and skills for quality patient care (in a word, "competence"). Simultaneously, quality of medical care, incompetent physicians, and consumer protection have become issues of broad concern on a national level. In response to the demand for quality measures and improvement, task forces were formed, including private and presidential commissions as well as an Institute of Medicine Committee, to examine the quality of health care in America. Dr. Kenneth Shine, President of the Institute of Medicine, has issued the message to America's physicians that demonstration of competence and verification of performance are the expectations for the future.

COMPETENCE AND MAINTENANCE OF CERTIFICATION

In 1993, the ABMS adopted as policy that "the goal of recertification is to evaluate the continuing competence of a diplomate in the specialty in which he/she was initially certified." In 1998, it followed with creation of a Task Force on Competence in recognition of the need to satisfy the public, the payers, other health care organizations, governmental agencies, and the profession itself that specialist physicians are competent and will maintain their competency throughout the span of their careers—in essence, in the words of then–ABMS President, Dr. Leo Dunn, "To do what we say we do."

The ABMS leadership espoused that recertification programs should transform from a minimum of periodic examination and meeting of CME requirements to a continuing process of updating and maintaining knowledge and skills through ongoing learning and improvement such that competence in practice is maintained. In March 2000, the ABMS member boards adopted a policy of commitment to evolve their current or planned programs of recertification into programs of Maintenance of Certification (MOC).

The competence movement has gained momentum during the past 4 years and been embraced in the policies of not only the ABMS but also the Accreditation Council of Graduate Medical Education (ACGME) and the Association of American Medical Colleges (AAMC). The expectation is that the training and acquisition of knowledge and skills for competence in medical practice, which begin in medical school, will be enhanced and honed to the specialty in residency training and maintained throughout the specialist's career.

Admittedly, the designation of "competence" has been troublesome for the member boards. All boards share the belief that their diplomates possess "requisite or adequate ability or qualities," but all boards and, particularly, their legal counsels are reluctant—indeed, unwilling—to accept the responsibility that certification verifies competence in all aspects of practice and at all times, as might be inferred by the legal definition (i.e., "legally qualified or adequate"). Indeed, the Task Force on Competence had trouble providing a simple definition of physician competence, necessitating a description as follows: The competent physician should possess the medical knowledge, judgment, professionalism, and clinical and communication skills to provide high quality patient care. Patient care encompasses the promotion of health, prevention of disease, and diagnosis, treatment and management of medical conditions with compassion and respect for patients and their families.

Maintenance of competence should be demonstrated throughout the physician's career by evidence of lifelong learning and ongoing improvement of practice.

In concert with the ACGME, six general competencies have been identified as key elements for the full spectrum of physician clinical competence. These six competencies, as appropriate to the specialty, will form the foundation for physician and resident training and the basis for credentialing, including individual certification and future MOC, and also for the accreditation of residency training programs by the ACGME and residency review committees as they assess resident teaching and performance against the six general competencies. The six general competencies include:

1. Medical knowledge,
2. Patient care,
3. Interpersonal and communication skills,
4. Professionalism,
5. Practice-based learning and improvement, and
6. Systems-based practice.

Examples of elements of these competencies that pertain to neurosurgical practice have been suggested:

1. *Medical Knowledge—General and Practice Specific:* Know and critically evaluate current medical information; understand and incorporate evidence-based decision making.
2. *Patient Care:* Medical interview and physical examination; synthesis of clinical data, performance skills.
3. *Interpersonal and Communication Skills:* Communicate effectively with patients and families; communicate effectively with other professionals and team members; maintain comprehensive, legible medical records.
4. *Professionalism:* Demonstrate self-awareness and knowledge of limits; demonstrate high standards of ethical and moral behavior;

demonstrate reliability and responsibility; demonstrate respect for patient's dignity and autonomy. (The American Board of Internal Medicine, in collaboration with the American College of Physicians and the European Federation of Internal Medicine, has elaborated the obligations for Medical Professionalism in a recent publication [4]).

5. *Practice-Based Learning and Improvement:* Engage in ongoing learning to improve knowledge and skills; analyze one's practice to recognize strengths and deficiencies; seek input to improve practice and quality care.
6. *Systems-Based Practice:* Promote patient safety within the system; provide value for patients through cost effective care; promote health and prevention of disease and injury; demonstrate effective practice management.

ABNS MAINTENANCE OF CERTIFICATION

The ABNS envisions that its initial certification program will remain as it is currently functioning, with verification of credentials, candidate evaluation by peers, 1 year's practice review, and an oral examination. Maintenance of certification programs for the ABNS as well as other ABMS member boards will necessarily conform to the model adopted by the ABMS, with assessment of four basic components:

1. Evidence of professional standing,
2. Evidence of commitment to lifelong learning and involvement in a periodic self-assessment process,
3. Evidence of cognitive expertise, and
4. Evidence of evaluation of performance in practice.

The ABNS and its Committee on Maintenance of Certification have been giving careful thought and study to the methodology of our MOC program, with the expectation that in approximately 1 year, we will be ready to submit our plan for assessment of the first components to the ABMS for review and approval. Certain principles governing our plan are already established, whereas others are just beginning to take shape. The overriding principles of the MOC program are that the process must evaluate in its spectrum the six basic competencies and will evolve into a continuous, rather than remain a periodic, process.

Concerning evidence of *professional standing*, it is agreed that all ABMS Boards will require an unrestricted license to practice medicine. The ABNS likely will also want to include input from peers and, perhaps coworkers or even patients as part of this component.

Evidence of *cognitive expertise* will be met by a periodic examination, undoubtedly a written, multiple-choice examination that will be administered at test centers around the country. It is the only part of the MOC program that will be pass/fail, but there will be no limit on the possibility for retakes of this examination. The ABNS Examination Committee, with input from the Joint Section memberships, is already assembling a bank of material that will generate questions for this examination, which will cover fundamental knowledge and, especially, practice-related current and clinically valid knowledge. Additionally, the neurosurgeon is expected to possess knowledge relating to the practice environment, such as quality assurance, safety, ethics, and economic issues. The requirement that the examination be practice related should allay fears regarding esoteric questions and also give the candidate options to be examined in those areas that relate to his or her practice and areas of expertise.

The requirement for evidence of participation in *lifelong learning and self-assessment* seems to be challenging. This is one area that we should welcome, however, because it is particularly aimed at practitioner improvement. Traditional CME will probably be part of this requirement but less weighty than practice-related self-study and analysis of one's practice. The Self-Assessment Examination in NeuroSurgery (SANS) holds promise for being one of the important elements in this component as well as having value in preparing the diplomate for the secure cognitive examination.

Involvement in a program of *practice assessment* also has the potential for bringing about significant improvement of practice. It seems implausible that both time and expense would permit an in-depth practice review such as that carried out for initial certification. Analysis of key cases relative to management methods or procedural outcomes, possibly Web-based, however, is conceivable. Focused record audits have been employed by other specialties. Methods for assessment and feedback relative to one's performance in the areas of the six competencies will undoubtedly evolve and, ultimately, may become the most meaningful. The ABNS will proceed slowly in developing these programs and looks to the cumulative experience of other surgical boards and the direction of the ABMS and our societies, particularly the Congress of Neurological Surgeons (CNS) and AANS, as we proceed.

GRANDFATHERING

Many neurosurgeons are concerned about "grandfathering" and those with non–time limited certificates are wondering if they will have to enter the MOC program. The simple answer is "No." Participation for these individuals will not be required by the ABNS, though it would be encouraged. For those diplomates with time-limited certificates, upon expiration of their current certificates and when recertified, it will be into the MOC program.

ROLE OF SOCIETIES

This review does not allow discussion of the critical role of our societies, especially the CNS and AANS, in this process. Their role is of paramount importance, however, because the major neurosurgical societies will be primary participants in developing the neurosurgical curriculum and in identifying the contemporary knowledge and skills as they pertain to each of the competencies. Furthermore, it will be the responsibility of the societies to carry out all educational aspects for MOC.

CONCLUSION

Many neurosurgeons will regard this MOC program with trepidation or even outright hostility, which is understandable. I would reassure you, however, that the ABNS is committed to the program, with the realization that "its time has come" and it is "the right thing to do" for our patients and our specialty. Neurosurgery MOC will be a "work in progress." It is our goal and expectation that in the end, it should not be onerous or expensive but, rather, will be meaningful and, more than ever, enhance our practice and competence as neurosurgeons.

REFERENCES

1. *ABMS Research & Education Foundation 2002 Annual Report & Reference Handbook.*
2. *ABMS Proceedings of the COBRE and Assembly 1999–2002.*
3. *American Board of Neurological Surgery Booklet of Information, June 2002.*
4. Medical Professionalism Project: ABIM Foundation, ACP-ASIM Foundation, European Federation of Internal Medicine. Medical Professionalism in the New Millennium: A Physician Charter. **Ann Intern Med** 136:243–246, 2002.

CHAPTER

18

Acoustic Tumors: Operation Versus Radiation—Making Sense of Opposing Viewpoints

STEVEN L. GIANNOTTA *VERSUS* DOUGLAS KONDZIOLKA

PART

I

Acoustic Neuroma: Decision Making with All the Tools

INDRO CHAKRABARTI, M.D., MICHAEL L.J. APUZZO, M.D., AND STEVEN L. GIANNOTA, M.D.

INTRODUCTION

"This is getting complicated," she says. She is a 48-year-old speech pathologist and part-time opera singer discovered to have a unilateral, 1.8-cm acoustic neuroma. During her first consultation, her physicians recommended a translabyrinthine removal, with the invariable loss of hearing. She has read about radiosurgery on several websites, but her first surgeon did not offer this technology. In fact, it was repudiated. Subsequently, she had talked to a number of Acoustic Neuroma Society members who were touting fractionated radiotherapy for its safety benefits. Her comment was prompted by the introduction of yet another alternative, namely a retrosigmoid approach for tumor removal with a 30% to 50% success rate for preserving useful hearing.

Admittedly, the decision making for treatment options in acoustic neuroma has taken on more complexity for both the physician and the patient. Surgical results, at least in experienced hands, have become highly commendable and provide a reasonable success rate to those looking for an excisional cure. Radiosurgical tumor control data, again in the best of hands, grows more impressive, now with 10 to 15 years of follow-up. Hypofractionated radiosurgery has a laudable safety record, although long-term efficacy data are lacking. In selected cases, avoidance of any treatment is also an effective strategy. Clearly, there is not one best way to treat a patient with an acoustic tumor. In the ideal situation, a simple comparison between efficacy and safety data from several different therapeutic options should be sufficient to make a decision. Besides the various treatment options that exist, however, other factors come into play, including patient preference, surgeon bias, cost, patient age, and lifestyle issues. A large support group, the Acoustic Neuroma Society, is available to advise those contemplating treatment and publishes helpful information to those suffering from the disabilities secondary to treatment.

The goal of this report is to review the optimal results of all three treatment options, to discuss the techniques that are instrumental in obtaining those results, and to outline the decision-making process in an institution at which all modalities are available and no competition exists among practitioners.

CONSERVATIVE MANAGEMENT

Many patients with newly diagnosed acoustic neuromas have minimal symptoms and are aware that this most often is a benign, slow-growing process. In selected cases, a logical strategy is simply to follow patients with surveillance imaging. Indeed, several studies concerning the natural history of acoustic neuroma behavior have bolstered this stance.

In Rosenberg's well-quoted study (1), conservatively monitored tumors over 4.8 years did not grow or regressed 42% of the time. Additionally, after surgery for subtotal resections, tumors did not grow or regressed in 68% of patients, and only 6% needed reoperation.

More studies have corroborated the value of the observational approach in selected cases with tenacious radiographic follow-up (2–9). The annual growth rates of untreated tumors have ranged from 0.15 to 4 mm. Rosenberg (1) demonstrated that after subtotal removal, the annual growth rate was 0.35 mm per year. Age, sex, initial symptoms, and initial tumor size did not reliably predict growth rates. A yearly growth rate of roughly 3 mm, however, is correlated with need for intervention (5). Our experience suggests that in younger patients, conservative management in the hopes of avoiding some form of therapeutic initiative in the future is usually futile.

SURGICAL MANAGEMENT

Microsurgery Results

SURGICAL EFFICACY

The gold standard for treatment of any benign tumor is curative total removal. The concept of complete removal without the need for lifelong surveillance is appealing to patients. Thus, a discussion of cure and recurrence rates is helpful for informed decision making. It is axiomatic that a microscopic total removal will result in surgical cure. Long-term follow-up data are available for selected surgical series. Reports by Samii, Sampath, Ebersold, Koos, and others cite recurrence rates of 1% or less (*Table 18.1(I)*). This represents data on more than 2,500 cases and strengthens the conclusion that in an experienced surgeon's hands, cure is a reasonable expectation.

Not all surgery results in total removal. Certain factors stand in the way of that technical feat. The two most important are lack of experience with the technical maneuvers necessary for safe removal and the compromise of those maneuvers for the purpose of cranial nerve preservation. Even subtotal removal, however, may well be associated with long-term tumor control. The regrowth of tumors requiring intervention in 49 subtotal resections that were followed for nearly 5 years was 6% in one analysis (1). With small intracanalicular residual tumors, the rate of clinically significant recurrence has been reported as zero in one study (10). Certainly, the larger the residual, the greater the likelihood of a symptomatic recurrence. Lesions left along the brain stem and, especially, large residuals in the internal canal

TABLE 18.1(I)
Surgical Results: Complications and Recurrence Rates (%)[a]

Series	CSF Leaks	Major Events	Mortality	Recurrence
Ebersold	10	2	0.8	1.1
Gjuric	2	0.3	0.4	0.2
Gormley	15	0.5	1	0.5
Harner	12	2	0.6	0.2
Samii	9	1	1.1	0.7
Sampath	25	1	0.16	0.8
Tos	11	0	2	1
Wiegand	11	9	—	7.8

[a]Data from large reports on complication and recurrence rates arising from surgery for acoustic neuromas. Major events include ataxia, hemiparesis, and lower cranial nerve palsy.

can gain sufficient blood supply to regrow. It seems that small residuals left along a cranial nerve are less likely to recur, suggesting a strategic alternative to the microscopic total removal standard (11, 12).

SAFETY

Long-term tumor control or cure is desirable to many patients, but at what price? Among the larger series, the surgical complication rates have become acceptably low (*Table 18.1*). The most common complication is cerebrospinal fluid (CSF) leaks, occurring in 2% to 25% of cases (13–16). Major morbidity, such as lower cranial nerve palsy, ataxia, or long-tract dysfunction, is also low, occurring 0% to 2% of the time (13–16). Mortality from surgery is rare, occurring in 0.4% to 2%. The two most important factors that relate to safety and efficacy are tumor size and surgeon experience. Strategies for maximizing surgical outcomes will be discussed subsequently.

FACIAL NERVE OUTCOMES

Of all potential negative factors, patients are most concerned about facial nerve function. In fact, this is clearly how the most accomplished practitioners of the surgical art keep score. It is important for the surgeon advising a patient to be familiar with state-of-the-art statistics and whether he or she can offer those same results. Most reports defined an "excellent" or "good" outcome as a House-Brackman (H-B) score of 1 or 2 (17).

A review of our results in 382 acoustic tumors of all sizes revealed a 79% H-B score of 1 or 2 facial nerve function rate. A number of much larger series exists in the literature (*Table 18.2(I)*). Samii and Mathies (14) reported the largest single-surgeon series, in which 1,000 cases are described. In this series the seventh facial nerve was preserved 93% of the time, with H-B score of 1 or 2 in 59% of patients. A number of groups have reported experiences ranging from 250 to more than 500 cases. These authors report a range of 64% to 90% good facial nerve results (13, 15, 18–27).

The Acoustic Neuroma Registry, started in the late 1980s, catalogues the national results of various surgeons through questionnaires and surveys. In a summary of 1,579 cases recorded in this registry between 1989 and 1994, Wiegand et al. (16) found in 92% of cases that surgeons felt the removal to be total, with 94% preservation of the facial nerve continuity. Of these, 69% had excellent facial nerve function after follow-up at 1 year.

Because tumor size is one of the most important determining factors in predicting surgical outcome, stratifying results in terms of size can be more instructive. A few authors specifically report their expe-

TABLE 18.2(I)
Facial Function after Surgery for Acoustic Neuromas: Summary of Large Series Reports[a]

Series	Cases (n)	"Good" Seventh Nerve Function (H-B 1–2; %)
Wiegand	1,579	69
Samii	1,000	59
Gjuric	735	92
Sampath	611	90
Sterkers	576	83
Wiet	504	78
Ojeman	410	77
Symon	392	64
Giannotta	381	79
Koos	364	90
Harner	335	81
Arriaga	315	80

[a]Summary of facial nerve outcomes from published surgical series. H-B 1–2 refers to the Houseman-Brackman facial nerve function score; grades 1 and 2 are largely considered to be acceptable of "good" results.

rience with large tumors (>3 cm). These statistics are particularly important, because very few treatment alternatives have a demonstrated efficacy rate. In well-practiced hands, facial nerve continuity rates of greater than 80% and good functional results of up to 70% can be accomplished even with tumors ranging from 3.5 to 6 cm (28–31).

Conversely, excellent results can be expected with the smallest of acoustic tumors. Purely intracanalicular tumors were addressed by Haines and Levine (32). All 14 patients had excellent nerve outcomes. The series of Nadol (33) and of Samii (14) also report 100% good facial scores for purely intracanalicular tumors. In an analysis of the retrosigmoid approach, Rowed and Nedzedlski (34) mention 96% of 26 intracanalicular tumors with good outcomes (34).

To attempt a more direct comparison between surgery and radiosurgery, we sifted through the various publications to identify those which stratified facial nerve results based on tumor size. Facial nerve outcomes after surgery for tumors less than 3 cm were tabulated (*Table 18.3(I)*), because single-fraction radiosurgery only addresses this subgroup of patients. As expected, these facial nerve outcomes are laudable, with favorable facial nerve outcomes in the 80% to 99% range (15, 18, 19, 23, 27, 35).

Another way to capture surgical results that can be compared with radiosurgical data is to look at cases in which the surgeon attempted to preserve hearing. The majority of theses lesions would be in the size range for single-fraction radiosurgery (*Table 18.4(I)*). Shelton et

TABLE 18.3(I)
House-Brackman Grades 1–2 in Small Tumors (<3 cm) after Surgery[a]

Series	Patients with House-Brackman Grades 1–2 (%)
Arriaga	92
Ebersold	99
Giannotta	90
Gjuric	92
Gormley	96
Koos	88
Lalwani	92
McElveen	99
Sampath	92
Slattery	95
Sterkers	83

[a]Facial nerve outcomes for tumors 3 cm or less in linear dimension. House-Brackman grades 1 and 2 are generally accepted as "good" outcomes.

al. (36) reported that 89% of their patients experienced good facial function in a series of 106 cases performed through the middle fossa approach. Other groups have elevated their surgical techniques to the point at which facial nerve preservation and cochlear nerve preservation are an expected outcome (25, 33, 37–39).

HEARING PRESERVATION

The data on hearing are a bit difficult to interpret, because patient outcomes are sometimes reported as simply at or near preoperative

TABLE 18.4(I)
Attempted Hearing Preservation: Rates after Surgery for Acoustic Neuroma[a]

Series	Cases (n)	Hearing Preservation (%)
Brackman	333	50
Slattery	150	68
Fischer	99	29.3
Rowed	94	35
Dornhoffer	93	45
Umezu	73	41
Giannotta	72	36
Torrens	62	32
Arriaga	60	67
Hecht	60	37
Post	56	52
Moffat	50	8

[a]Results from published reports on hearing preservation rates after surgery for acoustic neuroma. Outcomes were described as either unchanged from preoperative levels, Gardner-Robertson grade 1 or 2, or AAO-HNS class A or B.

levels. Per the Gardner-Robertson scale, however, a class I or II is considered to be serviceable or better hearing (40). In this scale, pure-tone average of 0 to 30 dB and speech discrimination of 70% to 100% corresponds to class 1 hearing. Class 2 hearing assumes a 31- to 50-dB pure-tone average and 50% to 69% speech discrimination. The AAO-HNS guidelines on the evaluation of hearing preservation also developed a system of classification, with class A or B generally indicating useful hearing (41). Class A hearing includes less than 30-dB pure-tone thresholds and more than 70% speech discrimination. Class B includes 30- to 50-dB pure-tone thresholds and more than more than >50% speech discrimination. Most reports use one of these two methods for recording hearing outcomes.

The data with regards to hearing preservation among the large series are somewhat variable. Good hearing can range from 24% to 60% depending on the series (13, 14, 18–20, 23, 27, 30, 33, 35). It is noteworthy that the Acoustic Neuroma Registry data described by Wiegand et al. (16) reports a 22% hearing preservation rate (*Table 18.4(I)*).

A cursory look at data from groups who report large series of middle fossa approaches would suggest that this strategy might be more effective in terms of hearing preservation. Most accomplished groups report good hearing rates in the range of 50% (25, 32, 34, 36, 38, 39, 42, 43, 44); however, these series are all biased towards the smallest of tumors.

Maximizing Results

Before one can reasonably offer a patient the option of total surgical removal, the requisite psychomotor skills must be mastered to approximate results that have been publicized and used for comparison to other nonsurgical modalities. Despite the myriad of potential complications that can occur from posterior fossa surgery, cranial nerve injury and vascular complication cause the most disability. Thus, small vessel and cranial nerve preservation is the key to successful results. Those skills are developed in the same way as other highly sophisticated techniques. Foremost is the availability of a mentor with highly evolved technical facility and a proven track record. Time spent observing successful maneuvers, usually during residency or fellowship training, is equally as important as the ability to mimic these techniques. The "learning curve" for surgical mastery of acoustic neuroma cases has been pointed out by several authors (18, 20, 45, 46).

Repetition of highly stylized maneuvers is mandatory for mastery of skills. This implies a ready source of patients to take advantage of the learning curve. A query of the California state databank for the years 1999 and 2000 suggests that 85% of the operative treatment for acoustic neuromas occurs in 1.7% of the state's hospitals (47). Also, according to the acoustic neuroma registry, 26.1% of catalogued operative cases have come from two centers (16). The opportunity to hone one's skills with a large number of cases is thus limited unless one works in an environment that has developed referral sources.

Unfortunately, very little overlap exists, especially in terms of cranial nerve manipulation, with other neurosurgical procedures to boost skill levels when acoustic tumors are not available. In this circumstance, a vascular and skull base practice can afford the opportunity to advance one's expertise. Manipulating small vessels around aneurysms or removal of AVMs may strengthen the techniques necessary to dissect branches of PICA and AICA during acoustic removal. Dissection of facial and cochlear nerves during removal of petrotentorial or clival meningiomas, although not nearly as demanding as in the case of acoustic tumors, allows for some basic skills application.

For cranial nerve preservation, some form of sharp or semisharp dissection, whether by scissors, knives, or hooks, usually produces the best results. When dealing with facial or cochlear nerves, three cues are important to observe: The nerve must remain slack, wet, and vascularized. Dissection of the nerve in a direction that minimizes traction will maintain the EMG monitor in its quietest mode. Strategies must be learned to limit heavy tumor fragments from hanging on the nerve. Nerves must remain moist throughout the dissection process, either by irrigation or bathing in CSF. Avoidance of the sitting position is the easiest way to obviate drying out of the relevant cranial nerves during protracted dissection. Resistance to the use of bipolar cautery around the facial and cochlear nerves will lessen ischemic injury from heat transmission. Ignoring it, if possible, or irrigation with the gentle application of hemostatic agents best manages bleeding on the nerve surface. Cranial nerve monitoring facilitates the accrual of requisite skills by providing timely feedback to ill-advised surgical maneuvers. Several studies have documented the improvement of surgical results by comparing outcomes before and after employment of EMG and BAER monitoring (42, 48, 49). Such adjuncts are highly advised while ascending the learning curve. Mastery of these techniques will assure that what is offered to a nervous and confused patient is commensurate with results found in the literature.

SURGICAL APPROACHES

Each of the three traditional approaches to the CP angle have there own putative strategic advantages. The translabyrinthine approach minimizes retraction, maximizes exposure of the internal auditory canal, and facilitates defining the facial nerve within the canal. The retrosigmoid approach has the advantage of being stereotypical for most neurosurgeons while enabling preservation of the hearing apparatus. The middle fossa approach, while admittedly for smaller tumors, also facilitates exposure of the lateral most extent of the internal auditory canal. Proponents of each approach are able to post impressive numbers in terms of safety and cure rates. Many studies have looked at outcomes based on approach, and no discernible advantage has been documented for one approach over another (15, 25). For purely intracanalicular tumors, however, several reports have shown that the middle fossa approach is safer than the retrosigmoid approach for hearing preservation (19, 34, 38). A cursory review of the literature would suggest no way to resolve controversies that may emerge regarding the best approach for a given situation. Hearing preservation, facial nerve function, and incidence of total removal seem to be practitioner or team related as opposed to approach related. This suggests that technical expertise and strategic operative decision making can negate most disadvantages related to the various approach strategies.

A retrospective review of our institution's last 50 cases of retrosigmoid resections was compared to the last 50 translabyrinthine resections. Tumors were included that were 3 cm or less, and results were categorized in terms of facial nerve outcome, incidence of total resection, and major complications. At discharge, 37 of the patients with retrosigmoid resections had an H-B score of 1, as compared to 28 of the patients with translabyrinthine resections. Combining H-B 1 and 2 scores showed 82% with the retrosigmoid cases and 70% of the translabyrinthine cases. This did not reach statistical significance. One major neurological complication occurred in the retrosigmoid group, and none occurred in the translabyrinthine group. Three cases of subtotal removal resided in each group. Long-term follow-up of these patients showed even less of a difference in facial nerve function. This suggests that surgical technique may be more important than approach strategies in terms of outcome for acoustic tumors.

Ideally, each practitioner should have a working knowledge of all approaches. This can instill the wary patient with some confidence that decision making is based on assessment of the patient's best interests. For those who are experiencing unacceptable results, altering approach strategy may show modest benefits, but doing such will not make up for deficiencies in surgical technique as it relates to the brain stem vascularity and cranial nerves.

RADIOSURGERY

The emergence of single dose, highly collimated radiation-delivery systems has yielded another alternative in the management of acoustic tumors. Data suggest that tumor control can be expected for as long as 5 to 10 years with currently fashionable doses in as much as 80% to 90% of cases (50). Although longer-term follow-up is desirable, it becomes less likely that a dramatic increase in regrowths will suddenly emerge after such a long interval. As mentioned in the *Introduction*, however, some patients have been known to harbor tumors with biological inactivity, thus calling into question the ultimate efficacy of radiosurgery in certain cases (1–3, 6–7). Although safety remains a concern, using total doses of 24 to 28 Gy with 12 to 14 Gy to the periphery and treating to the 50% isodose line, morbidity matches that of the best surgical series, with hearing preservation rates in the short run that exceed those of microsurgery. Despite the automated nature and user-friendliness of the radiation-delivery systems available today, are these results reproducible? As with surgical skills, experience and adherence to a strict paradigm will allow practitioners to approach results quoted in the literature.

Radiosurgical Results

EFFICACY

The Karolinska experience is based on more than 900 treated patients. They report 95% tumor control rate. Also, hearing was preserved in 70%, with a 5% to 10% incidence of facial nerve palsy (51). The Pittsburgh group also has extensive experience with radiosurgery for acoustic neuromas (*Table 18.5(I)*). A comparison of 78 patients treated radiosurgically with a matched group treated microsurgically achieved a 94% tumor control rate, with 75% (6/8) having preserved hearing and an 8% rate of facial nerve palsy at 1 year (52). With 5-year follow-up, another report on 162 patients showed 98% tumor control rates, 51% hearing preservation, 15% seventh nerve palsy, and 16% fifth nerve palsy (50). In 20 patients with useful hearing pretreatment, 95% had tumor control, 45% had useful hearing at 2 years, 10% had seventh nerve palsies, and 25% had fifth nerve dysfunction (53). After dose reduction to the tumor margin to 11 to 13 Gy, no cases of fifth or seventh nerve palsies occurred (54). In a recent manuscript, 5-year outcomes with gamma knife on 190 patients were reported to have 97% tumor control, 71% hearing preservation, 1.1% fifth nerve palsy, and 2.6% fifth nerve palsy (55). Finally, a group of more than 130 patients followed for 10 to 15 years was reported at the 2002 Congress of Neurological Surgeons (CNS) meeting with 97% control (Kondziolka, oral presentation, 2002 CNS).

TABLE 18.5(I)
Gamma Knife Radiosurgery Outcomes for Acoustic Neuroma[a]

Series	Cases (n)	Mean Follow-up (mo)	Tumor Control (%)	Hearing Preservation (%)	Seventh Nerve Palsy (%)	Fifth Nerve Palsy (%)
Noren	669	12	95	65–70	5–10	—
Flickinger	238	30	—	55	17.2	2.3
Kondziolka	162	60	98	51	15	16
Ito	125	37	—	58	36	25
Foote	108	34	93	—	5	2
Prasad	96	52	93	—	1.3	1.6
Kwon	88	52	95	66 (2/3)	8.8	—
Pollock	78	36	94	75 (6/8)	8	—
Andrews	69	30	98	33	2	5
Unger	56	62	89	61	7	—

[a]Summary of reports on the use of gamma knife stereotactic radiosurgery for acoustic neuroma.

Experience with linear acceleration (LINAC) has produced similar results (56–58). Tumor control has been documented in 85% to 98% of cases. Facial palsy rates were between 7% and 32%, and hearing was preserved in 19% to 71%.

In the search for improved cranial nerve preservation, hypofractionation of radiosurgically delivered energy has been used increasingly (59–63) (*Table 18.6(I)*). Long-term follow-up is lacking, but thus far, tumor control has been noted in 91% to 100% of cases. Hearing

TABLE 18.6(I)
Fractionated Stereotactic Radiosurgery Outcomes for Acoustic Neuroma[a]

Series	Cases (n)	Mean Follow-up or Range (mo)	Tumor Control (%)	Hearing Preservation (%)	Seventh Nerve Palsy (%)	Fifth Nerve Palsy (%)
Andrews	56	29	97	81	2	7
Shirato	54	30.5	98	—	0	0
Fuss	51	42	98	85	0	5
Lederman	38	27	100	94	0	0
Meijer	37	25	91	66	0	3
Poen	32	24	97	77	3	16
Song	31	6-44	100	75	0	0
Varlotto	12	26.5	100	92	0	0

[a]Use of fractionation of dose in stereotactic radiosurgery. A summary of current literature.

preservation rates have been impressive, with 33% to 94% success. Also, rates of facial nerve palsy are lower, with 0% to 3% being reported.

With experience has come increased wisdom as to tumor dosimetry and planning for radiosurgical treatment of acoustic neuroma. Decreasing the dose to the margin of the tumor and fractionation have yielded impressive results; however, the long-term outcomes remain to be seen.

MAXIMIZING RESULTS

Although some would question the term *radiosurgery* for this treatment modality, compulsion and attention to detail are necessary when using doses of radiation that will invariably produce necrosis if aimed directly at brain tissue. *Figure 18.1(I)* shows three treatment plans for

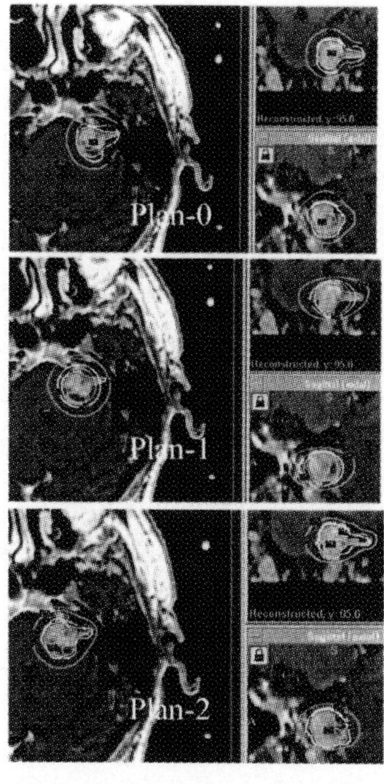

Plan Summary

Parameters	Plan-0	Plan-1	Plan-2
Tumor (cm^3)	2.9	2.9	2.9
Tumor Tx (%)	100	99	99
Total V Tx (cm^3)	4.4	5.9	3.9
TVT / TT	1.52	2.04	1.34
75% Hot Spot(cm^3)	0.30	3.70	1.20
Collimator(mm)/No	8/8	18/1	4/29
Tx Time (min)	34	12	159

Note: Rx = 14 Gy to 50 %

FIG. 18.1(I) Three potential gamma plans for stereotactic radiosurgery. Plan 1 uses a few large collimator beams to cover the tumor; however, the brain stem is needlessly covered as well. Plan 2 uses multiple small collimator shots to create a more tightly conformal plan. In this plan, however, the time of treatment is lengthy, and overlap of the beams creates hot spots. Finally, plan 0 uses different-size collimators to create a conformal plan covering the tumor morphology without hot spots and optimizing the gamma knife capabilities.

the gamma knife treatment of a 2-cm acoustic neuroma. At first glance, each looks to be acceptable; however, plan 1 uses only a single shot with an 18-mm collimator. The target is completely covered, but a portion of the brain stem is needlessly included. The relatively large treatment volume to tumor volume ratio (TVT/TT = 2.04) is evidence for this. The plan is quick and easy to produce but does not take advantage of the safety and efficacy of a tightly conformal paradigm, and it cannot be legitimately called *radiosurgery*. This plan produces nonuniform dosage, raising the possibility of inadequate treatment or hot spots that may increase cranial nerve morbidity.

Plan 2 uses many small collimator shots that uniformly cover the target, but the treatment time is long (159 min), making this a very inefficient strategy and not maximizing the radiosurgical potential of the gamma knife. Plan 0 has excellent coverage using different-sized collimators with excellent conformation to the tumor morphology. The target volume to treated volume ratio is acceptable (TVT/TT = 1.52), and the treatment time is reasonable. By treating to the 50% isodose line, reasonably uniform dosage across the target volume can be expected, reducing toxicity to adjacent cranial nerves and brain stem but maximizing the effectiveness of the prescription to the tumor edge. Thus, there seems to be both an art and a skill to the application of high-energy forms to strategically situated, benign lesions.

RADIOSURGICAL SAFETY

Initial experience with radiosurgery for acoustic tumors suggested acceptable tumor control, but cranial nerve toxicity was surprising. Series by Noren and others reported facial dysfunction rates of 10% to 36% and trigeminal symptoms in 7% to 25% (50, 51, 53, 56–58). By reducing the edge dose to 12 to 14 Gy, much improvement was seen in terms of toxicity, with rates falling to less than 2% in some series. With fractionation, hearing preservation rates have been reported as high as 94%.

One of the major appeals of radiosurgery is the seemingly nonexistent mortality rate. It is reasonable to assume that, with such large numbers of patients getting radiosurgery for benign conditions, malignant degeneration may occur; however, reports have been sparse. Yu et al. (64) reported the occurrence of a glioblastoma in the bed of a previously radiosurgically treated meningioma. This was discovered 7 years later. Kaido et al. (65) found a glioblastoma in the region of a previously treated AVM. In this case, the patient was treated with the gamma knife at age 14, and the tumor was discovered at age 20, both of which are ages at which the incidence of glioblastoma is uncommon. Similarly, Shamisa et al. (66) reported a glioblastoma in the area of a previously treated acoustic tumor. Perhaps the most compelling report comes from Shin et al. (67), who identified the malignant transformation of a residual acoustic neuroma treated with gamma knife radiosurgery. Again, the time interval between treatment and malignancy was approximately 6 years. Genotyping showed a TP-53 mutation in the malignant tumor that was not present in the surgically removed remnant. The oncogenetic effects of radiation to the brain are well established, lending further credence to the presumed finite rate of malignant induction of benign, radiosurgically treated targets.

DECISION MAKING

At our institution, the three traditional approaches for surgical excision of acoustic tumors are practiced. Furthermore, three technologies for radiosurgery (gamma knife, LINAC, and Cyberknife) are offered. The surgical decision making is less predicated on available technologies or reliance on a practiced single surgical approach than it is on patient age, tumor size, and need for hearing preservation.

Age and Size

For younger patients, the emphasis is on surgical removal. A surveillance strategy in this group is likely to be futile, because inevitably, the lesion will cause further symptoms and require treatment. Radiosurgery has a long follow-up period, and the window of vulnerability for recurrence is potentially wide. Reliable data concerning lifelong tumor control for patients in their thirties or forties are lacking. For patients in their fifties and sixties, single-fraction radiosurgery is an attractive alternative. Efficacy and safety statistics are available for this group and are highly acceptable. Patients in older age groups rarely need any therapy unless their tumor is large enough to be threatening.

For large lesions greater than 3 cm, single-fraction radiosurgery has no role. For these lesions, surgical removal or, in certain situations, subtotal removal, with follow-up radiosurgery, is advisable. Subtotal removal for a patient with a single tumor and good hearing in the other ear should be an unusual event. A small residual may be left behind in an effort to avoid a major complication, such as facial nerve sacrifice or brain stem injury. For younger patients with large tumors, surgical removal is the preferred strategy. The length of vulnerability for recurrence is too great for younger patients to rely on subtotal removal. Some further therapeutic endeavor will ultimately be necessary, thus multiplying the potential for complications.

Large lesions on older patients can present some strategic problems. This would seem like an ideal situation for hypofractionated radiosurgery. With lesions greater than 4 cm or somewhat smaller lesions with associated arachnoid cysts (*Fig. 18.2(I)*) usurping much of the

A

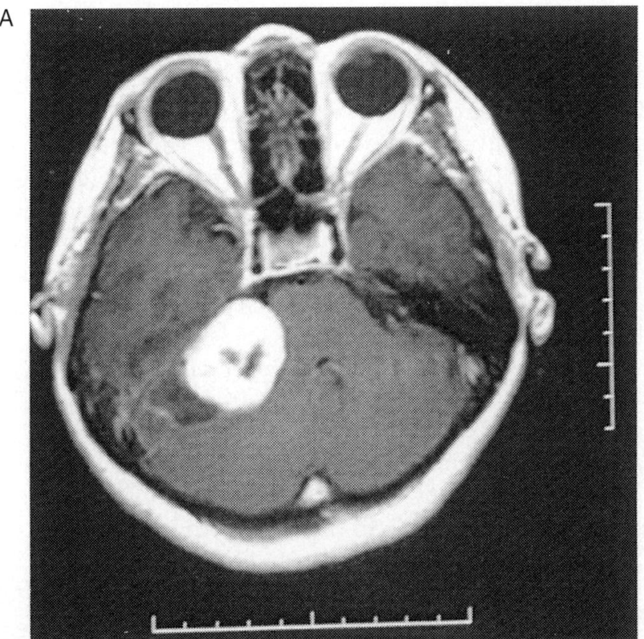

B

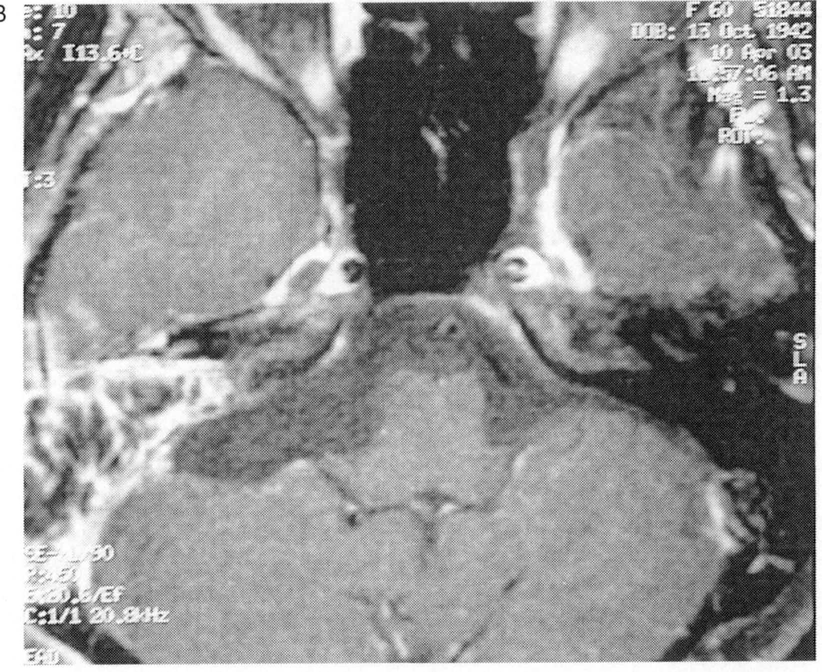

FIG. 18.2(I) Preoperative (*A*) and postoperative (*B*) MR images of a 60-year-old woman with a 3-cm acoustic neuroma in association with an arachnoid cyst. Surgical excision was chosen to avoid the potential for increased mass effect from radiation edema. No facial nerve morbidity resulted.

available reserve in the posterior fossa, however, radiosurgery with its attendant edema formation may produce unacceptable risks 6 to 12 mo posttreatment. Data are sorely lacking for this modality in larger tumors. Until better long-term studies are available, older patients in good health with large lesions should be offered the option of surgical removal. The decision for total versus subtotal removal is made at the time of surgery and is predicated on the likelihood of complications. Radiosurgery as an adjunct can be offered for any threatening residual. For tumors greater than 2.5 cm in older patients who are poor surgical risks, hypofractionated radiosurgery is a logical option.

Hearing Preservation

Hearing preservation in the context of surgical removal can be expected in experienced hands to be successful 50% of the time with intracanalicular tumors and 30% of the time with larger lesions that are generally under 3 cm. This presupposes good functional hearing to begin with. Attempts to save hearing in a marginal or poorly hearing ear will be unrewarding. That ear will be a constant source of distraction to the patient as it picks up unstructured background noise and reduces the overall functionality of the hearing. Thus, compromises in surgical strategy to preserve the function of a poorly hearing ear should be vigorously resisted.

Single-fraction radiosurgery is growing fast in popularity and may become the treatment of choice in the absence of an experienced surgeon with a proven track record of the safe and effective removal. For those lesions less than 3 cm, one can expect at least 50% hearing preservation or better assuming accepted, proven radiosurgical techniques are utilized. The major drawback in prescribing it for all small acoustic tumors is the lack of long-term efficacy data. For many patients, the need for continued surveillance and the thought of the continued presence of the lesion are negative satisfiers.

Other Factors

Unfortunately, other factors come into play as patients try to make their decisions. Socioeconomic and educational status may complicate decision making in patients who cannot understand a complex set of options. Patient and family biases either for or against surgery or radiation may direct the patient's thinking contrary to the physician's best judgment. Access to the Internet, influence from patients who have had one form of therapy or another, and loyalty to a particular institution may also be relevant factors in decision making.

One can guide the decision-making process by trying to simplify principles. Explaining away misconceptions is a place to start. Identifying patient and family biases and dealing with them in a forthright way will also help. If it is perceived that this discussion is simply a device to steer the decision toward the surgeon's or radiosurgeon's bias, confusion and mistrust can develop. If a patient harbors a tumor that may be amenable to either surgical removal or radiosurgery, a simple construct can be presented to the family and patient to facilitate their decision making. Does the patient insist that the tumor be gone? Benefits include diagnostic certainty and the lack of need for long-term surveillance. If the tumor's absence is not an overriding concern, radiosurgery is a highly acceptable alternative. Hypofractionated techniques, if they prove to have long-term effectiveness, may very well become the treatment of choice.

REFERENCES

1. Rosenberg S: Natural history of acoustic neuromas. **Laryngoscope** 110:497–508, 2000.
2. Tshudi DC, Linder TE, Fisch U: Conservative management of unilateral acoustic neuromas. **Am J Otol** 21:722–728, 2000.
3. Charabi S, Thomsen J, Mantoni M, et al.: Acoustic neuroma (vestibular schwannoma): Growth and surgical and nonsurgical consequences of the wait-and-see policy. **Otolaryngol Head Neck Surg** 113:5–14, 1995.
4. Charabi S, Tos M, Thomsen J, Charabi B, Mantoni M: Vestibular schwannoma growth—Long-term results. **Acta Otolaryngol Suppl** 543:7–10, 2000.
5. Deen HG, Ebersold MJ, Harner SG, et al.: Conservative management of acoustic neuroma: An outcome study. **Neurosurgery** 39:260–266, 1996.
6. Hoistad DL, Melnik G, Mamikoglu B, Battista R, O'Connor CA, Wiet RJ: Update on conservative management of acoustic neuroma. **Otol Neurotol** 22:682–285, 2001.
7. Levo H, Pyykko I, Blomstedt G: Nonsurgical treatment of vestibular schwannoma patients. **Acta Otolaryngol Suppl** 529:56–58, 1997.
8. Leutje CM: Spontaneous involution of acoustic tumors. **Am J Otol** 21:393–398, 2000.
9. Modugno GC, Pirodda A, Ferri GG, et al.: Small acoustic neuromas: Monitoring the growth rate by MRI. **Acta Neurochir (Wien)** 141:1063–1067, 1999.
10. Kameyana S, Tanaka R, Kawaguchi T, Honda Y, Yamazaki H, Hasegawa A: Long-term follow-up of the residual intracanalicular tumors after subtotal removal of acoustic neurinomas. **Acta Neurochir (Wien)** 138(2):206–209, 1996.
11. Silverstein H, Rosenberg SL, Flanzer JM, Wanamaker HH, Seidman MD: An algorithm for the management of acoustic neuromas regarding age, hearing, tumor size, and symptoms. **Otolaryngol Head Neck Surg** 108:1–10, 1993.
12. Van Leeuwen JP, Cremers CW, Theunissen EJ, Marres EH, Meyer E: Translabyrinthine and transotic surgery for acoustic neuroma. **Clin Otolaryngol** 19:491–495, 1994.
13. Gjuric M, Wigand ME, Wolf SR: Enlarged middle fossa vestibular schwannoma surgery: Experience with 735 cases. **Otol Neurotol** 22: 223–231, 2001.
14. Samii M, Matthies C: Management of 1000 vestibular schwannomas (acoustic neuromas): The facial nerve—Preservation and restitution of function. **Neurosurgery** 40:684–695, 1997.

15. Sampath P, Holiday MJ, Brem H, Niparko JK, Long DM: Facial nerve injury in acoustic neuroma (vestibular schwannoma) surgery: etiology and prevention. **J Neurosurg** 87:60–66, 1997.
16. Wiegand DA, Ojemann RG, Fickel V: Surgical treatment of acoustic neuroma (vestibular schwannoma) in the United States: Report from the Acoustic Neuroma Registry. **Laryngoscope** 106:58–66, 1996.
17. House JW, Brackman DE: Facial nerve grading system. **Otolaryngol Head Neck Surg** 93:146–147, 1985.
18. Wiet RJ, Mamikoglu B, Odom L, Hoistad D: Long-term results of the first 500 cases of acoustic neuroma surgery. **Otolaryngol Head Neck Surg** 124:645–651, 2001.
19. Sterkers JM, Morrison GAJ, Sterkers O, Badr El-Dine MMK: Preservation of facial, cochlear, and other nerve functions in acoustic neuroma treatment. **Otolaryngol Head Neck Surg** 110:146–155, 1994.
20. Tonn JC, Schalke HP, Goldbrunner R, Milewski C, Helms J, Roosen K: Acoustic neuroma surgery as an interdisciplinary approach: a neurosurgical series of 508 patients. **J Neurol Neurosurg Psychiatry** 69:161–166, 2000.
21. Ojemann RG: Management of acoustic neuromas (vestibular schwannomas) (Honored Guest Presentation). **Clin Neurosurg** 40:408–535, 1993.
22. Symon L, Bord LT, Compton JS, Sabin IH, Sayin E: Acoustic neuroma: A review of 392 cases. **Br J Neurosurg** 3:343–348, 1989.
23. Koos WT, Matula C, Kitz K: Microsurgery versus radiosurgery in the treatment of small acoustic neurinomas. **Acta Neurochir Suppl** 63:73–80, 1995.
24. Harner SG, Beatty CW, Ebersold MJ: Retrosigmoid removal of acoustic neuroma: Experience 1978–1988. **Otolaryngol Head Neck Surg** 103:40–45, 1990.
25. Arriaga MA, Chen DA, Fukushima T: Individualizing hearing preservation in acoustic neuroma surgery. **Laryngoscope** 107:1043–1047, 1997.
26. Tos M, Thomsen J, Harmsen A: Results of translabyrinthine removal of 300 acoustic neuromas related to tumor size. **Acta Otolaryngol (Stockh) Suppl** 452:38–51, 1988.
27. Ebersold MJ, Harner SG, Beatty CW, Harper CM, Quast LM: Current results of the retrosigmoid approach to acoustic neurinoma. **J Neurosurg** 76:901–909, 1992.
28. Jung S, Kang SS, Kim TS, et al.: Current surgical results of retrosigmoid approach in extralarge vestibular schwannomas. **Surg Neurol** 53:370–378, 2000.
29. Hardy DG, MacFarlane R, Baguley D, Moffat D: Surgery for acoustic neurinoma. An analysis of 100 translabyrinthine operations. **J Neurosurg** 71:799–804, 1989.
30. Sugita K, Kobayashi S: Technical and instrumental improvements in the surgical treatment of acoustic neurinomas. **J Neurosurg** 57:747–752, 1982.
31. Lanman TH, Brackman DE, Hitselberger WE, Subin B: Report of 190 consecutive cases of large acoustic tumors (vestibular schwannoma) removed via the translabyrinthine approach. **J Neurosurg** 90:617–623, 1999.
32. Haines SJ, Levine SC: Intracanalicular acoustic neuroma: Early surgery for preservation of hearing. **J Neurosurg** 79:515–520, 1993.
33. Nadol JB, Chiong CM, Ojemann RG, et al.: Preservation of hearing and facial nerve function in resection of acoustic neuroma. **Laryngoscope** 102:1153–1294, 1992.
34. Rowed DW, Nedzelski JM: Hearing preservation in the removal of intracanalicular acoustic neuromas via the retrosigmoid approach. **J Neurosurg** 86:456–461, 1997.
35. Gormley WB, Sekhar LN, Wright DC, Kamerer D, Schessel D: Acoustic neuromas: Results of current surgical management. **Neurosurgery** 41:50–60, 1997.
36. Shelton C, Brackman DE, House WF, Hitselberger WE: Middle fossa acoustic tumor surgery: Results in 106 cases. **Laryngoscope** 99:405–408, 1989.
37. Post KD, Eisenberg MB, Catalano PJ: Hearing preservation in vestibular schwannoma surgery: What factors influence outcome? **J Neurosurg** 83:191–196, 1995.

38. Irving RM, Jackler RK, Pitts LH: Hearing preservation in patients undergoing vestibular schwannoma surgery: Comparison of middle fossa and retrosigmoid approaches. **J Neurosurg** 88:840–845, 1998.
39. Slattery WH, Brackman DE, Hitselberger W: Middle fossa approach for hearing preservation with acoustic neuromas. **Am J Otol** 18:596–601, 1997.
40. Gardner G, Robertson JH: Hearing preservation in unilateral acoustic neuroma surgery. **Ann Otol Rhinol Laryngol** 97:55–66, 1988.
41. Committee on Hearing and Equilibrium guidelines for the evaluation of hearing preservation in acoustic neuroma (vestibular schwannoma). **Otolaryngol Head Neck Surg** 113:179–180, 1995.
42. Glasscock ME, Hays JW, Minor LB, Haynes DS, Carrasco VN: Preservation of hearing in surgery for acoustic neuromas. **J Neurosurg** 78:864–870, 1993.
43. Brackman DE, Owens RM, Friedman RA, et al: Prognostic factors for hearing preservation in vestibular schwannoma surgery. **Am J Otol** 21(3):417–424, 2000.
44. Friedman RA, Kesser BW, Slattery WH, Brackman DE, Hitselberger WE: Hearing preservation in patients with vestibular schwannomas with sudden sensorineural hearing loss. **Otolaryngol Head Neck Surg** 125(5):544–551, 2001.
45. Buchman CA, Chen DA, Flannagan P, Wilberger JE, Maroon JC: The learning curve for acoustic tumor surgery. **Laryngoscope** 106:1406–1411, 1996.
46. Symon L, Bordi LT, Compton JS, Sabin IH, Sayin E: Acoustic neuroma: A review of 392 cases. **Br J Neurosurg** 3:343–348, 1989.
47. California Office of Statewide Health and Planning Development, 1998–1999 statistics.
48. Lalwani AK, Butt FY, Jackler RK, Pitts LH, Yingling CD: Facial nerve outcome after acoustic neuroma surgery: A study from the era of cranial nerve monitoring. **Otolaryngol Head Neck Surg** 111:561–570, 1994.
49. Matthies C, Samii M: Management of vestibular schwannomas (acoustic neuromas): The value of neurophysiology for intraoperative monitoring of auditory function in 200 cases. **Neurosurgery** 40:459–468, 1997.
50. Kondziolka D, Lundsford LD, McLaughlin MR, Flickinger JC: Long-term outcomes after radiosurgery for acoustic neuromas. **N Engl J Med** 339(20):1426–1433, 1998.
51. Noren G: Long-term complications following gamma knife radiosurgery of vestibular schwannomas. **Sterotact Funct Neurosurg** 70(suppl):65–73, 1998.
52. Pollock BE, Lunsford LD, Kondziolka D, et al.: Outcome analysis of acoustic neuroma management: A comparison of microsurgery and stereotactic radiosurgery. **Neurosurgery** 36:215–229, 1995.
53. Ogurinde OK, Lunsford LD, Flickinger JC, Kondziolka D: Stereotactic radiosurgery for acoustic nerve tumors in patients with useful preoperative hearing: Results at 2-year follow-up examination. **J Neurosurg** 80:1011–1017, 1994.
54. Flickinger JC, Kondziolka D, Lunsford LD: Dose and diameter relationships for facial, trigeminal, and acoustic neuropathies following acoustic neuroma radiosurgery. **Radiother Oncol** 41:215–219, 1996.
55. Flickinger JC, Kondziolka D, Niranjan A, Lunsford LD: Results of acoustic neuroma radiosurgery: An analysis of 5 years' experience using current methods. **J Neursurg** 94:1–6, 2001.
56. Suh JH, Barnett GH, Sohn JW, Kupelian PA, Cohen BH: Results of linear accelerator-based stereotactic radiosurgery for recurrent and newly diagnosed acoustic neuromas. **Int J Cancer** 90:145–151, 2000.
57. Mendenhall WM, Friedman WA, Buatti JM, Bova FJ: Preliminary results of linear accelerator radiosurgery for acoustic schwannomas. **J Neurosurg** 85:1013–1019, 1996.
58. Spiegelman R, Lidar Z, Gofman J, Alezra D, Hadani M, Pfeffer R: Linear accelerator radiosurgery for vestibular schwannoma. **J Neurosurg** 94:7–13, 2001.

59. Song DY, Williams J: Fractionated stereotactic radiosurgery for treatment of acoustic neuromas. **Stereotact Funct Neurosurg** 73:45–49, 1999.
60. Lederman G, Lowry J, Wertheim S, et al.: Acoustic neuroma: Potential benefits of fractionated stereotactic radiosurgery. **Sterotact Funct Neurosurg** 69:175–182, 1997.
61. Andrews DW, Suarez O, Goldman HW, et al: Stereotactic radiosurgery and fractionated stereotactic radiotherapy for the treatment of acoustic schwannomas: Comparative observations of 125 patients treated at one institution. **Int J Radiat Oncol Biol Phys** 50(5):1265–1278, 2001.
62. Meijer OWM, Wolberg JG, Baayen JC, Slotman BJ: Fractionated stereotactic radiation therapy and single high-dose radiosurgery for acoustic neuroma: Early results of a prospective clinical study. **Int J Radiat Oncol Biol Phys** 46(1):45–49, 2000.
63. Varlotto JM, Shrieve DC, Alexander E, Kooy HM, Black PM, Loeffler JS: Fractionated stereotactic radiotherapy for the treatment of acoustic neuromas: Preliminary results. **Int J Radiat Oncol Biol Phys** 36(1):141–145, 1996.
64. Yu JS, Yong WH, Wilson D, Black K: Glioblastoma induction after radiosurgery for meningioma. **Lancet** 356:1576–1577, 2000.
65. Kaido T, Hoshida T, Uranishi R, et al.: Radiosurgery-induced brain tumor. **J Neurosurg** 95:710–713, 2001.
66. Shamisa A, Bance M, Nag S, et al.: Glioblastoma multiforme occurring in a patient treated with gamma knife surgery. **J Neurosurg** 94:816–821, 2001.
67. Shin M, Ueki K, Kurita H, Kirino T: Malignant transformation of a vestibular schwannoma after gamma knife radiosurgery. **Lancet** 360:309–310, 2002.

PART

II

Acoustic Neuromas: Sorting Out Management Options

DOUGLAS KONDZIOLKA, M.D., M.Sc., F.R.C.S.(C.), F.A.C.S., L. DADE LUNSFORD, M.D., F.A.C.S., AND JOHN C. FLICKINGER, M.D., F.A.C.R.

Patients with acoustic neuromas have several treatment options, including observation, surgical resection, stereotactic radiosurgery, and perhaps, fractionated radiotherapy. Resection is indicated for patients with larger tumors that have caused major neurologic deficits from brain compression. Surgeons perform stereotactic radiosurgery as primary treatment, with the goals of preserved neurologic function and prevention of tumor growth. The long-term outcomes of radiosurgery, particularly with the gamma knife technique, have proven its role in the primary or adjuvant management of this tumor. Fractionated radiotherapy has been suggested as an alternative for selected patients with larger tumors for whom microsurgery may not be feasible. Patients with neurofibromatosis type 2 (NF-2) pose specific challenges, particularly in regard to preservation of hearing and other cranial nerve function. Many patients choose between radiosurgery and resection based on their own specific goals and their understanding of possible results. The decision can be difficult, and it depends on the sources and strengths of information given to the patient. These include discussions with surgeons and other physicians, written material from peer-reviewed medical journals, handouts from support groups, Internet-based reports (of variable reliability), and discussions between patients.

The primary clinical issues include avoiding tumor- or treatment-related mortality, prevention of further tumor-related neurologic disability, minimizing treatment risks (e.g., spinal fluid leakage, infections, and cardiopulmonary complications), maintaining regional cranial nerve function (facial, trigeminal, cochlear, and glossopharyngeal/vagal), avoiding hydrocephalus, maintaining quality of life and employment, and reducing cost. All treatment choices should strive to meet all of these goals.

MANAGEMENT

Surgical Resection

For decades, resection of an acoustic neuroma has been the mainstay of treatment (1). Many years ago, the goal was simple debulking of the tumor (which was often large) and relief of regional brain stem compression and hydrocephalus. The goal was life saving. Neurologic deficits, such as hearing loss, facial weakness, or balance disorders, were tolerated as simply part of the expected result. During the 1970s, introduction of the operating microscope facilitated meticulous dissection of the tumor so that attempts at cranial nerve preservation could be made. Over the next 20 years, preservation of facial nerve continuity became more common than not. During the 1990s, hearing preservation became an achievable goal in selected cases. At the same time, improvements in anesthetic technique and wound closure reduced the risk of cerebellar infarction, meningitis, and leakage of cerebral spinal fluid. Nevertheless, these problems continue to exist, and cerebral spinal fluid leakage remains a significant problem after resection (2).

At present, there are three main routes for resection of an acoustic neuroma. These approaches are chosen based upon educational bias, surgical experience, and the specific goals of the operation. The suboccipital retrosigmoid approach is the oldest and remains widely used, particularly when hearing preservation is attempted. The translabyrinthine approach destroys hearing but provides direct exposure of the tumor without cerebellar retraction. Even large tumors can be removed through this route. The "middle fossa" approach is performed by a temporal craniotomy but requires elevation of the temporal lobe and drilling of the temporal bone to expose the auditory canal from above. Using this route, hearing preservation can be attempted. It is usually chosen for patients with intracanalicular tumors.

Stereotactic Radiosurgery

Stereotactic radiosurgery has become a common therapeutic choice for patients with acoustic tumors (vestibular schwannomas). During the late 1980s and early 1990s, patients and their doctors chose radiosurgery or resection based mainly on data regarding early outcomes in limited patient series (3–10). In 1987, we began a prospective assessment of the response of patients with acoustic tumors to gamma knife radiosurgery. Both early and later (5–10 year) outcomes were determined through the use of serial imaging studies, hearing and facial function examinations, and physician-based evaluations (11). Because expected outcomes may be different for patients with solitary tumors or those with NF-2, we have analyzed these patient populations separately.

PATIENT CHARACTERISTICS: UNIVERSITY OF PITTSBURGH

Over a 15-year interval, 787 patients underwent stereotactic radiosurgery for an acoustic tumor (vestibular schwannoma) at the University of Pittsburgh. These included 726 patients with solitary tumors and 61 with NF-2.

A resection had been performed in 158 patients (20%). Twenty-eight patients had two previous resections, eight patients had three resections, and four patients had four resections. Although normal facial function (House-Brackman grade 1) was present in 70% of patients, others had grade 2 function (5%), grade 3 function (5%), grade 4 function (2.3%), grade 5 function (1.7%), or grade 6 function (3%) (12). The Gardner-Robertson scale was used to code hearing function (13). "Useful" hearing before radiosurgery was noted by 33% of patients.

In our last review of 45 patients with NF-2, previous resection had been performed in 13 (16). Multiple resections were performed in four patients. Normal facial function before radiosurgery was present in 74%, normal trigeminal function in 75%, and useful hearing (Gardner-Robertson grades 1+2) in 31%.

TECHNIQUE OF GAMMA KNIFE RADIOSURGERY

All patients underwent stereotactic radiosurgery using the Gamma Knife (Elekta Instruments, Atlanta, GA) supplemented with local anesthesia and intravenous sedation as necessary. Children under the age of 12 years with NF-2 had radiosurgery under general anesthesia. Radiosurgery was performed with CT scanning between 1987 and 1991. Subsequent patients underwent radiosurgery using MR imaging after a prospective, comparison study confirmed the accuracy of MR imaging–based stereotactic targeting (14). Multiple irradiation isocenters were used to conform the radiation margin to the intracanalicular and extracanalicular tumor components (7) (*Fig. 18.1(II)*). The 50% isodose line was used to cover the tumor margin in 696 patients with solitary tumors (88%). An initial tumor margin dose of 18 to 20 Gy was selected based on the initial experience from the Karolinska group in Stockholm (8). This dose was decreased to between 16 and 18 Gy within the first 2 years and, by 1992, to a margin dose of 14 to 16 Gy. Repeated reevaluations of the cranial nerve response prompted additional small decreases in dose to preserve cranial nerve function (7, 15). The mean dose delivered to the margin of both non-NF-2 and NF-2 tumors was 14 Gy. The most commonly prescribed margin dose at the present time is 13 Gy, and this dose has been fairly constant for the past nine years

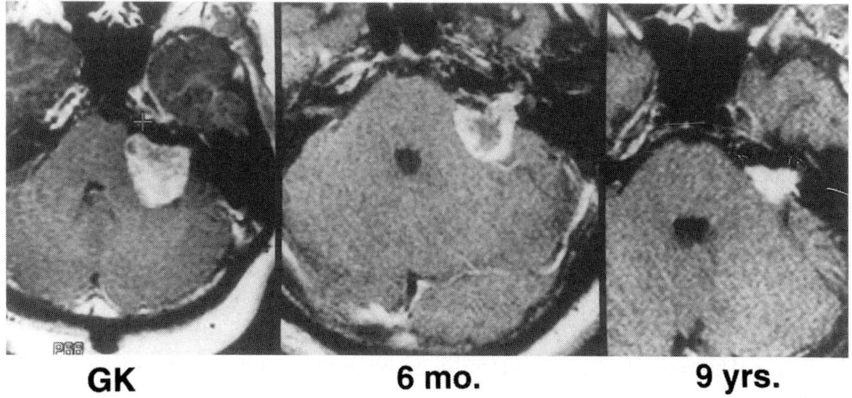

FIG. 18.1(II) Serial axial MR images at radiosurgery (*left*), 6 mo later (*middle*), and 9 years later (*right*). This 44-year-old man was treated with an 11 isocenter gamma knife plan to a margin dose of 14 Gy. He maintains normal facial nerve function and had marked return of his energy level within several months of the procedure.

(16, 17). Dose selection in individual patients was based on the factors of tumor volume, surgical history, hearing status, facial motor function, and patient desires. After radiosurgery, all patients received a single 40-mg dose of intravenous methylprednisolone and were discharged from hospital the next morning.

FOLLOW-UP EVALUATIONS

Serial imaging studies (MR imaging, or CT when MR imaging was contraindicated) were requested every 6 mo for the first 2 years, annually for the next 2 years, and biannually thereafter. Serial audiograms were obtained at 6- to 12-mo intervals in patients with hearing. Contrast-enhanced imaging studies were used to define the tumor response and to identify any peritumoral imaging changes. Before and after radiosurgery, each tumor was measured in five separate dimensions (three extracanalicular and two intracanalicular) using a method previously reported (1). A significant imaging change using this caliper technique was defined as a difference of ± 2 mm.

INITIAL EXPERIENCE WITH SOLITARY TUMORS

A comprehensive evaluation was made of all patients managed before 1992 with a minimum 5 years of clinical follow-up (n = 162). This study represented results of our initial techniques (11). The results of all imaging studies were entered into a database and compared over time according to the tumor size being decreased, unchanged, or increased. The majority of irradiated acoustic tumors decreased in size over time (*Fig. 18.1(II)*). At the 1-year evaluation, only 26% of tumors had decreased in size, but by 3 years, 59% of patients had smaller tumors. Of patients evaluated between the fifth and tenth years, 72% had a decrease in tumor volume, and 28% had no change in the size of their tumor. Nine patients had tumors that increased in size, and all were identified within the first 3 years after radiosurgery (11). Enlargement represented either true neoplastic tumor growth (n = 4) or tumor death with an expansion of the tumor margins as the central portion of the tumor became necrotic. In the latter patients (n = 5), subsequent imaging studies confirmed tumor volume regression. Four patients underwent resection. No further increase in tumor volume was identified in any patient from years 4 to 10 after radiosurgery (15).

Occasional patients had a transient headache after removal of the stereotactic frame. There were no infections or systemic complications. Patients returned to their routine activities immediately. In our 5- to 10-year review, three patients developed hydrocephalus and required a ventriculoperitoneal shunt (11).

All new or worsened postradiosurgery deficits occurred within 28 mo of radiosurgery, and no patient described a new neurologic problem after the third year. Planning with CT was followed by a higher rate of cranial neuropathy (5, 11).

CURRENT EXPERIENCE WITH SOLITARY TUMORS

Refinements in technique followed a continued review of results. In 1991, we began to use MR imaging–based stereotactic planning, because CT-based planning did not show well the intracanalicular portion of the tumor. With MR imaging, we could image the tumor and regional neural structures in greater detail. This facilitated the use of multiple small irradiation isocenters for more conformal radiosurgery. With this type of radiosurgery, cranial nerve morbidity dropped precipitously. Similarly, our analysis of hearing preservation in patients with NF-2 patients (see below) showed significant gains.

Between 1992 and 1997, 192 patients had radiosurgery and were eligible for extended follow-up (15). The maximum follow-up in this cohort was 65 mo. The median tumor margin dose was 13 Gy.

The actuarial 5-year clinical tumor control rate (no need for any additional treatment) was 97%. One patient underwent a resection 6 mo after radiosurgery. The 5-year actuarial rates of any facial weakness, facial numbness, hearing level preservation, and preservation of testable speech discrimination were 1.1% ± 0.8%, 2.6% ± 1.2%, and 71% ± 4.7%, and 91% ± 2.6%, respectively. At a tumor margin dose of 13 Gy or less, the rate of facial neuropathy was 0%, and at greater than 13 Gy, the rate of facial neuropathy was 2.5% (usually mild and transient). Tumor diameter did not significantly affect results. Reports from other centers have shown similar results (37).

NEUROFIBROMATOSIS TYPE 2

Serial imaging studies of 45 tumors over a median 36 mo of follow-up (range, 6–120 mo) found that 16 tumors (36%) had regressed, 28 (62%) had remained unchanged in size, and 1 (2%) had demonstrated progression (16). Loss of central contrast within tumor was frequently, but inconsistently, observed and thought to reflect tumor necrosis. The single patient demonstrating tumor progression despite radiosurgery was treated early in our experience (1988), without the benefit of MR imaging for planning, and ultimately underwent surgical resection. The cumulative tumor control rate was 98%.

The mean period of clinical follow-up was 41 mo (range, 6–120 mo). No patient demonstrated improvement in their clinical examination after radiosurgery. Thirty patients (67%) maintained a stable examination, and 15 (33%) demonstrated some degree of clinical deterioration. Two patients (4%) died during the follow-up period secondary to unrelated illnesses. The median Karnofsky score after radiosurgery was 80. Thirty-five patients (78%) were able to carry out normal daily activities at the time of the last examination (Karnofsky score, ≥80).

Of the 14 tumors associated with useful hearing (Gardner-Robertson grades 1 or 2) at the time of radiosurgery, 6 (43%) demonstrated no change in hearing class during the follow-up period. Eight other patients lost all functional hearing (defined as absent speech discrimination) at a mean of 6 mo from radiosurgery (range, 3–15 mo). The overall rate of hearing preservation in the series was 43%. In 1992, we began to use MR imaging–guided stereotactic planning with increasing numbers of smaller isocenters. By specifically dividing the population into those patients treated before 1992 and those treated after 1992, the difference in hearing preservation again becomes apparent. Before 1992, five patients with useful hearing (grade 1 or 2) were treated. All patients subsequently lost speech discrimination. After 1992, nine patients with useful hearing underwent radiosurgery. Six of the patients (67%) had hearing preservation at the time of last examination (16). Thirty-one tumors (67%) were associated with intact facial nerve function (House-Brackman grade 1) at the time of radiosurgery. The overall rate of facial nerve preservation (grade 1) was 81%. Thirty-six of the treated tumors were associated with intact trigeminal nerve function. Three patients (8%) experienced trigeminal distribution sensory loss at a mean of 5 mo (range, 4–5 mo) from radiosurgery. One patient subsequently recovered all trigeminal function, and two patients manifest residual deficits. The overall rate of trigeminal nerve preservation was 94%.

TUMOR RESECTION OR RADIOSURGERY?

Survey responses from 541 patient members of the Acoustic Neuroma Association provided data concerning tumor resection between 1973 and 1983 (18). The problems of facial weakness were reported in 62% of these patients, eye-related problems in 84%, depression in 38%, sleep disturbance in 26%, and speech or swallowing difficulties in 16%. More recently, a larger survey of 1,579 resections performed between 1989 and 1994 found improved results, which included a 44% rate of facial weakness, an 11% rate of cerebrospinal fluid leakage, and persistent balance problems in 9%. Approximately 8% had recurrent or residual tumor on follow-up imaging (19).

Better results following resection have been documented since that time. Samii et al. (20) and Gormley et al. (2) found that complete tumor removal was a frequent outcome; however, neurologic and systemic morbidity remained present, with 1% mortality rates and cerebrospinal fluid fistula rates of 9.2% and 15%, respectively. Experienced surgical teams report significant reductions in postresection complication rates, although the incidence of specific problems, such as cerebrospinal fluid leakage, have remained unchanged (32). Brennan et al. (32) reported that translabyrinthine approach–related leaks had a higher incidence of surgical repair than retrosigmoid approach-related leaks. For patients with large acoustic tumors (>3 cm in extracanalicular diameter) and those with progressive neurologic deficits that require brainstem decompression, however, surgical resection (total or subtotal) is the preferred option. We believe that a complete resection should be performed in such patients if possible—but not at the expense of lost neurologic function. Stereotactic radiosurgery can be considered for patients with intracanalicular, small or medium-sized acoustic tumors, because most such patients do not have a rapidly progressive neurologic syndrome. The initial symptoms caused by most acoustic tumors are not improved by resection (21).

A recent report by Martin et al. (33) evaluated quality of life in patients after tumor resection. They found a disparity between the patients' report and the physicians' assessment of function, with decreases in physical functioning, general health, and social functioning after surgery. More severe balance functions led to worse social functioning.

The long-term effects of both resection and radiosurgery must be documented to assist physician and patient decision making. Surprisingly little information has been published concerning long-term imaging after resection, despite long-term use. A report by Cerullo et al. (22) noted a 10% recurrence rate by 10 years following resection. Mazzoni et al. (23) reported their series of more than 100 patients with attempted hearing preservation; the overall tumor recurrence rate was 8.1%. Post et al. (24) found that 4 of 56 patients (7%) had an incomplete resection in their attempted hearing preservation series and that 3 patients developed regrowth within 3 years. In the largest series, Samii et al. (20) reported a complete resection in 98% of patients and found later recurrence in 6 of 880 who did not have NF-2. In our radiosurgery series, 98% of patients required no further surgery, and 94% had imaging confirmation of persistent tumor control. Tumors that increased in size during the first year or two after radiosurgery did so usually in association with central tumor necrosis, with a small expansion of the tumor capsule. Most such tumors then regressed in size to below baseline with longer follow-up. Such transient expansion may be associated with transient retroauricular pain, perhaps from regional dural inflammation. Recurrence or continued tumor growth may follow resection or radiosurgery (25, 26), and periodic neuroimaging should be obtained in all patients.

Similar results were found for patients with solitary or NF-2 tumors. After 3 years of postradiosurgery follow-up, regardless of tumor type, we found no instance of delayed tumor enlargement, with most patients demonstrating further tumor reduction. Nevertheless, we continue to follow all our patients with imaging studies every 2 to 3 years once they pass the -year mark after radiosurgery.

We believe that all patients with newly diagnosed, residual, or recurrent acoustic tumors (<3 cm in extracanalicular diameter) are now suitable radiosurgery candidates (11, 15). Radiobiology studies showed that the doses used caused tumor regression in a human xenograft model (27). Patients with larger tumors are not as good candidates because of the dose reduction necessary to reduce the rate of potential radiation-related side effects. Younger patients with good hearing should have attempted hearing preservation, either with radiosurgery or resection (28). During our first 3 years of experience, we accepted elderly patients, those with concomitant medical problems that argued against resection, patients with residual or recurrent tumors after resection, and patients with preserved hearing function. By 1991, we began to offer radiosurgery to all patients with acoustic tumors regardless of age, surgical history, or symptoms. We continued to observe older patients (>70 years) with small and minimally symptomatic tumors and recommended management only for imaging-defined tumor growth or progressive symptoms (29–31).

When we evaluate patients with acoustic tumors, many of them ask the following two questions: First, is the tumor more difficult to resect if radiosurgery fails? The answer to this is not clear. Few patients have required resection, and the opinions of the surgeons we have asked indicate that some tumors were less difficult, some about the same, and some more difficult. In a report on this issue that included 13 patients who had resection after radiosurgery, 8 were thought to be more difficult. Five of these eight patients, however, had failed resection *before* they had radiosurgery.

Second, patients inquire about the risk of delayed malignant transformation. Malignant schwannomas are rare, but have been reported de novo, after prior resection (34), and after irradiation. We answer that this is always a risk after irradiation, but that the risk should be very low. We have not seen this yet in any of our 5,200 patients during our first 15 years of experience with radiosurgery, but we quote the patients a risk between 1 in 1,000 and 1 in 20,000. We reported one patient with a malignant mesenchymal tumor of the cerebellopontine angle that resembled an acoustic tumor (36). One report from Japan found a malignant tumor 4 years after resection and 6 mo following radiosurgery (34). The time interval after irradiation was too short to be causative. A second report noted the development of a temporal lobe glioblastoma 7.5 years after radiosurgery for a nearby acoustic neuroma (35). The temporal lobe had received a low radiation dose. In contrast, we have a patient who had initial management of a frontal lobe astrocytoma and years later developed an acoustic neuroma. Was the development of these tumors related in some oncogenetic way, or were they radiation related? We believe the risk of developing a tumor years after radiosurgery is much less than the risk of mortality immediately after a resection—and likely less than the risk of the patient developing another tumor on their own in another body location.

FRACTIONATED RADIOTHERAPY

During the last several years, a number of groups have used fractionated radiation therapy to treat patients with acoustic neuromas. This technique developed when several centers who used linear accelerator irradiation technology were not satisfied with the results or accuracy after single fraction irradiation (radiosurgery). To decrease the cranial nerve morbidities they were observing, they began to deliver radiation over multiple sessions (fractionation). The goal of this approach is to weaken the effect of each radiation administration and maintain brain or nerve function. Correspondingly, this also weakens the effect of the radiation on the tumor target. Little data concerning this approach are available in the peer reviewed literature that includes diligent outcomes and follow-up. Williams et al. reported 80 patients who had fractionated stereotactic radiotherapy (Congress of Neurological Surgeons meeting, San Antonio, TX, October 2001). Mean follow-up after radiotherapy was 1.1 years. Seventy patients received 25 Gy in five fractions, and 10 patients received 30 Gy in 10 fractions. The treatment was delivered using CT targeting, which is limited in evaluating the intracanalicular portion of the tumor. Only 9 of 80 patients had Gardner-Robertson grade 1 or 2 hearing at the time of treatment. Hearing levels were preserved in six of nine patients. Two patients had transient trigeminal neuropathies, and no patient had a significant facial neuropathy. In a separate oral report, Lederman et al. provided results from the Staten Island group at the 2001 meeting of the International Stereotactic Radiosurgery Society. They provided no treatment planning images or cranial nerve outcome data using the accepted grading systems, and they did not define "hearing preservation." They did describe that hearing was preserved at a rate "above" 90%, but the quality of hearing was not reported.

In a more comprehensive report, Andrews et al. (38) reported 69 patients who had gamma knife radiosurgery and 56 patients who had linear accelerator based radiotherapy. Tumor control rates were high (97%) in early follow-up and cranial nerve morbidities low in both groups. With their technique, they found a higher rate of early hearing preservation after radiotherapy, but both treatments had median follow-up times of less than 10 mo. Their rate of hearing preservation after radiosurgery (33%) was lower than reported by others. The main drawback of this report is the lack of randomization. Patients were allocated to either treatment according to "strong physician preferences."

Optimally, appropriate doses of radiation should be delivered precisely to the tumor, and the regional brain structures should be spared of radiation. This is not the case with fractionated techniques, in which larger volumes of regional tissue are irradiated. We believe that any advantage of fractionation in limiting toxicity only makes sense if the target volume contains normal brain or nerve. Sophisticated stereotactic radiosurgical instruments allow regional brain or nerve to be spared through frame-based, single-session image guidance. We do not believe that fractionation provides any useful advantage over radiosurgical techniques that have been in use for the last 10 years.

A SURVEY OF NEUROSURGEONS ON ACOUSTIC NEUROMA MANAGEMENT

A survey was mailed to members of the Congress of Neurological Surgeons in July 2002, and 663 (30%) surgeons responded. The survey was mailed with four questions written on one page. Forty one

TABLE 18.1(II)
Response from a Survey of Neurosurgeons (n = 662) on Acoustic Neuroma Management

Neurosurgeon Age (years)	n	%
30–40	122	19
40–50	269	41
50–60	178	27
60–70	86	13
>70	7	1

percent of responders were between the ages of 40 and 50 (*Table 18.1 (II)*). Eighty percent of neurosurgeons surveyed had either performed radiosurgery on a patient with an acoustic neuroma or had referred a patient for neurosurgery (n = 530).

Survey Case One

QUESTION

You are a 37-year-old neurosurgeon who presents with mild decreased hearing on one side. You have no tinnitus and no balance problems. Facial function is normal. An MR image depicts an intracanalicular acoustic neuroma, and serial images have depicted a small amount of growth. Which management strategy would you choose for yourself? (Observation; surgical resection; stereotactic radiosurgery; fractionated radiotherapy) (*Fig. 18.2(II)*).

RESPONSE

The majority of surgeons stated that they would choose stereotactic radiosurgery for management of their small acoustic tumor (n = 283; 43%). Only 122 surgeons stated that they would choose surgical resection of their tumor (18%). Fractionated radiotherapy was chosen by 2% of responders. Interestingly, 240 surgeons stated that they would continue to observe their tumor (36%) rather than undergo any specific treatment at the present time. It had been stated in the case presentation that serial scans had already shown a small amount of growth. This tumor had been observed and was increasing in volume. Nevertheless, approximately one-third of responders continued to choose observation for a 37-year-old patient with a small but growing tumor (*Table 18.2(II)*).

We evaluated the age of the responding surgeon and compared this to the treatment chosen by that surgeon (*Table 18.3(II)*). Across the age groups between 30 and 70 years, at least twice as many neurosurgeons chose radiosurgery rather than resection for their tumor.

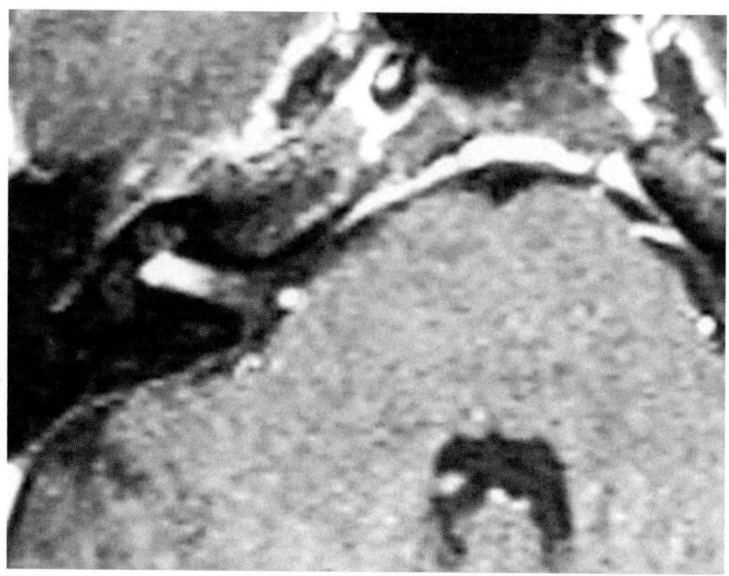

FIG. 18.2(II) Axial MR image of a 37-year-old man with a right intracanalicular acoustic neuroma (see *Survey Case One*).

This was most pronounced in the younger surgeon age group (30–40 years), in which four times the number of surgeons chose radiosurgery rather than resection. Observation, however, continued to be chosen by many. One might think than an older person might choose radiosurgery over resection simply to avoid the risks of general anesthesia or the surgical exposure, but this did not necessarily appear to be true.

This case reflected the care of an actual neurosurgeon who had gamma knife radiosurgery. He remains well at 18 mo following his procedure and maintains a full practice. He has had no facial weakness or change in hearing.

TABLE 18.2(II)
Choice of Treatment in a Survey of Neurosurgeons

	Case 1		Case 2	
	n	%	n	%
Observation	240	36	37	6
Resection	121	18	347	52
Radiosurgery	283	43	260	39
Radiotherapy	16	2	18	3

TABLE 18.3(II)
Survey of Neurosurgeons

	Surgeon Age (years)				
	30–40	40–50	50–60	60–70	>70
Case One					
Observation	45	106	64	4	1
Resection	15	47	36	20	3
Radiosurgery	60	104	74	42	3
Radiotherapy	1	11	4	0	0
Case Two					
Observation	6	7	13	10	1
Resection	69	148	92	36	2
Radiosurgery	46	102	68	40	4
Radiotherapy	1	12	5	0	0

Survey Case Two

QUESTION

You are a 50-year-old neurosurgeon who presents with mild decreased hearing on one side. You have tinnitus but no balance problems. Facial function is normal. An MR image shows a left acoustic neuroma. Which management strategy would you choose for yourself? (Observation; surgical resection; stereotactic radiosurgery; fractionated radiotherapy) (*Fig. 18.3(II)*).

RESPONSE

In this scenario, the neurosurgeon had a medium-sized acoustic tumor that indented the middle cerebellar peduncle but without compression of the fourth ventricle. The tumor measured 22 mm in the maximum diameter. The minority of surgeons recommended continued observation for a tumor of this size (6%). Surgical resection was recommended by 347 surgeons (52%), whereas radiosurgery was chosen by 261 surgeons (39%). Fractionated radiotherapy was only chosen by 3%. When the results were stratified by age, resection was the most popular choice across the groups between the ages of 30 and 60 years. Radiosurgery, however, became more popular with advancing age of the survey group, passing resection as the most popular choice when the neurosurgeon was older than age 60. It appears that surgeons chose to have a resection because of the larger volume of the tumor with indentation of the lateral surface of the brain stem.

This patient was also a real neurosurgeon who had radiosurgery. He remains well at 18 mo after the procedure, with a decrease in the size of the tumor. Facial function remains normal.

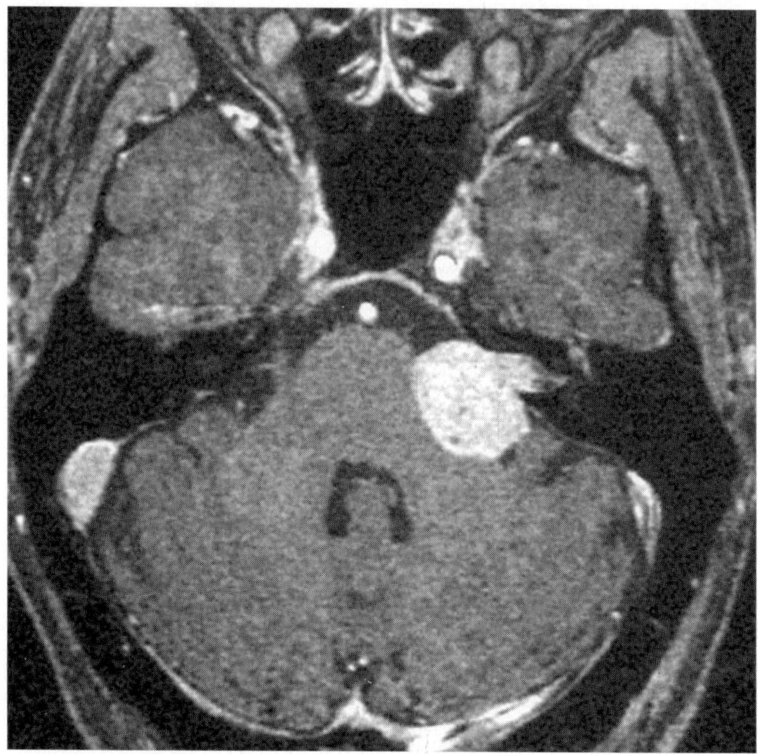

FIG. 18.3(II) Axial MR image of a man with a left acoustic neuroma (see *Survey Case Two*).

SUMMARY

Patients with acoustic neuromas have several options available to them. Large tumors with significant brain stem compression usually require surgical resection. For patients with small or medium-sized tumors, radiosurgery has become a common treatment, with excellent long-term results being reported. Patients must be comfortable with the concept of tumor control rather than tumor removal. Most seem to be satisfied with this concept if it allows them to avoid brain surgery. Surgeons should strive to educate their patients with information from the peer-reviewed literature. Confusion exists among patients, because the information from Internet sources, newsletters, support groups, and physicians has not always been validated and supported by outcomes data. Although we are asked to provide our opinions, our comments should not be based on myth, conjecture, training bias, or socioeconomic concerns.

REFERENCES

1. Linskey ME, Lunsford LD, Flickinger JC: Neuroimaging of acoustic nerve sheath tumors after stereotaxic radiosurgery. **AJNR Am J Neuroradiol** 12:1165–1175, 1991.
2. Gormley WB, Sekhar LN, Wright D, et al.: Acoustic neuromas: Results of current surgical management. **Neurosurgery** 41:50–60, 1997.
3. Foote RL, Coffey RJ, Swanson J, et al.: Stereotactic radiosurgery using the gamma knife for acoustic neuromas. **Int J Radiat Oncol Biol Phys** 32:1153–1160, 1995.
4. Flickinger JC, Kondziolka D, Lunsford LD: Dose and diameter relationships for facial, trigeminal, and acoustic neuropathies following acoustic neuroma radiosurgery. **Radiother Oncol** 41:215–219, 1996.
5. Flickinger JC, Kondziolka D, Lunsford LD, et al.: Evolution in technique for vestibular schwannoma radiosurgery and effect on outcome. **Int J Radiat Oncol Biol Phys** 36:275–280, 1996.
6. Flickinger JC, Lunsford LD, Linskey ME, et al.: Gamma knife radiosurgery for acoustic tumors: Multivariate analysis of four year results. **Radiother Oncol** 27:91–98, 1993.
7. Flickinger JC, Lunsford LD, Wu A, et al.: Treatment planning for gamma knife radiosurgery with multiple isocenters. **Int J Radiat Oncol Biol Phys** 18:1495–1501, 1990.
8. Norén G, Arndt J, Hindmarsh T: Stereotactic radiosurgery in cases of acoustic neurinoma: Further experiences. **Neurosurgery** 13:12–22, 1983.
9. Ogunrinde OK, Lunsford LD, Flickinger JC, Kondziolka D: Cranial nerve preservation after stereotactic radiosurgery of small acoustic tumors. **Arch Neurol** 52:73–79, 1995.
10. Ogunrinde OK, Lunsford LD, Flickinger JC, et al.: Stereotactic radiosurgery for acoustic tumors in patients with useful preoperative hearing: Results at two years. **J Neurosurg** 80:1011–1017, 1994.
11. Kondziolka D, Lunsford LD, McLaughlin M, et al.: Long-term outcomes ater acoustic tumor radiosurgery. The physicians and patients perspective. **N Engl J Med** 339:1426–1433, 1998.
12. House JW, Brackmann DE: Facial nerve grading system. **Otolaryngol Head Neck Surg** 93:146–147, 1985.
13. Gardner G, Robertson JH: Hearing preservation in unilateral acoustic neuroma surgery. **Ann Otol Rhinol Laryngol** 97:55–66, 1988.
14. Kondziolka D, Dempsey PK, Lunsford LD, et al.: A comparison between magnetic resonance imaging and computed tomography for stereotactic coordinate determination. **Neurosurgery** 30:402–407, 1992.
15. Flickinger JC, Kondziolka D, Niranjan A, Lunsford LD: Results of acoustic neuroma radiosurgery: An analysis of 5 years experience using current methods. **J Neurosurg** 94:1–6, 2001.
16. Subach B, Kondziolka D, Lunsford LD, Bissonette D, Flickinger JC, Maitz A: Stereotactic radiosurgery in the management of acoustic neuromas associated with neurofibromatosis type II. **J Neurosurg** 90:815–822, 1999.
17. Linskey M, Lunsford LD, Flickinger JC: Tumor control after stereotactic radiosurgery in neurofibromatosis patients with bilateral acoustic tumors. **Neurosurgery** 31:829–832, 1992.
18. Wiegand DA, Fickel V: Acoustic neuroma—The patients perspective: Subjective assessment of symptoms, diagnosis, therapy, and outcome in 541 patients. **Laryngoscope** 99:179–187, 1989.
19. Wiegand DA, Ojemann R, Fickel V: Surgical treatment of acoustic neuroma (vestibu-

lar schwannoma) in the United States: Report from the Acoustic Neuroma Registry. **Laryngoscope** 106:58–66, 1996.

20. Samii M, Matthies C: Management of 1000 vestibular schwannomas (acoustic neuromas): Surgical management and results with an emphasis on complications and how to avoid them. **Neurosurgery** 40:11–23, 1997.
21. Pollock BE, Lunsford LD, Kondziolka D, et al.: Outcome analysis of acoustic neuroma management: A comparison of microsurgery and stereotactic radiosurgery. **Neurosurgery** 36:215–229, 1995.
22. Cerullo LJ, Grutsch JF, Heiferman K, et al.: The preservation of hearing and facial nerve function in a consecutive series of unilateral vestibular nerve schwannoma surgical patients. **Surg Neurol** 39:485–493, 1993.
23. Mazzoni A, Calabrese V, Moschini L: Residual and recurrent acoustic neuroma in hearing preservation procedures: Neuroradiologic and surgical findings. **Skull Base Surg** 6:105–112, 1996.
24. Post KD, Eisenberg MB, Catalano PJ: Hearing preservation in vestibular schwannoma surgery: What factors influence outcome? **J Neurosurg** 83:191–196, 1995.
25. Pollock B, Lunsford LD, Flickinger J, Clyde B, Kondziolka D: Vestibular schwannoma management. Part I. Failed microsurgery and the role of delayed stereotactic radiosurgery. **J Neurosurg** 89:944–948, 1998.
26. Pollock B, Lunsford LD, Kondziolka D, et al.: Vestibular schwannoma management. Part II. Failed radiosurgery and the role of delayed microsurgery. **J Neurosurg** 89:949–955, 1998.
27. Linskey ME, Martinez AS, Kondziolka D, et al.: The radiobiology of human acoustic schwannoma xenografts after stereotactic radiosurgery evaluated in the subrenal capsule of athymic mice. **J Neurosurg** 78:645–653, 1993.
28. Rowed DW, Nedzelski JM: Hearing preservation in the removal of intracanalicular acoustic neuromas via the retrosigmoid approach. **J Neurosurg** 86:456–461, 1997.
29. Bederson JB, von Ammon K, Wichmann W, et al.: Conservative treatment of patients with acoustic tumors. **Neurosurgery** 28:646–651, 1991.
30. Samii M, Tatagiba M, Matthies C: Acoustic neurinoma in the elderly: Factors predictive of postoperative outcome. **Neurosurgery** 31:615–620, 1992.
31. Yamamoto M, Hagiwara S, Ide M, et al.: Conservative management of acoustic neurinomas: Prospective study of long-term changes in tumor volume and auditory function. **Min Invasive Neurosurg** 41:86–92, 1998.
32. Brennan JW, Rowed D, Nedzelski J, Chen J: Cerebrospinal fluid leak after acoustic neuroma surgery: Influence of tumor size and surgical approach on incidence and response to treatment. **J Neurosurg** 94:217–233, 2001.
33. Martin HC, Sethi J, Lang D, et al.: Patient-assessed outcomes after excision of acoustic neuroma: Postoperative symptoms and quality of life. **J Neurosurg** 94:211–216, 2001.
34. Hanabusa K, Morikawa A, Murata T, Taki W: Acoustic neuroma with malignant transformation. Case report. **J Neurosurg** 95:518–521, 2001.
35. Shamisa A, Bance M, Nag S, et al.: Glioblastoma multiforme occurring in a patient treated with gamma knife surgery. Case report. **J Neurosurg** 94:816–821, 2001.
36. Comey C, McLaughlin M, Jho H, et al.: Death from a malignant cerebellopontine angle triton tumor despite stereotactic radiosurgery. **J Neurosurg** 89:653–658, 1998.
37. Petit JH, Hudes RS, Chen T, et al.: Reduced dose radiosurgery for vestibular schwannomas. **Neurosurgery** 49:1299–1307, 2001.
38. Andrews DW, Suarez O, Goldman HW, et al.: Stereotactic radiosurgery and fractionated radiotherapy for the treatment of acoustic schwannomas: Comparative observations of 125 patients treated at one institution. **Int J Radiat Oncol Biol Phys** 50:1265–1278, 2001.

CHAPTER

19

Honored Guest Presentation: The Neurosurgeon as Mentor and Student

VOLKER K.H. SONNTAG, M.D.

The term *mentor* derives from a character by that name in Homer's *Odyssey*. Mentor was the loyal friend, counselor, and teacher of Odysseus' son, Telemachus, while Odysseus made his long journey back from the Trojan War. Apparently, the goddess Athena (the goddess with the flashing eyes), who was infatuated with Odysseus, assumed the form of Mentor while watching over Telemachus (5, 7). So, it is unclear if Mentor represented an actual person or if Mentor was the goddess Athena, who had transformed herself into a human being. To quote from the *Odyssey*, "she [Athena] assumed the appearance of Mentor and seemed so like him as to deceive both eye and ear"(10). The names *mentes* and *mentor*, along with the word *mental*, stem from the Greek word for mind (*menos*), a marvelously flexible word that can mean intention, force, or purpose as well as mind, spirit, remembrance, or courage.

One of the greatest mentors in antiquity was the centaur Chiron. Centaurs were half-man and half-horse. Most centaurs were more like beasts than men and, as a rule, wild and savage creatures. Chiron, however, was an unusually kind and peaceful centaur who mentored many of the Greek leaders. Chiron had the energy and constitution of his wild nature, but he gentled and redirected it to teaching. He was the bridge between humans and the higher powers of nature and the universe. Chiron was a foster father and trainer to an army of Greek heroes, including Hercules, Achilles, Actaeon, Peleus, and Aesculapius, the greatest surgeon of antiquity (7). Chiron also taught the use of herbs, gentle incantations, and cooling potions. As a mentor, Chiron led his heroes-in-training through their threshold of manhood by patiently teaching them the skills of archery, poetry, and surgery. Chiron received the highest distinction the Greeks could bestow. Zeus

Adapted from Sonntag VKH: Athena, Aesculapius, and beyond: The art of mentoring. 2001 North American Spine Society Presidential Address. **The Spine Journal** 2:5–9, 2002; with permission from Elsevier Sciences, Inc.

transformed him into a constellation in the rising Zodiac: Sagittarius, a centaur firing a bow.

Medicine can trace its lineage to the legendary mentor Aesculapius, one of Chiron's pupils. Aesculapius became Greece's god of medicine and was able to help all types of maladies. He delivered all, whether suffering from wounded limbs or bodies wasted away with disease, even those who were sick unto death, from their torment. Apparently, he raised Theseus' son from death, an act that led to Aesculapius' death. Zeus would not allow a mortal to exercise such power over the dead, and he struck Aesculapius with a thunderbolt and killed him (7).

Throughout antiquity, temples to Aesculapius, the equivalent in Egyptian mythology of Imenhotep, were common throughout the Mediterranean and, for hundreds of years, attracted patients seeking miraculous cures. In these temples, the sick and maimed prayed and made sacrifices. During sleep, Aesculapius revealed to the patients how they would be cured. Snakes were considered to be sacred servants of Aesculapius and played a significant part in cures. This association is most likely why the most recognized emblem of medicine, the caduceus, also known as the staff of Aesculapius, is a serpent entwined around a staff. Followers of Aesculapius, known as Aesculapiads, practiced in temples ministering to the sick (15, 21).

One follower of Aesculapius, Hippocrates (460–377 BC), changed the practice of medicine from an art involving the sacred to a discipline based on observation, reasoning, and experiments. Two of the most brilliant ancient philosophers, Plato and Aristotle, mentioned Hippocrates' name with obvious admiration and respect. Plato called him "Aesculapiad," and Aristotle referred to him as the "leader of the Aesculapiads" (17). Hippocrates rejected the long-standing concept that illness was caused by divine powers. He attributed disease to natural causes and believed that treatment should be based on observation, reasoning, and experience. This radical departure from convention earned Hippocrates the title of "the father of medicine" (16). According to Hippocrates, the ideal physician was concerned primarily with the patient, not only with the disease.

Hippocrates also could be called the father of spine surgery. In his book *On Joints* (24), Hippocrates described anatomy and diseases of the spine and suggested treatment for patients with spinal deformities. He considered knowledge of spinal anatomy to be essential for physicians: "[O]ne first should get the knowledge of the structure of the spine; for this is also a requisite for many diseases" (16). Hippocrates described the segments of the human spine in the *On Nature of Bones* (9, 16) and classified diseases of the spine into five groups:

1. Kyphosis,
2. Scoliosis,
3. Concussion of the spinal cord,
4. Dislocation of the vertebrae, and
5. Fracture of the spinous processes.

These abnormalities were treated by correcting the abnormal curvature and by reducing the dislocation. He used what is now known as Hippocrates' ladder and Hippocrates' boards to help achieve these goals. He also described cranial procedures. Hippocrates used trephining to treat skull fractures, epilepsy, blindness, and headaches (1). His instructions for the use of trephination were precise (1): The opening should not be made over the cranial sutures, because the dura, which adheres to the skull in this area, would likely be damaged. The region of the temple was to be avoided for fear of damaging a vessel—possibly he was referring to the middle meningeal artery—and such damage might lead to convulsions on the opposite side of the body. The trephine was to be removed repeatedly from the skull, cooling the burr hole with water intermittently. The opening was to be examined to ensure that the dura was not yet reached. He advocated leaving a thin shell of the inner table to protect the dura, which would later extrude itself as suppuration developed.

Hippocrates also knew that extradural bleeding could result from a blow to the head (1, 11) and that the presence of a skull fracture was a matter of grave concern that required immediate attention. If left untreated, it could cause fevers "7 days in summer or 14 days in winter," followed by local changes in the wound, convulsion, and death (1). Hippocrates rejected the idea that convulsions were of sacred or divine origin and attributed the notion to charlatans, conjurers, and excessively religious persons who used the concept to hide their own ignorance.

Hippocrates was respected not only as a great physician but also as an inspired teacher—that is, as a *mentor*. One of his followers was Galen (129–200 AD) (15, 21). At an early age, Galen received intensive instruction from his father, who exposed him to the importance of anatomy, empiricism, and the doctrines of Hippocrates. Galen's contribution to medicine were staggering. He wrote extensively: 9 books on anatomy, 17 on physiology, 6 on pathology, 14 on therapeutics, and 30 on pharmacology. Galen's views dominated European medicine for 15 centuries, until the time of Andreas Vesalius (1514–1564) and William Harvey (1578–1657).

Not until the seventeenth century, the "age of scientific revolution," did a major turning point in the history of medicine occur. Instead of asking *why* things occurred, scientists began to ask *how* things occurred. The seventeenth century, however, was not an innovative period in medical education. In universities and medical societies, teaching was, at best, haphazard and depended on the works of antiquity or the writings of Arabic authors such as Avicenna.

Throughout the seventeenth and eighteenth centuries and for most of the nineteenth century, medicine was taught at medical centers that greatly benefited from the charismatic presence of a single teacher or mentor. Alexander Monro (1697–1767), who was succeeded by his son and grandson of the same name, was a master anatomist who made Edinburgh the principle center of medical instruction for the English-speaking world (15, 21). Morgagni (1682–1771) did the same for the university of Padua when he disposed of the ancient humoral theory of a single morbid cause for all diseases. Many giants, including Harvey, Hunter, Magendie, Virchow, Vesalius, Billroth, and Horsley, contributed to medical education by teaching admiring student apprentices. Formal education of budding physicians before and after receiving their medical degree was nonexistent. Admission requirements for medical schools were minimal. Usually, a high school or equivalent education was all that was needed. Annual sessions were short and often a repetition of previous years (12).

In the United States, a few medical schools, such as Harvard, Michigan, and Pennsylvania, were attempting to establish university standards and faculties. In 1893, the establishment of Johns Hopkins University School of Medicine, headed by William Welch and William Osler, was a bold, inspired departure in medical education. Welch, a pathologist, first introduced microscopy and bacteriology to the United States. Osler was a firm advocate of extensive bedside training for medical students. These two giants, joined by William Halsted, changed American medical education and established a pattern that persists today (12).

Two surgeons who were most responsible for making neurosurgery a subspecialty—as well as being master surgeons, educators, and mentors themselves—also had strong connections to Johns Hopkins. Harvey Cushing trained under Halsted at Johns Hopkins starting in the fall of 1896 and stayed as a faculty member until 1912, establishing himself as a "brain surgeon" in his early years (4, 23). Cushing also established the Hunterian Laboratory of Experimental Medicine at the medical school. He, of course, continued his brilliant career in Boston. As a surgeon, Cushing's persistent inquiry gave birth to the modern science of neurosurgery. As a teacher, he was a relentless and sometimes hard taskmaster, yet he unfailingly won the lasting respect and affection of his pupils. He also was a generous man and established scholarships for the study of medicine at both Harvard and Yale University.

Walter Dandy started his training at Johns Hopkins as a second-year medical student in the fall of 1907. After graduation, Dandy became the sixth of Cushing's Hunterian appointees (1910–1911). At that time, Dandy claimed that "Cushing was a dramatically good teacher" (22). Dandy remained at Johns Hopkins Medical University for the rest of his illustrious career. Initially Cushing's pupil, Dandy became a giant in neurosurgery, rivaling Cushing himself. Dandy advanced the specialty of neurosurgery by continually questioning how, what, and why. His curiosity was combined with the courage to break new ground: "Not content with existing procedures when these seemed to be inadequate, his keen observation and deduction often led to a solution which meant the saving of a life in an apparently hopeless situation" (20). In addition, "Dandy was an unlikely and largely reluctant hero, but a hero for all that, to the young physicians and the many patients that came within his orbit" (2). His loyalty to the Johns Hopkins Medical Institution is legendary.

Johns Hopkins required a college degree as a prerequisite for admission. The university provided a 4-year curriculum, made extensive use of laboratories for teaching, and integrated the hospital and college facilities to provide clinical training to advanced students. In 1904, Halsted's resident training program, modeled after the German *Oberartz* system, consisted of serving as an assistant for 6 years in preparation for 2 years as house surgeon (similar to the contemporary chief resident) (6, 12). The trainees received extensive clinical experience and were expected to engage in research. In 1954, this pattern of training was formalized by the Committee on Graduate Surgical Training (now the Resident Review Committee in Surgery).

Although the education of medical students and residents at Johns Hopkins was somewhat structured, the training of most medical students was still seeded with corruption, profiteering, fraud, and malpractice. In 1910, the Flexner report (commissioned by the Carnegie Foundation for the Advancement of Teaching) on medical education in the United States and Canada helped to introduce the standard medical curriculum, which persists, largely unmodified, today. Before the report, the primary problem with medical education centered on the motivation to profit from educating physicians and a concomitant disregard for libraries, laboratory facilities, admission standards, or even knowledgeable faculty. It led to an epidemic of iatrogenic morbidity and mortality (8).

Besides emphasizing biomedical teaching and standards, Flexner stressed that budding physicians needed "a varied and enlarging culture experience" (3). Consequently, medical educators in the latter half of the twentieth century turned their attention to training humane physicians to treat illnesses not only with technology and pharmacology but also with attentive listening and empathy. For a variety of reasons, in the beginning—and even now—this move to teach humanities to future physicians was and is quite slow. Students were and are infatuated with high technology (i.e., computers). Financial incentives often overshadow appropriate and correct patient care. An ingredient appears to be missing, an ingredient that is needed to transform brilliant biomechanical technicians into effective healers. Perhaps incorporating a humanitarian curriculum into medical schools—or even earlier, in high schools or college—could reverse this tendency. The days of subjecting medical students to overwork, abuse, demeaning attitudes, and unrealistic demands must end. Physician-teachers who apply scientific and humanistic views to the marvelous technology of contemporary medicine and, through it, to healing need to serve as actual mentors to foster this mindset.

During the last half-century, the medical world has become bureaucratized, depolarized, and yes, specialized, yet the popular expectation of medicine remains, in part, traditional—that is, to receive excellent care from caring, devoted physicians. Nevertheless, almost all Americans also want that excellent care to include the latest breakthroughs and high-technology procedures or techniques. With these conflicting changes and demands, how can the learning process be structured to avoid becoming depersonalized, boring, procedural, and ultimately, unsuccessful?

The greatest challenge to improving medical education is to modify the internal culture of the academic health center to reinforce the scientific and humanistic values that medical educators wish to impart. At present, this is no small task, because the managed care revolution has caused medical schools and teaching hospitals to become less friendly to patients and students, thus contributing to the deterioration of bedside clinical skills and to the demoralization of faculty. Perhaps it has affected the quality of care adversely (13). Managed care is a business that survives, in part, by its ability to deny customers the product they want, a product that can be the difference between life and death. A patient's bill of rights, presently under consideration by the U.S. Congress, should provide the right of a second opinion, prohibit health plans from paying bonuses to administrators for denying care, guarantee access to emergency care and specialties, and establish procedures for timely internal and external review.

The emphasis on the bottom line has eroded the quality of the clinical learning environment, particularly by reducing the time that is available for teachers to teach and for students to learn (13, 14). One might wonder about the long-term consequences of educating the nation's physicians in today's commercial atmosphere, in which a good visit is a short visit, patients are "consumers," and institutional officials more often speak about the financial sheets than about service and relief of patients' suffering. This attitude challenges the altruism and idealism that students typically bring to the study of medicine (13, 14).

To make the culture of teaching centers less commercial and more service-oriented requires not only attention to formal didactic teaching but also active faculty mentoring. This combination can help to create competent residents and physicians.

This competency should continue throughout a physician's career. In 1910, Flexner recommended that physicians pursue lifelong learning and critical teaching skills (19). Until recently, Flexner's educational recommendation had not been implemented. Acquiring competency during medical school and residency is mandatory, and maintaining that competency is just as crucial. The American Board of Medical Specialties (ABMS) appointed a task force on competence in March 1998. The ABMS is the umbrella organization for 24 member boards, including the American Board of Neurological Surgeons (ABNS).

Board certification signifies that diplomates have met their board standards through education, training, knowledge, skills, and experience. The public, hospitals, health plans, and other organizations recognize these certification credentials as attainment of high standards. Nevertheless, the ABMS and its member boards recognize that board certification does not necessarily guarantee that a diplomate will practice competently after the certification process. The public has come to understand this point as well. Recertification by most boards every 10 years or so is designed to stimulate diplomates to "keep up" with new knowledge by testing, usually by taking a written examination.

Unfortunately, simply passing a written examination also does not connote competency in contemporary medical practice. Medicine, especially highly technical specialties such as neurosurgery, changes more often than every 10 years. In fact, changes occur almost daily. Neither the appropriate and skillful use of these changing technologies nor desirable characteristics such as professionalism and communication skills can be assessed adequately by a written examination.

Consequently, the ABMS and Accreditation Council of Graduate Medical Education (ACGME) have agreed on six general competencies that both residents and practicing physicians should display (18):

1. Patient care,
2. Medical knowledge,

3. Practice-based learning and improvement,
4. Interpersonal and communication skills,
5. Professionalism, and
6. System-based practices.

Most of these competencies are self-explanatory. System-based practice, however, needs further explanation.

Competency in a system-based practice means how a physician practices cost-effective care, understands the interaction of practice in a larger system, and acts as an advocate for patients within the health care system. These general competencies were introduced to the accreditation of residency programs on July 1, 2002. The six general competencies can differ, depending on the specialty. For example, the communication skills needed by a neurosurgeon differ from those of a pathologist. Medical knowledge and patient care also differ among specialties. Despite these differences, however, competencies should be measurable, teachable, and learnable.

Besides the six general competencies, the ABMS and its member boards agreed that four primary elements are required to maintain certification (18):

1. Evidence of professional standing,
2. Evidence of commitment to lifelong learning and involvement in periodic self-assessment,
3. Cognitive expertise, and
4. Practice performance.

Being competent in these four elements will assure that a physician is a "lifelong" learner (i.e., a lifelong student).

The ABNS has adopted the ABMS definition of evidence of professional standing. The physician must hold an unrestricted license to practice medicine in at least one jurisdiction in the United States, its territories, or Canada. If licenses are held in more than one jurisdiction, all licenses held by a physician should meet the requirement. Letters of concern or reprimand shall not be considered a restriction.

Lifelong learning might consist of an open-book examination every 2 years, CME hours, or both. The cognitive examination most likely will be a proctored, closed-book examination that is taken at a computer center and is based on questions from the open-book examinations.

Practice performance might consist of key case submissions (i.e., 10 consecutive anterior cervical discectomy cases for spine specialists or 10 consecutive clippings of a supratentorial aneurysm for vascular specialists). These analyses would be submitted every 2 years. The second component of practice performance could consist of analyzing all consecutive operative cases during 1 year, that year being from 1 to 2 years before the physician takes the cognitive examination. The analysis of these cases is not punitive; rather, it is educational, with the hope of improving patient care by comparing data from one period to another.

Physicians and teachers should be mentors to medical students, residents, younger colleagues, and even to peers. They have a chance to influence budding or new physicians. They need to devote the extra time and effort to impart knowledge and skills and to guide and counsel them. Their excitement and enthusiasm should be visible. They should share their failures as well as their successes—but the students' role in success and the teachers' role in failures should be emphasized.

Patients not only seek relief from pain, suffering, disease, or disorders, they also seek counseling and guidance—that is, *mentoring*. The physician's primary professional duty and responsibility is the appropriate and compassionate treatment of patients. This duty should be performed with integrity, honor, and respect. It should never be driven by self-serving, greedy, or financial goals.

From the heroes in Greek mythology to Hippocrates to Halsted, Flexner, Welch, Osler, Cushing, Dandy, and others, we in neurosurgery have had the good fortune to have enjoyed great mentors. A mentor is someone who cares; someone who is competent and gives of himself or herself freely; someone who values respect, knowledge, and fairness. All physicians can be such a mentor. All physicians *should* be such a mentor, whether to colleagues, students, patients, or their own children.

Medicine is at a crossroads, with pressures related to financial management, high technology, litigation, and endless paperwork—all of which erode the humanistic, caring way in which we want to treat our patients and in which our patients want to be treated. Being a competent physician means being a mentor and a student, creating an environment that emphasizes excellence and healthy morale. In this way, we can hope to navigate safely through the difficult terrain ahead so that, at the end of the day, we have the respect not only of those around us but also, more importantly, our own.

REFERENCES

1. Adams F: *The Genuine Works of Hippocrates*. London: Sydeham Society, 1849.
2. Austin LL: Capon Springs, WV. Interview with the author, Sept. 29, 1966. In Turner TB (ed): *Heritage of Excellence: The Johns Hopkins Medical Institutions, 1914–1947*. Baltimore: Johns Hopkins University Press, 1974, p 411.
3. Flexner A: Medical education in the United States and Canada: A report to the

Carnegie Foundation for the Advancement of Teaching. **Carnegie Foundation for the Advancement of Teaching** 4, 1910.

4. Fulton JF: *Harvey Cushing: A Biography*. Springfield, IL: Charles C Thomas, 1946, p 256.
5. Grant M: *Myths of the Greeks and Romans*. New York: New American Library, 1964.
6. Halsted WS: The training of the surgeon. **Am Med** 8:69–75, 1904.
7. Hamilton E: *Mythology: Timeless Tales of Gods and Heros*. New York: The New American Library, 1942.
8. Herren GE: Motivation for medical education reform: The post-Flexner era. **The Pharos** (Winter):25–32, 1999.
9. Hippocrates: On nature of bones. In Littre PE (ed): *Oeuvres Completes d'Hippocrate*. Amsterdam: AM Hakkert, 1982, pp 162–197.
10. Burcher SH, Lang A (transl): *The Odyssey*. New York: PF Collier and Son, 1937, p 12.
11. Littrè E: *Hippocrates: Oeuvres Complètes d'Hippocrates*. Paris: JB Baillière, 1853.
12. Longmire WP Jr: The Halstedian influence goes west: Personal and historical remarks. **The Pharos** (Summer):19–24, 1999.
13. Ludmerer KM: Instilling professionalism in medical education. **J Am Med Assoc** 282:881–882, 1999.
14. Ludmerer KM: *Time to Heal: American Medical Education from the Turn of the Century to the Era of Managed Care*. New York: Oxford University Press, 1999.
15. Lyons AS, Petrucelli RJ: *Medicine: An Illustrated History*. New York: Harry N. Abrams, 1987.
16. Marketos SG, Skiadas PK: Hippocrates. The father of spine surgery. **Spine** 24:1381–1387, 1999.
17. Marketos SG, Skiadas PK: The modern Hippocratic tradition. Some messages for contemporary medicine. **Spine** 24:1159–1163, 1999.
18. Nahrwold DL: The Competence Movement: A report on the activities of the American Board of Medical Specialties. **Bulletin of the American College of Surgeons** 85:14–18, 2000.
19. Regan-Smith MG: Commentary on Flexner's impact—Then and now: A profound effect on medical education, research, practice. **The Pharos** (Winter):31, 1999.
20. Reichert FL: An appreciation. **Surgery** 19:580, 1946.
21. Rutkow IM: *Surgery: An Illustrated History*. St. Louis: Mosby-Year Book, 1993.
22. Stone HB: Harvey B. Stone, MD, Baltimore, Interview with the author, May 25. 1967.
23. Thomson EH: *Harvey Cushing: Surgeon, Author, Artist*. New York: Collier Books, 1961.
24. Withington ET (transl): Hippocrates. On joints. In Capps E, Page T III, Rouse WHD (eds): *Hippocrates: The Loeb Classical Library*. London: W. Heinemann, 1927, pp 200–397.

Resident and Young Investigator Awards

CHAPTER

20

CNS Resident Award: Role of the Lateral Premotor Cortex in Articulation

NITIN TANDON, M.D., SHALINI NARAYANA, Ph.D., JACK L. LANCASTER, Ph.D., STEVEN BROWN, Ph.D., STEPHEN DODD, Ph.D., DENNIS G. VOLLMER, M.D., ROGER INGHAM, Ph.D., JANIS INGHAM, Ph.D., MARIO LIOTTI, M.D., AND PETER T. FOX, M.D.

AIMS

The preservation of language function is a compelling directive during surgery for tumors or epilepsy in the dominant hemisphere. Language production may be viewed as the integrated output of two systems: the semantic/syntactic system and the phonatory/articulatory system. The articulation (speech) system has been widely studied in patients with lesions (strokes/resections) and by cortical stimulation mapping (CSM). These studies have led to a rich body of literature that details the importance of the inferior frontal gyrus (Broca's area), primary face and laryngeal motor cortex, the anterior insula (2), and several subcortical regions (11) in articulation. The primary modality for localization of eloquent speech areas in the neurosurgical population, CSM relies on the production of a transient cortical lesion by focal cortical depolarization (6, 8). Unaltered task performance in the presence of this focal depolarization suggests that a given region of the brain is not crucial to the task being studied and may be resected with a low risk of long-term dysfunction of a particular process. In terms of the function studied, CSM is time intensive and usually produces results that are "all or none." Given its invasive nature, it is not a strategy that can be applied to the scientific study of speech function in normal humans.

It has recently become possible to produce transient, virtual cortical lesions noninvasively using transcranial magnetic stimulation (TMS), which can be carried out in normal subjects, can be repeated many times, and can be performed in conjunction with precise behavioral measurements. Studies on TMS-induced speech disruption in the past have principally used stimulation at high frequencies and intensities, a strategy that is painful and unsafe (potentially inducing seizures) (7, 10). Also, speech arrest, an "all-or-none" response, precludes closer characterization of the nature of the articulatory defect produced in response to the region stimulated. We sought to produce articulatory disruption in normal subjects in a safe, painless manner with lower frequencies of TMS, both to characterize the speech disruption produced and to localize the cortical region responsible for the behaviors observed.

METHODS

Characterization of TMS Effects

The study was carried out in eight normal English speakers (six right-handed and two left-handed). The TMS was delivered using a water-cooled, figure-8 coil (Cadwell, Inc., Kennewick, Washington) powered by a Cadwell HSMS unit. The Cadwell HSMS unit delivers a triphasic electric pulse with a total duration of 240 μs and a peak electric field (E-field) of 500 V/m at 100% of machine output at the coil surface. The location of the left hemispheric primary hand motor cortex was determined by delivering TMS to localize the region where stimulation produced contractions of the first dorsal interosseous (FDI) muscle. The intensity of machine output that elicited barely palpable contractions in approximately half the trials was used to define the motor threshold. The location on the skullcap under the portion of the coil where the induced E-field was highest, where FDI contractions were just barely elicited with threshold-level stimulation, was defined as the location for M1-hand. For localization, subjects were first fitted with an elastic nylon cap (Electro-Cap International, Inc., Eaton, OH) that they wore during the entire study. During the characterization of the speech disruption, the subject's head was held immobile with the use of a custom-molded, thermoplastic face mask (*Fig. 20.1*).

With the coil handheld, TMS at 4 Hz was delivered to both lateral frontal lobes with the subjects reading unfamiliar material; subjects were observed closely for effects on speech fluency. Speech disruption following stimulation of regions that also resulted in face or lip movements (primary face motor cortical regions) was not considered as relevant to the study (3). Speech disruption that was accompanied by pain (areas overlaid by temporalis muscle) was also excluded from further study given the confounding effects of pain on verbal fluency. In all eight individuals, we were able to localize a region where TMS at 4 Hz resulted in a profound disruption of speech that was not associated with pain or with face or lip movement. This region consistently was approximately 2 cm anterior and ventral to the location of primary hand motor cortex (M1-hand), between the locations for electrode contacts D3 and D5 (10–20 electrode convention). This region was found on the left side in seven (six right-handed and one left-handed) subjects and on the right side in one (left-handed) subject.

The scalp location of the site of stimulation was marked with a fiducial. A symmetric "homologous" location on the opposite side was used as a control site. Characterization of the speech disruption was done with the subjects performing a variety of tasks during concomitant stimulation of the site of speech disruption (TMS) or of the control site (sham TMS) or during no stimulation (baseline). Stimulation was carried out at 4 Hz for 5 sec at 110% of motor threshold. During behavioral characterization, the TMS coil over the site of speech disruption was held in position with a NeuroMate neurosurgical robot to facilitate optimal positioning and to ensure coil immobility throughout the study. Sham stimulation was delivered to the homologous contralateral location using a second figure-8 coil held by a custom-made, malleable gooseneck holder (*Fig. 20.1*).

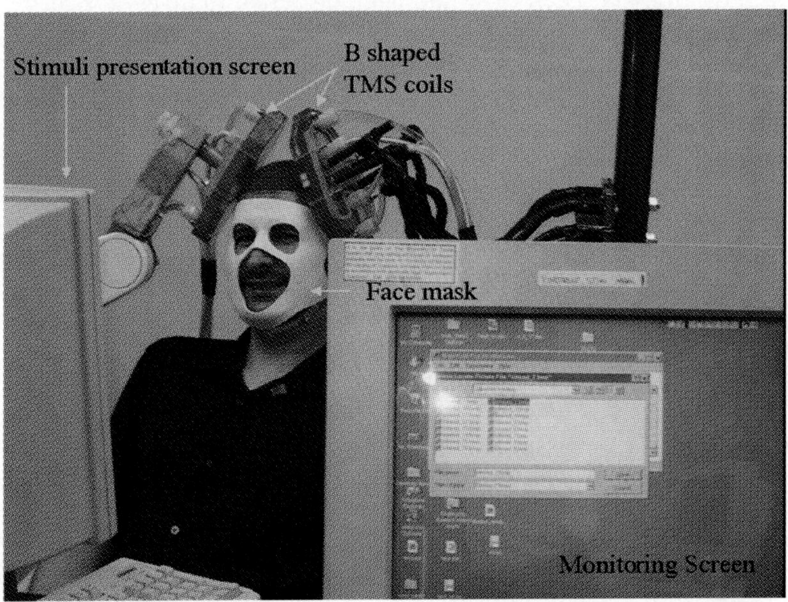

FIG. 20.1 Experimental setup. The subject is facing a computer screen, where stimuli are presented. Two TMS coils are positioned on his head: one over the region where speech disruption was found and one over its contralateral homologue. The thermoplastic face mask holds the subjects head immobile for the duration of the experiment. A second computer monitor faces the researchers, and the video camera that is used to record the session.

Subjects performed 11 tasks. The TMS trains (20 pulses at 4-Hz stimulation for 5 sec) were delivered in a randomized manner to the location for speech disruption or to the contralateral sham TMS region during these tasks. Baseline (no TMS) measurements were made between TMS pulses. In this manner, eight baseline and eight TMS measurements were made per subject per task. Tasks performed were as follows: overt reading of unfamiliar text; silent reading of unfamiliar text; articulation of serial additives of number 3 (e.g., 15, 18, 21, etc.); overt singing an overlearned song (e.g., "Happy Birthday"); overt humming of a nonlyrical tune (e.g., "Col. Bogey's March," from *Bridge on the River Kwai*); repetitive, self-paced articulation of the syllables Pa-Ta-Ka; lingual praxis (self-paced, side-to-side tongue movement); labial praxis (self-paced, alternating smiling and lip pursing); verb generation to nouns (reported *after* each block); right-hand typing ("LKJ" typed repeatedly, in sequence); and left-hand typing ("SDF" typed repeatedly, in sequence).

Videotapes, audio recordings, and where appropriate, records of keyboard strikes for each task were made and used to score the behavioral measure that each task had been designed to disrupt. Scoring of video and audio recordings was carried out by a specialist in speech research who was blinded to the test conditions (real or control TMS). Measures from real TMS (speech-arrest location) and sham TMS (contralateral location) were compared with each other (two tailed t-test assuming unequal variances). This comparison between TMS effects from real versus control stimulation eliminated extraneous effects from phenomena such as the TMS click and cutaneous/muscular stimulation by the induced E-field that could confound comparisons made solely between TMS and baseline states.

Custom robotic guidance software was developed in-house for the purpose of delivering TMS precisely using the NeuroMate robot and for mapping the induced E-field directly onto the cortical surface of each subject. This overlay allows for the accurate determination of the cortical region where the E-field is highest and the effects of stimulation most likely to manifest. This technique was used to compute the location of the site of stimulation that resulted in disruption of articulation per subject. An average of these loci was computed to calculate the mean location of the site of speech disruption by TMS.

MR Imaging

All subjects underwent a high-resolution anatomical MR (aMR) imaging and functional MR (fMR) imaging. The aMR images were obtained with fiducials marking the location of the site of motor stimulation and the site of speech disruption. The fMR images were obtained using a Elscint 2T MR scanner. The fMR imaging data were collected during covert (silent) generation of verbs to nouns, during overt articulation through clenched jaws (to minimize motion), during self-paced opening and closing movements of the hand contralateral to the hemisphere where speech disruption was produced (right hand in seven subjects and left hand in one), and during rest. All imaging data were spatially normalized, and then contrast images of verb generation versus rest and of overt articulation versus rest were generated and t maps computed and overlaid onto the aMR image.

RESULTS

Characterization of TMS Effects

The number of correct syllables (measure of articulatory fluency) produced during the overt speech—reading of text, serial additions, internally cued syllable production (Pa-Ta-Ka), and singing tasks—were all markedly diminished ($P < 0.0001$) during TMS of the frontal lobe on the side where speech disruption was determined to occur (left hemisphere in seven subjects and right hemisphere in one) (*Fig. 20.2*).

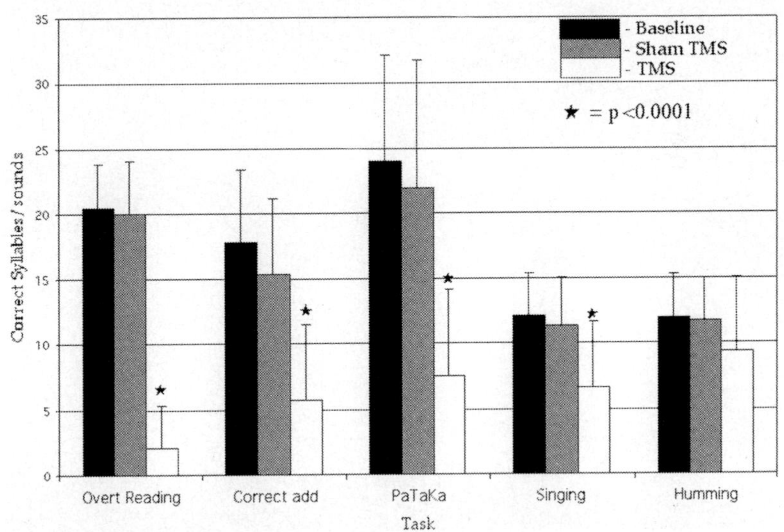

FIG. 20.2 Effects of TMS on tasks: The numbers of correct syllables/sounds produced per 5-sec block during TMS of the premotor region in the dominant hemisphere were compared with no TMS (baseline) and with TMS of the contralateral hemisphere (sham TMS). Highly significant differences ($P < 0.0001$) were seen with intrinsically or extrinsically cued syllable production but not with production of a nonverbal melody.

In contrast, there was no effect on the number of syllables read silently without articulation, typing with either hand, or the silent generation of verbs. There was also an effect on humming, but this was not pronounced and barely reached significance ($P = 0.04$). Interesting results were seen with the analysis of self-paced labial and lingual movements. Analysis of the entire group revealed small disruptions ($P = 0.04$ and 0.01, respectively) on the production of correct lip and tongue excursions, yet these effects appeared to stem from three subjects in whom the overt speech disruptive effect, though present, was not as pronounced. A subgroup analysis excluding these three subjects with an "atypical" behavioral response revealed no statistically significant effects on labial or lingual function ($P = 0.4$ and 0.3, respectively).

The location on the cortical surface that was subjected to the highest intensity of the E-field, determined by registering the coil location into the imaging space, was assumed to be the site responsible for the articulatory function being disrupted (*Fig. 20.3*). The average location

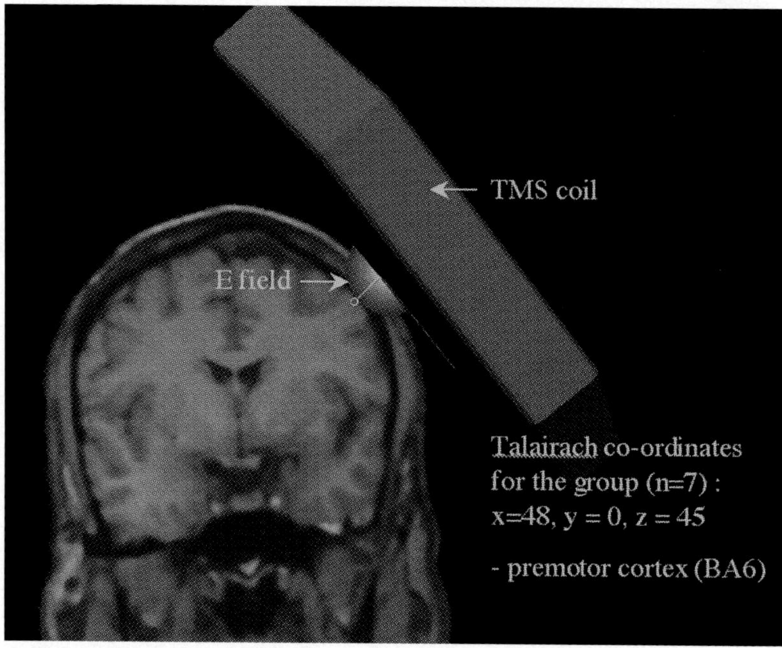

FIG. 20.3 Localization of the site of stimulation. The three-dimensional aMR image is stereotactically registered to the subjects' head and to the location of the TMS coil. The E-field produced by the coil is mapped onto the image, and the spot where it interacts with the cortex is localized and reported in standardized space. The average location of the TMS effect for the group (n = 7) is listed.

for all seven subjects who had a left hemispheric speech disruption was computed and given by the Talairach coordinates: $x = 48$, $y = 0$, and $z = 45$. This corresponds to a region in Brodmann area 6 (lateral premotor cortex, based on the Talairach atlas).

fMR Images

Contrasts between whispered reading and rest, covert verb generation and rest, and hand movement and rest were examined for local maxima. The first of these contrasts was of the most interest and revealed a clear region of activation of the lateral premotor cortex (BA6), with overt articulation, directly under the average position of fiducial marker that had been placed at the site if TMS induced speech disruption (*Fig. 20.4*). All subjects who had a left hemispheric speech disruption were noted to have left hemispheric dominance on the language tasks by fMR imaging. The single subject with a right-sided

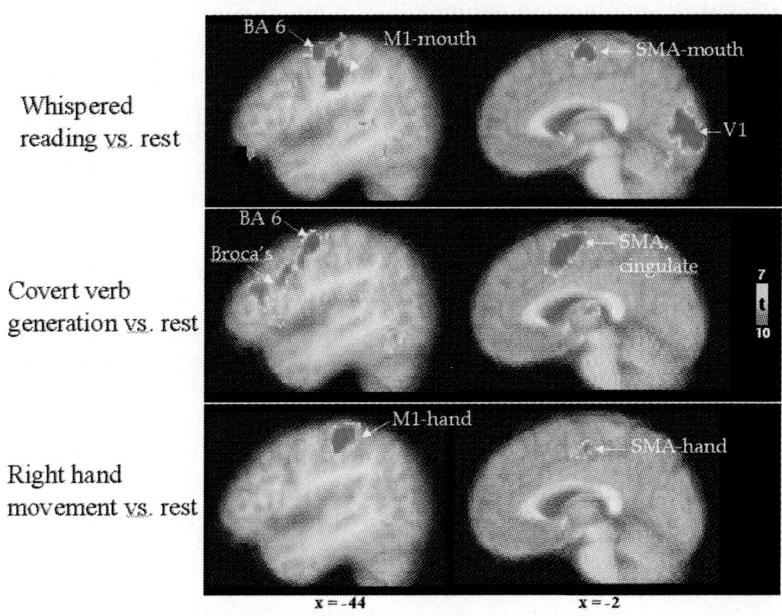

FIG. 20.4 Results of fMR imaging. Overt (whispered) reading shows activation of the primary motor cortex and of the lateral premotor region. The premotor region also shows activation during covert verb generation, presumably reflecting its involvement in the generation of an articulatory plan. It lies one gyrus anterior to the primary motor cortex. Movement of the right hand (a control task) shows activation of the hand motor cortex and the SMA. As expected the location of SMA-mouth is more rostral than that for SMA-hand.

locus for speech disruption was noted to be markedly right hemisphere lateralized by functional imaging. The center of mass of the premotor activation was situated at the Talairach coordinates of $x = 48$, $y = -6$, and $z = 50$. Thus, the functionally activated region correlates well with the region subjected to the highest intensity of the E-field. This corroborates our notion that the speech disruption produced here results from transient dysfunction induced in the lateral premotor cortex by suprathreshold TMS pulses.

DISCUSSION

We have shown that the lateral premotor cortex is significantly involved in articulatory plan generation/execution. The lateral premotor region was found to be activated distinct from the primary mouth motor cortex in a whispered-speech paradigm. The average location of the cortical region across subjects, stimulation (and, therefore, disorganized depolarization) of which induces a profound articulatory impediment, essentially overlaps with this region of functional activation. Other functions, such as silent reading, verbal working memory, and face and tongue motor function, are insignificantly unaffected by this induced dysfunction. The region is functionally and anatomically distinct from the Broca's area and from the face motor cortex. There is some individual variability in the location of this region and a slight divergence in the phenomenology of the response to TMS of the premotor region.

Recently, functional imaging studies (fMR imaging, positron-emission tomography [PET], and magnetoencephalography have been used to localize eloquent cortex in efforts to minimize the need to map the cortex intraoperatively or by using subdural electrodes. These studies have yielded results that show variable degrees of concordance between both the number of and the center of mass of activations seen by functional imaging techniques. The mismatch between these observations likely reflects the fact that functional images reveal all regions involved in task-related processing but do not comment on their essential nature (1, 4, 5, 9). For this reason, preoperative functional language mapping data are unable to completely inform surgical decisions around language sites; a continued dependence on intraoperative electrical stimulation mapping remains the norm. Transient "virtual" lesion production using TMS-PET provides a measure of whether the region is essential rather than "involved" in task performance. Having access to a single essential region of the speech motor pathway may provide us with an avenue to construct a connectivity map of this system using concurrent TMS-PET. It is also likely to be of use in assessing language laterality in a noninvasive fashion, spatiotemporal sequencing of articulatory plan generation and execution, and exploration of gender differences in speech motor planning.

REFERENCES

1. Bookheimer SY, Zeffiro TA, Blaxton T, et al.: A direct comparison of PET activation and electrocortical stimulation mapping for language localization. **Neurology** 48:1056–1065, 1997.
2. Dronkers NF: A new brain region for coordinating speech articulation. **Nature** 384:159–161, 1996.
3. Epstein CM, Meador KJ, Loring DW, et al.: Localization and characterization of speech arrest during transcranial magnetic stimulation. **Clin Neurophysiol** 110:1073–1079, 1999.
4. FitzGerald DB, Cosgrove GR, Ronner S, et al.: Location of language in cortex: A comparison between functional MR imaging and electrocortical stimulation. **AJNR Am J Neuroradiol** 18:1529–1539, 1997.
5. Herholz K, Reulen H-J, von Stockhausen H-M, et al.: Preoperative activation and intraoperative stimulation of language-related areas in patients with glioma. **Neurosurgery** 41:1253–1262, 1997.
6. Ojemann G, Ojemann J, Lettich E, Berger M: Cortical language localization in left, dominant hemisphere. **J Neurosurg** 71:316–326, 1989.
7. Pascual-Leone A, Gates JR, Dhuna A: Induction of speech arrest and counting errors with rapid rate transcranial magnetic stimulation. **Neurology** 41: 697–702, 1991.
8. Penfield W, Boldrey E: Somatic motor and sensory representation in the cerebral cortex of man as studied by electrical stimulation. **Brain** 60: 389–443, 1937.
9. Simos GS, Papanicolaou, Breier JI, et al.: Localization of language-specific cortex by using magnetic source imaging and electrical stimulation mapping. **J Neurosurg** 91:787–796, 1999.
10. Wassermann EM: Risk and safety of repetitive transcranial magnetic stimulation: report and suggested guidelines from the International Workshop on the Safety of Repetitive Transcranial Magnetic Stimulation, June 5–7, 1996. **Electroencephalo Clin Neurophys** 108: 1–16, 1998.
11. Wise RJS, Greene J, Buchel C, Scott SK: Brain regions involved in articulation. **Lancet** 353:1057–1061, 1999.

CHAPTER

21

Tumor Young Investigator Award: Induction of Glioblastoma Multiforme in Primates after Fractionated Whole-Brain Irradiation in the Therapeutic Dose Range

RUSSELL R. LONSER, M.D., STUART WALBRIDGE, B.S., ALEXANDER O. VORTMEYER, M.D., SVETLANA D. PACK, Ph.D., TUNG T. NGUYEN, M.D., NITIN GOGATE, M.D., JEFFERY J. OLSON, M.D., AYTAC AKBASAK, M.D., R. HUNT BOBO, M.D., THOMAS GOFFMAN, M.D., ZHENGPING ZHUANG, M.D., Ph.D., AND EDWARD H. OLDFIELD, M.D.

INTRODUCTION

Radiation therapy is an effective method for treatment of many types of tumors in the central nervous system (CNS). Unfortunately, a significant number of well-established side effects can be associated with this therapeutic modality. These reactions have typically been divided into three categories based on when they occur: *early acute* reactions, which occur during radiation; *early delayed* reactions, which are delayed by days or weeks after irradiation; and *late delayed* reactions, which are delayed by months to years after irradiation (25). Early acute reactions typically include tissue edema, skin reactions, hair loss, and fatigue. Early delayed reactions can include lethargy, tissue edema, and focal demyelination. Late delayed reactions characteristically manifest as focal or diffuse necrosis (characterized by vascular changes, edema, and demyelination), gliosis, tissue calcification, and atrophy. In addition, sporadic reports have recently begun to suggest that delayed tumor formation may occasionally occur after a delay of several years after irradiation.

We report the outcome of a long-term study concerning the results of a clinically relevant dose of whole-brain irradiation in rhesus monkeys. The clinical, laboratory, radiographic, molecular, and histologic analyses of these animals up to 10 years after irradiation is described.

MATERIALS AND METHODS

Animals Groups

All animal experiments were performed in accordance with the National Institutes of Health guidelines on the use of animals in research and were approved by the Animal Care and Use Committee of the National Institute of Neurological Disorders and Stroke.

We used a total of 12 male primates (*Macaca mulatta*; age, 3 years). All animals underwent fractionated whole-brain irradiation (see *Radiation* below) while sedated. Previous work in our laboratory had demonstrated that pentobarbital is radioprotective against the early acute and early delayed reactions in the rat whole-brain irradiation model (37, 39, 40). However, the effect of barbiturates on late delayed reactions, which cause severe late radiation syndromes, was unknown. It is this late delayed toxicity that limits the cumulative dose of radiation and, therefore, tumor control. To determine the potential radioprotective effects of barbiturates in primates, the animals were divided into two groups based on whether they received barbiturates during irradiation. The control group ($n = 6$) was sedated with ketamine (25 mg/kg im) during each radiation session, and the barbiturate experimental group ($n = 6$) was sedated with pentobarbital (25 mg/kg iv) during each radiation session. The animals were allowed to awaken at the completion of each session.

Radiation

Fractionated whole-brain irradiation was given at 350 cGy/day for 10 days (5 days a week for 2 weeks; total dose, 3,500 cGy). The treatments were performed with a bilateral exposure replicating human treatment (cobalt-60 unit) of the whole brain while shielding the mouth, pharynx, and body at a source-to-target (midsagittal plane) distance of 50 cm and at a rate of 70 cGy/min.

Clinical Follow-Up

Animals were carefully followed for medical or neurologic difficulties over the study period (up to 10 years). Animals underwent serial (every 6 mo) blood analysis, including complete blood count and chemistry panels (including liver function studies).

Radiographic Follow-Up

Animals underwent MR imaging (T_1-weighted with and without contrast enhancement and T_2-weighted images; 1.5 Tesla) 1 to 3 mo before irradiation. After the completion of irradiation, animals underwent MR imaging (T_1-weighted with and without contrast enhancement and T_2-weighted images; 1.5 Tesla) serially at 6-mo intervals for the first 2 years and then at serial intervals of approximately 6 to 12 mo after that. Supplemental MR imaging was also performed upon development of neurologic symptoms.

Tissue Histologic Analysis

Animals were sacrificed when they developed severe medical problems, neurologic symptoms, parenchymal lesions on MR imaging, or at the completion of the study. All animals were euthanized by barbiturate overdose. Immediately after sacrifice, the animals' brains were either removed and frozen at −80°C or placed in 10% formalin. The brains were then cut coronally in serial sections (thickness, 10–40 μm). Tissue sections were cut through areas of enhancement and/or increased T_2-weighted signal on MR imaging (to examine for lesion pathology) and regions away from obvious tumor (to examine for evidence of radiation injury and distant tumor spread not evident by MR imaging). Sections were stained with hematoxylin and eosin. Immunohistochemistry for glial fibrillary acidic protein was performed on some tumors (nine tumors in six separate animals).

Tumor Comparative Genomic Hybridization

To determine what genetic alterations existed between tumor and normal tissues and how these differences corresponded within the human genome, we analyzed primate normal brain and tumor tissues using a novel interspecies comparative genomic hybridization (CGH) technique. The details of this technique are described in full elsewhere (S. Pack et al., submitted) and are summarized below.

Briefly, tumor and normal brain tissues from three animals were collected immediately after euthanization. The tissues (tumor and normal brain) then underwent mincing, alkaline lysis, and alcohol extraction (per the manufacturer's instructions; Qiagen, Inc., Valencia, CA). Extracted normal brain DNA was labeled with digoxygenin-11-dUTP, and tumor DNA was labeled with biotin-16-dUTP by nick translation. The labeled normal brain and tumor DNA probes were then simultaneously hybridized to healthy human male metaphase spreads. Red florescence labeling of normal DNA was then performed with antidigoxigenin Fab fragments conjugated to rhodamine, and green florescence labeling of tumor DNA was performed with fluorescein isothiocyanate conjugated to avidin.

Florescent images were then digitally captured and analyzed using the Quips CGH software (Downers Grove, IL) to determine the average ratio of green (tumor) to red (normal) florescence. The definition of altered regions was based on the cut-off levels of tumor to normal fluorescence ratios of 0.80 and 1.20. Regions in which the ratio was lower or exceeded these threshold levels were considered to be either a loss or a gain, respectively. Heterochromatic regions of chromosomes 1, 9, 13, 14, 15, 16, 19, 21, and 22 and the entire Y chromosome were excluded from the analysis.

Statistical Analysis

Statistical analysis was performed on Stat View 5.0 (Abacus Concepts, Berkeley, CA). Statistical tests were used as defined in the text.

RESULTS

Animal Outcome

CLINICAL EFFECTS

All animals tolerated fractionated whole-brain radiation without problems and completed the course of treatment as described. One animal died from a pulmonary abscess and sepsis 2.5 years after irradiation, leaving 11 animals available for long-term evaluation and comparison. There were no detectable differences (clinical, laboratory, or otherwise) between animal groups (control vs pentobarbital) in their response to radiation over the course of the study. Thus, all animals will be considered together for presentation of results.

There were no significant problems related to radiation in either group until 2.9 years after treatment, when one animal (animal 1) (*Table 21.1*) developed progressive (over 2–3 weeks) gait difficulties and was unable to feed itself. Magnetic resonance imaging was performed and depicted contrast-enhancing lesions in the brain stem and cerebellum, and the animal was sacrificed. The pathology at those sites was consistent with glioblastoma multiforme (GBM) (*Fig. 21.1*). Over the course of the next several years (up to 8.3 years after irradiation), eight additional animals developed contrast-enhancing cerebral lesions that were found initially on routine serial MR imaging ($n = 3$) or were discovered on MR imaging after neurologic deterioration (similar to animal 1) prompted supplemental scanning ($n = 5$). Neurologic symptoms related to GBMs corresponded with the imaged location of the tumor, peritumoral edema, and mass effect (*Table 21.1*). Seven animals with GBMs were sacrificed upon initial discovery of enhancing lesions on MR imaging. The remaining two animals with GBMs were followed clinically and radiographically for 1 to 2 mo after the initial discovery of enhancing tumor on MR imaging (animals 7 and 8) (*Table 21.1*). The mean latency to discovery of tumors in the nine animals (82% of the 11 animals with long-term follow-up) that developed GBMs (either by neurologic deterioration or incidental finding on MR imaging) was 5.4 ± 2.1 years (mean $\pm$ SD).

The remaining 2 animals that did not develop lesions depicted on MR images or neurologic deficits were euthanized at the study completion (10 years). These animals and the animal that died early (2.5 years after irradiation) had no gross or microscopic evidence of CNS disease.

TABLE 21.1

Summary of the Nine Animals that Developed GBM

Animal	Latency to Tumor (years)	Focality[a]	Cranial Region(s)[b]	Symptoms	Region(s) of Tumor[c]
1	2.9	M	I	Progressive gait difficulties and unable to feed over 2–3 weeks	Brain stem and cerebellum
2	3.4	M	S	Progressive visual difficulties over 10 days	Right parietooccipital, left occipital, and right anterior temporal
3	3.8	M	S	Progressive right arm weakness	Left temporal and right frontal
4	4.3	U	S	Progressive visual difficulties and not eating	Left occipital pole
5	4.4	M	B	Progressive blindness and difficulties feeding	Bilateral parietooccipital, left parietal, right frontal, and brain stem
6	5.8	M	S	Left arm weakness	Large right posterior temporal and smaller left parietooccipital
7	7.4	U	S	Discovered on imaging then increasing left arm and leg weakness	Right frontal
8	7.9	U	S	Discovered on imaging, then increasing lethargy and inability to care for itself over 1 mo	Bilateral frontoparietal (transcallosal)
9	8.3	M	I	Discovered on imaging	Left and medial cerebellum

[a]M, multifocal; U, unifocal.

[b]I, infratentorial, S, supratentorial; B, both.

[c]In all cases, the lesions identified on MR images were consistent with gross findings. These imaging foci were confirmed to be GBM in all cases.

Reprinted with permission from Lonser RR, Walbridge S, Vortmeyer AO, et al.: Glioblastoma multiforme formation after primate irradiation in the therapeutic dose range. *J Neurosurg* 97:1378–1389, 2002.

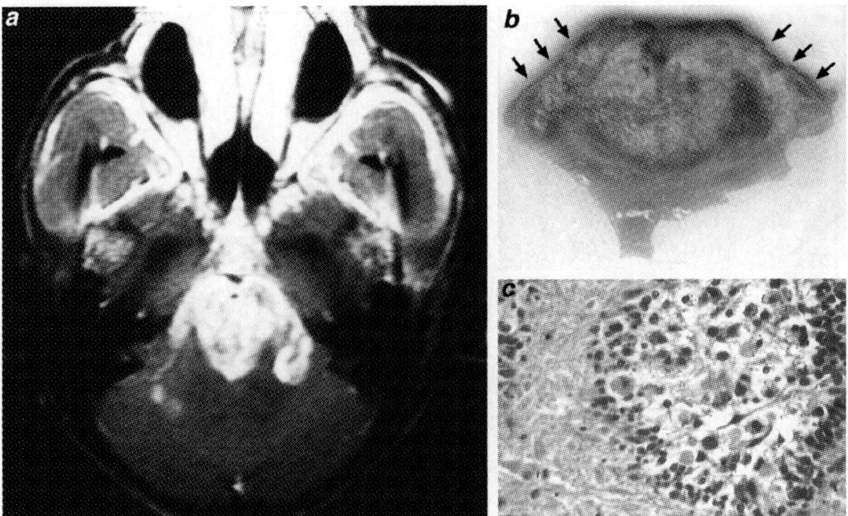

FIG. 21.1 Axial T_1-wieghted postcontrast MR image (*a*) through the pontocerebellar region of animal 1 (see *Table 21.1*) showing extensive enhancement of the pons and cerebellar peduncles. Imaging was performed after the animal began experiencing progressive eating and gait difficulties 2.9 years after irradiation. (*b*) Axial section through the corresponding region of the brain stem (tissue removed on day of imaging) showing gross invasion of the pons and cerebellar peduncles (arrows) by GBM. (*c*) Hematoxylin and eosin–stained section through brain stem regions of MR-enhancing tumor revealed histologic features consistent with GBM, including pseudopallisading cells with areas of necrosis. [Reprinted with permission from Lonser RR, Walbridge S, Vortmeyer AO, et al.: Glioblastoma multiforme formation after primate irradiation in the therapeutic dose range. **J Neurosurg** 97:1378–1389, 2002.]

IMAGING CHARACTERISTICS IN ANIMALS WITH GBM

Magnetic resonance imaging revealed unifocal (n = 3) or multifocal (n = 6) contrast-enhancing lesions located in the supratentorial (n = 6), infratentorial (n = 2), or both (n = 1) cranial regions (*Table 21.1 and Fig. 21.2*). All lesions evident on MR images correlated accurately with the location of GBM in gross morphology (*Figs. 21.1 and 21.3*). Magnetic resonance imaging in the two animals (animals 7 and 8) that were followed after the initial discovery of enhancing lesions revealed rapid progression in the size of the tumors and surrounding edema. This coincided with the development of progressive neurologic symptoms, which prompted euthanization at 1 mo (animal 8) and 2 mo (animal 7) after tumor discovery (*Figs. 21.4 and 21.5*). In the nine animals that developed GBMs, there was no evidence of tumor on the MR images obtained immediately before (10.8 ± 4.7 mo before; range, 6–20 mo) the first MR image revealing tumor.

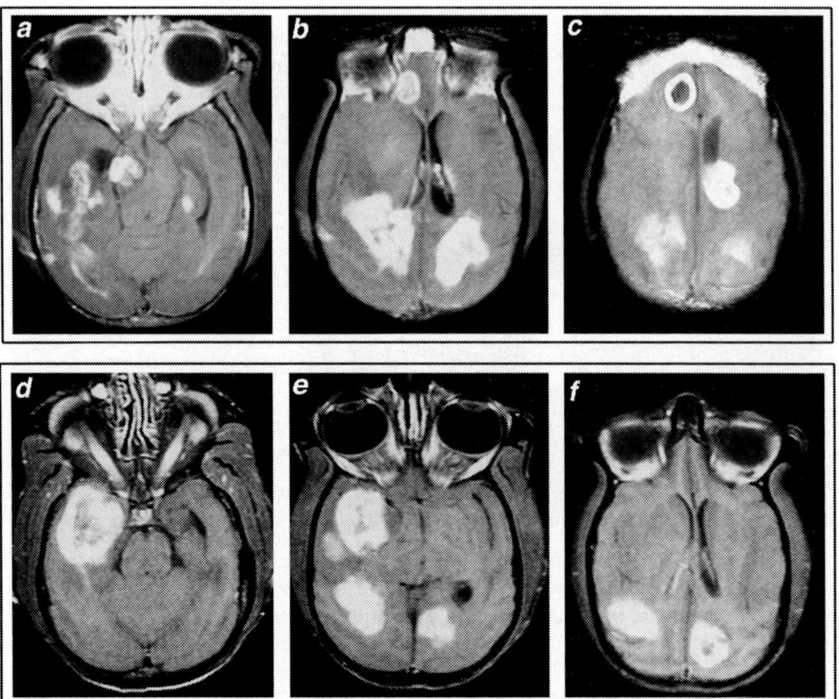

FIG. 21.2 The majority of animals (67%) with radiation-induced GBM had multifocal disease. (*a–c*) Axial postcontrast T_1-weighted MR images of animal 5 (see *Table 21.1*) 4.4 years after irradiation. Multifocal contrast-enhancing lesions were located in the brain stem (*a*) and cerebral hemispheres bilaterally (*b* and *c*) and were confirmed at autopsy to be GBM. (*d–f*) Axial postcontrast T_1-weighted MR images of animal 2 (see *Table 21.1*) 3.4 years after irradiation. Multifocal contrast-enhancing lesions (*d–f*) were seen in the cerebral hemispheres bilaterally and were confirmed at autopsy to be GBM. [Reprinted with permission from Lonser RR, Walbridge S, Vortmeyer AO, et al.: Glioblastoma multiforme formation after primate irradiation in the therapeutic dose range. **J Neurosurg** 97:1378–1389, 2002.]

Histologic Analysis

Histologic analysis of all contrast-enhancing lesions on MR images was consistent with GBM (nine animals, 18 enhancing lesions). Diagnosis of GBM was based on characteristic histologic findings (29), including marked hypercellularity, cellular pleomorphism, neovascularity, mitoses, and pseudopallisading necrosis (*Figs. 21.1, 21.3, 21.6, and 21.7*). Histologic analysis of the regions surrounding the tumor revealed extensive "finger-like" invasion of the immediately adjacent tissues (*Fig. 21.6*) and diffuse, noncontiguous distal spread of tumor cells

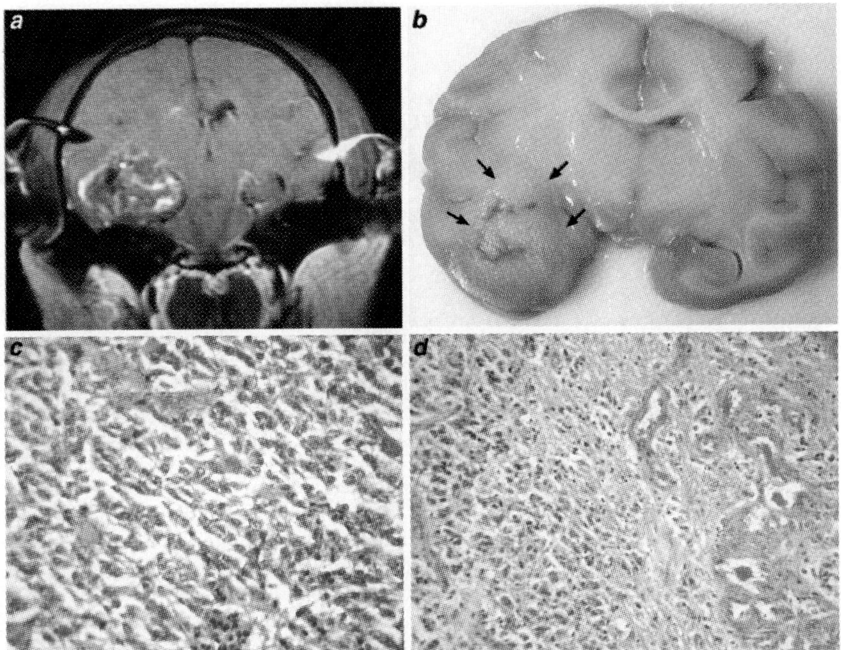

FIG. 21.3 (*a*) Coronal T_1-weighted postcontrast MR image shows a large, enhancing lesion in the left temporal region of animal 3 (see *Table 21.1*) 3.8 years after irradiation. (*b*) Corresponding coronal whole-brain section through the same region shows gross tumor (arrows). Before imaging, the animal had developed progressive right arm weakness. The animal was euthanized on the day of imaging, and histology revealed the lesion to be GBM. (*c* and *d*) Hematoxylin and eosin–stained sections through the left temporal region of MR-enhancing tumor reveal histologic features consistent with GBM, including marked endothelial proliferation (*c*) with areas of pseudopallisading and necrosis (*d*). [Reprinted with permission from Lonser RR, Walbridge S, Vortmeyer AO, et al.: Glioblastoma multiforme formation after primate irradiation in the therapeutic dose range. **J Neurosurg** 97:1378–1389, 2002.]

preferentially within the white matter (*Fig. 21.7*). Distant tumor cells were found well beyond regions that showed evidence of tumor on MR images (either T_1-weighted postcontrast or T_2-weighted studies) or that could be seen on gross examination (*Figs. 21.6 and 21.7*). Histologic analysis of nontumorous tissues revealed no evidence of radiation necrosis or other irradiation-induced brain injury. The neoplastic cells in sites of solid GBM (nine tumors in six animals) stained uniformly positive for glial fibrillary acidic protein in three tumors, had scattered sites of positive staining in four tumors, and were negative in two tumors (*Fig. 21.8*).

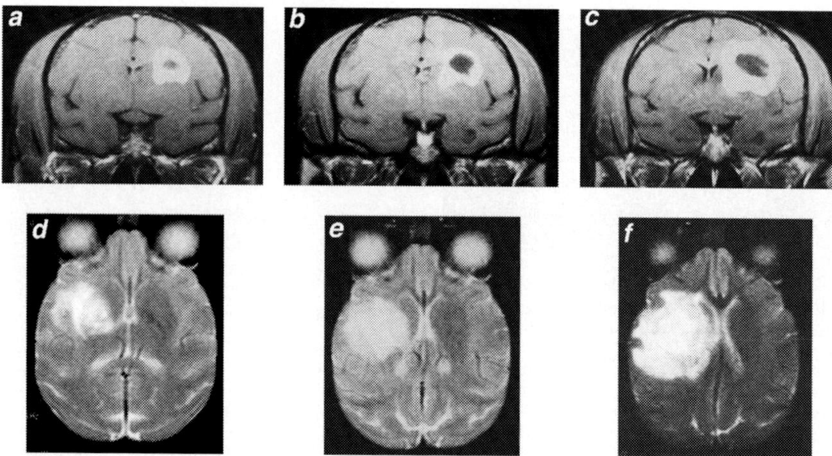

FIG. 21.4 Coronal T_1-wieghted, contrast-enhanced MR images show the rapid progression of GBM in a nonhuman primate 7.4 years after irradiation (animal 7) (see *Table 21.1*). There was rapid growth of the ring-enhancing lesion from 2 mo before sacrifice (*a*) to 1 mo before sacrifice (*b*) and 1 day before sacrifice (*c*). Axial T_2-weighted, non–contrast enhanced MR images show progression of peritumoral edema 2 months prior to sacrifice (*d*), 1 month prior to sacrifice (*e*), and 1 day prior to sacrifice (*f*). The animal exhibited progressive weakness of the left extremities over the 2 mo before euthanization. [Reprinted with permission from Lonser RR, Walbridge S, Vortmeyer AO, et al.: Glioblastoma multiforme formation after primate irradiation in the therapeutic dose range. **J Neurosurg** 97:1378–1389, 2002.]

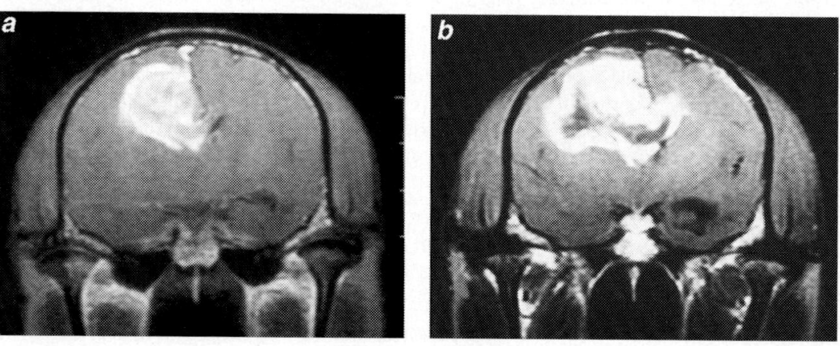

FIG. 21.5 (*a*) Coronal T_1-weighted postcontrast MR image shows enhancing tumor in the left frontoparietal region 1 month before sacrifice and 7.9 years after irradiation (animal 8) (see *Table 21.1*). (*b*) Coronal T_1-weighted postcontrast MR image shows expansion of left frontoparietal enhancing tumor through the corpus callosum and into the right frontoparietal region on the day of sacrifice. The animal experienced progressive weakness of the right extremities in the 1-mo interval between these images. [Reprinted with permission from Lonser RR, Walbridge S, Vortmeyer AO, et al.: Glioblastoma multiforme formation after primate irradiation in the therapeutic dose range. **J Neurosurg** 97:1378–1389, 2002.

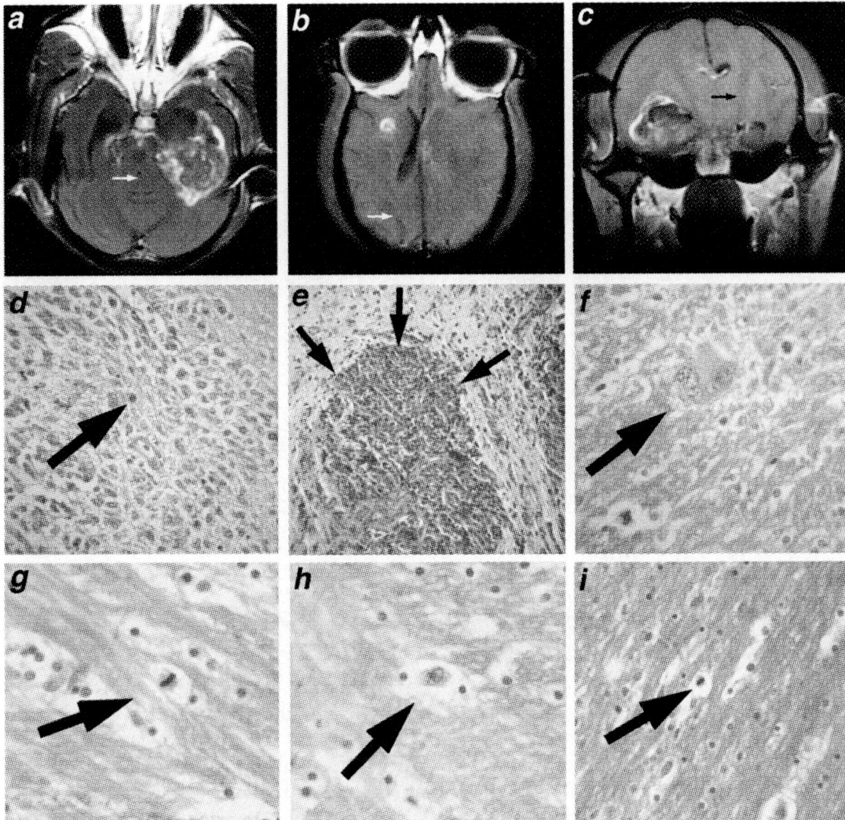

FIG. 21.6 Magnetic resonance images and corresponding histologic sections demonstrate the extent of tumor spread and variable cellular morphology that occurred in the tumor foci of animal 3 (3.8 years after irradiation) (see *Table 21.1*). Postcontrast, T_1-weighted axial (*a* and *b*) and coronal (*c*) MR images through various regions of the cerebrum in this animal are shown. Postcontrast imaging revealed two enhancing lesions. The larger of the two enhancing lesions was located in the left temporal region (*a* and *c*); the smaller lesion was located in the right frontal region (*b*). Hematoxylin and eosin–stained sections from the brain stem and supratentorial regions (*d–i*). Neoplastic cells (arrow in *d*) not evident on contrast-enhanced (*a–c*) or T_2-weighted (not shown) MR images were found directly posterior to the cerebral aqueduct (corresponding to white arrow in *a*). Tumor cells from the left temporal MR-enhancing region (*a* and *c*) had predominantly small cell morphology with finger-like invasion (arrows in *e*) into the immediately adjacent white matter. In contrast, tumor cells from the MR-enhancing right frontal lesion (*b*) had predominantly giant cell morphology (arrow in *f*). Hematoxylin and eosin–stained sections from various regions revealed diffuse, noncontiguous tumor cell invasion along white matter tracts distant to MR imaging evidence of neoplasia (arrows in *g–i*). Neoplastic cells were found in the fibers of the (*g*) corpus callosum, (*h*) internal capsule (corresponding to black arrow in *c*), and (*i*) occipital regions (corresponding to white arrow in *b*). [Reprinted with permission from Lonser RR, Walbridge S, Vortmeyer AO, et al.: Glioblastoma multiforme formation after primate irradiation in the therapeutic dose range. **J Neurosurg** 97:1378–1389, 2002.]

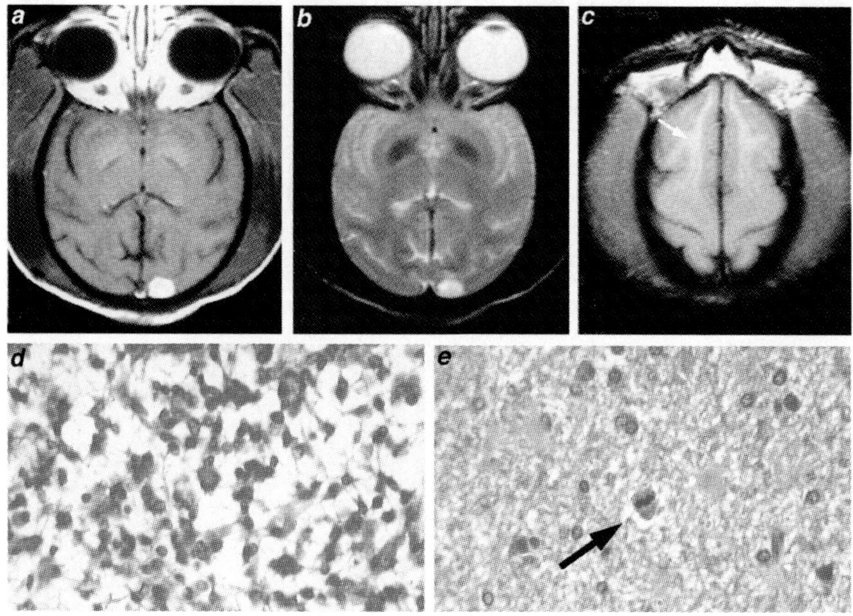

FIG. 21.7 Magnetic resonance images and corresponding histologic sections demonstrate the extent of tumor invasion in animal 4 (4.3 years after irradiation). Both T_1-weighted postcontrast (*a* and *c*) and T_2-weighted (*b*) axial MR images through supratentorial region are shown. Imaging revealed only one enhancing lesion (*a*), which was located in the left occipital region and had minimal surrounding edema (*b*). Hematoxylin and eosin–stained sections of MR-enhancing tumor (*a*) revealed pleomorphic neoplastic cells with glial differentiation (*d*). Noncontiguous neoplastic cells (arrow in *e*) with surrounding reactive astrocytes (pale pink cytoplasm) were found as distant as the right frontal region (corresponding to the white arrow in *c*) within white matter tracts. [Reprinted with permission from Lonser RR, Walbridge S, Vortmeyer AO, et al.: Glioblastoma multiforme formation after primate irradiation in the therapeutic dose range. **J Neurosurg** 97:1378–1389, 2002.]

Comparative Genomic Hybridization

To ascertain what chromosomal differences exist between the radiation-induced tumors and normal tissue as well as how these differences correspond within the human genome, we analyzed primate normal brain and tumor tissues using an interspecies CGH technique ($n = 3$). Successful hybridization was performed in three tumors studied from three separate animals (animals 7–9) (*Table 21.1 and Fig. 21.9*).

Numerous and variable chromosome and chromosomal region alterations were detected in all three tumors. *Figure 21.9* demonstrates the extensive chromosomal losses and gains that occurred in the various tumors. Loss of part or all of corresponding human chromosome

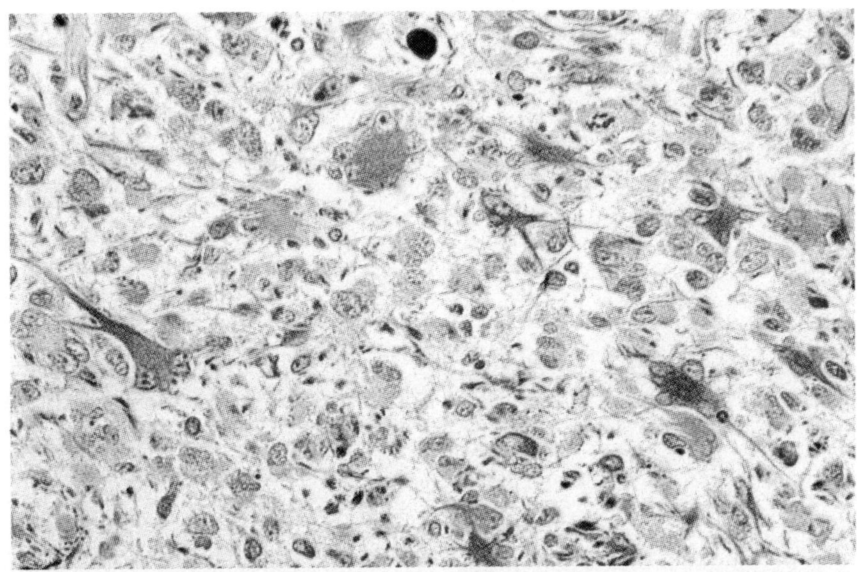

FIG. 21.8 Glial fibrillary acidic protein (GFAP) immunohistochemistry was performed on nine tumors from six separate animals. Three tumors were uniformly positive of GFAP, four showed scattered positive cells, and two were negative. Shown here is positive GFAP staining of tumor cells from animal 2. Original magnification ×40. [Reprinted with permission from Lonser RR, Walbridge S, Vortmeyer AO, et al.: Glioblastoma multiforme formation after primate irradiation in the therapeutic dose range. **J Neurosurg** 97:1378–1389, 2002.]

9 occurred in all tumors (*Fig. 21.10*). Deletions of the chromosomal regions corresponding to human chromosomes 17p (p53 gene), 5q31 (epidermal growth response factor, interleukin-5, and interleukin-6 genes), as well as 14 and 15 (both present in Robertsonian fusion as chromosome 7 in monkey) were found in two of three tumors (*Fig. 21.10*). Gains of the chromosomal regions corresponding to the human chromosome 8q (c-*myc* oncogene) were detected in two of three tumors (*Fig. 21.10*).

DISCUSSION

Current Study

CLINICAL FINDINGS

The initial purpose of this study was to determine the effects of whole-brain radiation, with and without barbiturate radioprotection during radiation treatment, in a primate model. Later in the study,

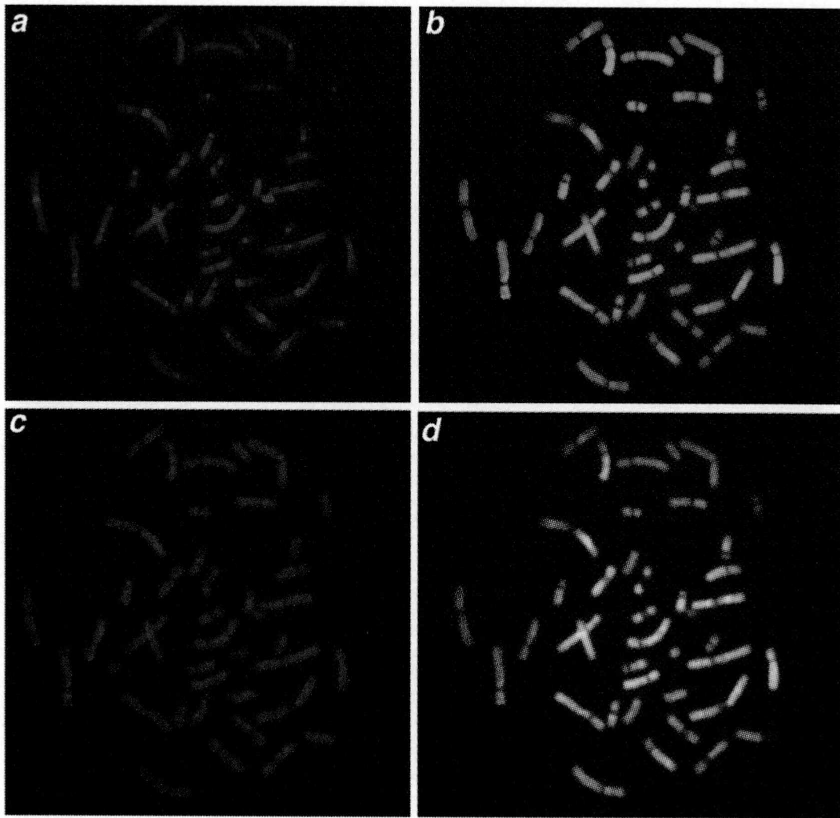

FIG. 21.9 Using CGH techniques, nonhuman primate (*Macaca mulatta*) DNA from a radiation-induced GBM (green fluorescence) and normal monkey brain tissue (red fluorescence) was successfully hybridized to corresponding human chromosomes. Shown is the hybridization pattern of the tumor from animal 7 (see *Table 21.1*). (*a*) 4,6-Diamidino-2-phenylindole image of the normal human metaphase spread used as the hybridization template. (*b*) Hybridization of the animal's tumor DNA (fluorescein isothiocyanate image). (*c*) The animal's normal reference DNA (rhodamine image) on the normal human metaphase spread. (*d*) The three fluorochrome colors merged. [Reprinted with permission from Lonser RR, Walbridge S, Vortmeyer AO, et al.: Glioblastoma multiforme formation after primate irradiation in the therapeutic dose range. **J Neurosurg** 97:1378–1389, 2002.]

when it became evident that there were no apparent clinical or laboratory differences between animal groups (barbiturate vs control) with this dosing scheme of radiation therapy and animals began developing GBMs, the goal of this study became analyzing the occurrence, distribution, and nature of radiation-induced tumors.

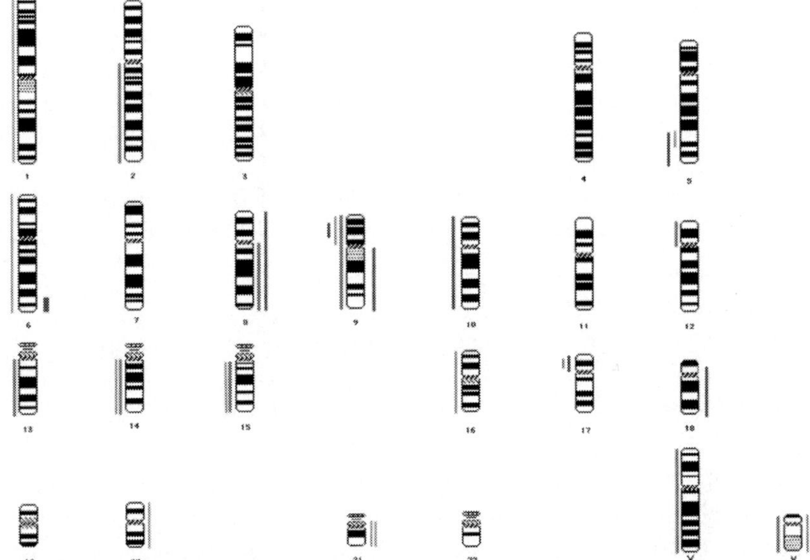

FIG. 21.10 Summary of the genetic changes detected in the three GBMs from the three nonhuman primates (animals 7–9) (see *Table 21.1*) by interspecies CGH projected to the homologous human chromosomes. The extent and specific chromosomal alterations are demonstrated by colored lines next to the affected chromosome. Lines to the left of the chromosomes represent chromosomal or chromosome region losses. Lines to the right of the chromosomes represent chromosomal or chromosome region gains. Specifically, the green line represents genomic alterations in the tumor of animal 7, the red lines alterations in tumor from animal 8, and the blue lines alteration in tumor from animal 9 (see *Table 21.1*). [Reprinted with permission from Lonser RR, Walbridge S, Vortmeyer AO, et al.: Glioblastoma multiforme formation after primate irradiation in the therapeutic dose range. **J Neurosurg** 97:1378–1389, 2002.]

All the animals tolerated the fractionated radiation treatments and were able to complete the course of therapy as described (total radiation dose, 3,500 cGy in 10 fractions over 2 weeks). One animal died from a pulmonary abscess and sepsis 2.5 years after irradiation, leaving 11 animals available for long-term evaluation and comparative analysis. None of the remaining 11 animals had apparent adverse reactions to radiation until 2.9 years after the completion of irradiation, when one animal developed neurologic symptoms and MR imaging depicted contrast-enhancing lesions that were pathologically confirmed to be GBM. After that point in time, an additional eight animals (nine total animals, or 82%; latency, 3.4–8.3 years in these animals) developed contrast-enhancing lesions as depicted on MR images (with and without neurologic symptoms) that at autopsy were confirmed to be GBMs. The remaining two animals that did not develop GBMs were sacrificed at the completion of the study (10 years after irradiation). These animals and the animal that died early during the study from abscess and sepsis (2.5 years after irradiation) had no imaging, gross, or microscopic evidence of CNS disease.

In the nine animals (82%) that developed GBMs, the criteria for being a radiation-induced tumor were met. These criteria (7, 46) include:

1. The tumor was not present before irradiation.
2. The tumor appears in an irradiated area.
3. A latent period must elapse between irradiation and appearance of the tumor.
4. The existence of the radiation-induced tumor must be histologically proven.

Preoperative MR imaging was performed in all animals and revealed no evidence of tumors before irradiation. All tumors appeared within the radiated area after a 2.9- to 8.3-year latency period. All tumors that developed were histologically confirmed to be GBM. Moreover, the large percent of the primates in this series that developed radiation-induced GBMs is especially striking when you consider that the incidence of spontaneous CNS malignancies in large primate autopsy series is extremely low (0–0.004%) (16, 27, 36).

IMAGING AND GROSS ANATOMIC FINDINGS

The MR imaging and gross anatomic findings in the animals that developed GBMs in this series give several powerful insights regarding the nature of radiation-induced tumors. First, MR imaging and gross tissue examination revealed that the majority of animals with GBMs had multifocal lesions (67%). This is similar to the findings in a small series of three patients by Fontana et al. (17), which suggested that perhaps a higher rate of multifocal lesions are seen with radiation-induced gliomas compared to those that occur spontaneously (~20% in human GBMs [44]). Second, the anatomic distribution of the radio-induced GBMs in our series was also unique. Typically, spontaneously occurring GBMs arise in the frontoparietal regions, but in this series, two animals (22%) developed GBMs in the cerebellum, which rarely occurs spontaneously in humans (*Table 21.1*). This distribution of GBMs appears to correspond with the volume of cerebral tissue that is irradiated (supratentorial vs infratentorial). Third, the serial MR imaging used to detect the tumor early and to follow GBM growth in two animals confirmed the aggressive nature of these tumors and showed rapid expansion of the tumors and surrounding edema over a short interval of time (*Figs. 21.4 and 21.5*). These imaging findings coincided with the rapid development and progression of neurologic symptoms that prompted euthanization 1 and 2 mo after the tumor was discovered. Finally, in all nine animals with GBMs, the presence of tumor was confirmed or discovered on MR images (either after neurologic symptoms developed or incidentally on serial imaging). Review of the MR images immediately before (mean, 10.8 mo before) the initial detection of tumor on imaging revealed no evidence of tumor, which suggests that these tumors were de novo GBMs, because it seems unlikely that they evolved from lower-grade astrocytomas, which would theoretically take longer (years) to develop and, subsequently, would be discovered on earlier imaging procedures.

HISTOLOGICAL FINDINGS

The histologic findings in the animals with radiation-induced GBMs reveal several critical insights regarding the nature of, and what might be necessary for successful treatment of, these and spontaneously occurring GBMs. First, neoplastic cells were found far beyond the region(s) of tumor presence predicted by MR imaging (either T_1-weighted contrast enhancement or T_2-weighted hyperintensity) (*Figs. 21.6* and *21.7*). This confirms that MR imaging, at least its current stage of development, cannot demonstrate the entire extent of tumor spread and that diffuse neoplastic infiltration has already occurred by the time that MR imaging detects tumor (*Fig. 21.7*). Second, the widespread distribution of microscopic tumor coupled with the frequent multifocality seen on MR images of these tumors suggest either that these tumors arise from a single cell clone that subsequently disseminates throughout the cerebrum or that these neoplasms arise from multiple cells in different regions of the CNS. The contemporaneous development of multifocal tumors, the frequent occurrence of similarly sized individual foci in multifocal tumors (*Fig. 21.2*), and the widespread distribution of neoplastic cells in multifocal and unifocal GBMs, combined with previous studies showing that motility is directly proportional to tumor grade (10, 11, 18), suggest that these neoplasms can arise from a single high-grade clone that disseminated rapidly throughout the brain. Third, the noncontiguous spread of neoplastic cells within the white matter might make some regional therapeutic strategies ineffective (*Figs. 21.6 and 21.7*). Specifically, because tumor-targeted gene therapy depends on distribution of a therapeutic gene by a replicating virus requires cell-to-cell contact of the tumor cells, the presence of noncontiguous neoplastic cells would render these therapies noncurative. Fourth, the preferential invasion of white matter by tumor cells confirms previous findings that these anatomic regions or environment provide a route for rapid spread of these cells (31, 44, 52). The preferential spread of neoplastic cells in these regions, however, may provide an ideal situation for certain regional therapies (52). Specifically, the increased hydraulic conductivity found in fibers of passage provide an excellent anatomic situation to use interstitial bulk flow delivery methods for widespread distribution of putative therapeutic agents (4, 34). Previous data have shown that white matter tracts provide the ideal mechanical properties to safely, reliably, and homogeneously distribute small and large molecules over large volumes using convection-enhanced delivery techniques (33).

COMPARATIVE GENOMIC HYBRIDIZATION

A powerful cytogenetic technique, CGH has been used to successfully determine genetic differences between normal and tumorous tissue in humans (24). Because of the interspecies homology between humans and nonhuman primates, we were able to apply novel CGH methods (S. Pack et al., submitted) to detect and localize chromosomal alterations in these primate radiation-induced tumors and to establish the corresponding human genomic differences. The large number of chromosomal losses and gains seen in these tumors reveals the mutagenic potential of radiation therapy, but the single difference common to all the tumors analyzed was genetic loss corresponding to human chromosome 9 (*Fig. 21.10*). Similar losses of chromosome 9 are found in de novo gliomas in humans (45), which support the theory that these radiation-induced GBMs are molecularly similar to spontaneously occurring GBMs in humans.

Previously, Olopade et al. (38) found molecular evidence of deletion in 9p in 10 of 15 glioma-derived cell lines and in 13 of 35 primary gliomas. The shortest region of overlap of these deletions mapped to the interval between the centromeric end of the interferon gene cluster and the methylthioadenosine phosphorylase locus. Bigner et al. (3) found chromosome abnormalities in 12 of 54 malignant gliomas. Structural abnormalities of 9p and 19q were increased to a statistically significant degree, but they concluded that the most frequent chromosomal changes in malignant gliomas are gains of chromosome 7 and losses of chromosome 10. Chromosome 10 was also implicated in GBMs by Fujimoto et al. (19), who found loss of constitutional heterozygosity in tumor samples from 10 of 13 patients in whom paired tumor and lymphocyte DNA samples were screened. Only one of three primate GBMs had loss of the chromosome corresponding to human chromosome 10.

Of special interest is the result of the interstitial 5q31 deletions in two of three tumors. This region was found to be deleted in patients with a secondary leukemia acquired after a therapeutic radiation treatment for other cancers, suggesting the presence of a radiation-sensitive region containing important tumor-suppressor genes (T. Knutsen et al., submitted). Acquired interstitial deletions of 5q have been found in a variety of secondary myeloid disorders, but no single critical gene has been identified as the sole underlying cause of these pathologic changes. Thus, it is possible that several genes may act as tumor suppressors in such cases. Among the candidates genes from the commonly deleted region are interleukin genes, interferon response factor I, colony-stimulating factor I receptor, and epidermal growth response factor (5).

Previous Reports of Glioblastoma Multiforme after Irradiation

ANIMAL STUDIES

Kent and Pickering (28) reported the first instance of GBM formation in a nonhuman primate (one animal) after whole-head irradiation (thermal neutron) in 1958. Since then, the development of brain tumors and other malignancies after irradiation in primates has primarily been observed in animals that underwent whole-body irradiation. Dalrymple et al. (14) and others (30, 51, 54) reported on a large series of rhesus monkeys that were treated with whole-body surface irradiation using nonfractionated schedules and lower doses (ionizing energies that would simulate the space radiation spectrum) than were used in this study. The animals were followed over an extended period of time (up to 24 years). Nine of 71 animals (12%) exposed to 55-MeV proton radiation (total dose range, 400–800 cGy) developed GBMs, with latent periods of 13 mo to 20 years. Likewise, Haymaker et al. (20) found that 3 of 10 rhesus monkeys that received 55-MeV proton, single-dose, whole-body surface irradiation (total dose range, 600–800 cGy) developed GBMs 3 to 5 years after treatment.

Previous reports by Caveness and his colleagues (8, 35, 53) on primates (*M. mulatta*) that received fractionated whole-brain radiation in the therapeutic dose range and were studied routinely at autopsy revealed some of the delayed effects of radiation in the primate, which correlate closely with observations in humans. They found dose-dependent pathologic responses in normal primate brains subjected to fractionated exposure of 200 cGy/day for total doses of 4,000, 6,000, and 8,000 cGy. Animals exposed to a total dose of 4,000 cGy had no adverse clinical effects and negligible pathologic findings. Animals exposed to a total dose of 6,000 cGy had evidence of increased intracranial pressure (papilledema) and widely scattered necrotic lesions evident as early as 26 weeks. Animals in the highest-exposure group

(8,000 cGy) also developed papilledema and had profound histologic changes in the radiated region, which included extensive focal and coalescing necrosis with significant brain destruction starting 26 weeks after irradiation. None of the animals reported in this series developed tumors.

The proportion of primates developing GBMs (82%) in our study is much higher than in previous animal studies, whether they received whole-body, single-dose exposure (12–30% of animals [7, 54]) or underwent fractionated whole-brain irradiation (0% [8, 35, 53]). One likely reason for the lower percentage of animals developing GBMs after radiation in whole-body, single-dose irradiated animals is that a direct relationship exists between total dose of radiation and tumor formation. Animals in those studies were irradiated with considerably lower total doses of radiation (total dose range, 400–800 cGy) compared to the current study (total dose, 3,500 cGy). The difference in tumor-induction rate in this series, compared to the Caveness series of fractionated, whole-brain irradiated animals is probably related to length of follow-up. All animals were sacrificed 2 years or less after radiation therapy in the Caveness series. The first animal in the present series developed a GBM 2.9 years after radiation.

HUMAN REPORTS

A number of sporadic reports in the literature implicate radiation in the induction of high-grade glial CNS tumors in humans (6, 13, 17, 23, 26, 32, 42, 43, 47–49, 55, 56). In 1990, Cavin et al. (9) summarized 56 previously published cases and added their institution's four cases of CNS tumor induction after radiotherapy. They found that patients who underwent cranial radiation for acute lymphoblastic leukemia (ALL; mean dose, 2,389 cGy), CNS neoplasms (4,544 cGy), or benign disease (313 cGy) were at a significantly higher risk (relative risk 125 in ALL group) for developing intra-axial brain tumors. These radiation-induced tumors were identified as GBMs (73%), astrocytomas (22%), ependymomas (3%), or other (2%). The mean latency to tumor induction for the ALL, CNS neoplasm, and benign disease irradiation groups was 7.5, 11.0, and 9.9 years, respectively.

The rate of GBM formation in this series of primates is much higher than would be expected after reviewing human irradiation literature. Several factors may underlie this difference. First, there might exist an interspecies variation in which nonhuman primates are more susceptible to the tumor-inductive effects of radiation. Second, it is possible that these animals were infected with known oncogenic viruses endemic to the nonhuman primate population, such as simian virus 40 (associated with simian immunodeficiency virus–infected monkeys) or JC virus (12, 22). A subsequent infection by these viruses could predispose the study primates to developing gliomas. This seems unlikely to be the predisposing cause of tumor development in this study, however, because none of the animals had serology positive for the simian immunodeficiency virus or was immunocompromised. Third, animals in this study underwent whole-brain irradiation, which may have a higher incidence of tumor development because of the larger volume of tissue that is irradiated compared to more focused irradiation therapies such as stereotactic radiosurgery. Recently, radiation-induced malignant cranial tumors have been reported after stereotactic radiosurgery (23, 30,55), suggesting that despite the reduction of the radiation-exposed tissue, it remains a potential complication of this form of radiation therapy. The induction of tumors after stereotactic radiosurgery could be the result of either malignant progression of a lower-grade tumor or de novo tumor formation in the rim of irradiated tissue at the tumor margin. Fourth, because of the long latency to tumor formation, many patients with poor-grade CNS neoplasms undergoing irradiation die before developing radiation-induced neoplasms. Alternatively, as the number of young patients who are irradiated for benign cranial tumors (i.e., vestibular schwannomas, meningiomas) and other disease processes (i.e., Parkinson's disease, seizures, trigeminal neuralgia, intractable pain) increases, there will be a large enough cohort with prolonged follow-up (≥10 years) to get a better estimate regarding the true incidence of radiation-induced tumors in humans (including those undergoing stereotactic radiosurgery). Fifth, patients undergoing radiation for glial neoplasms that later develop a higher-grade tumor in the irradiated field may be occasionally misclassified as having a recurrence rather than a radio-induced tumor. In any case, our findings and an increasing number of published clinical reports suggest that induction of neoplasms, particularly high-grade tumors, should be considered a possible long-term complication of therapeutic irradiation and that patients should be monitored for tumor induction over long latency periods.

Potential Mechanisms of Radiation-Induced Tumorigenesis

The mutagenic effects of radiation in these animals seem to be the most plausible explanation for the development of these tumors. Recently, Holland et al. (21) discovered evidence that genetic alterations of pluripotent stem cells, not differentiated glial cells, may be the underlying precursor in GBM formation. They induced GBM formation in mice after tissue-specific transfer of activated tumorigenic genes into neuroprogenitor cells but were unable to do so in terminally differentiated astrocytes. The development of GBMs in our monkeys may result from radiation-induced genetic alterations or the radiation-induced impairment of DNA repair mechanisms within a CNS neuroprogenitor cell(s) that trigger the transformation and subsequent development of the cells into neoplasms.

The hypothesis of a neuroprogenitor precursor is intriguing, because it could explain some of findings in the present and previous studies and provide direction for further investigation. First, naturally occurring neuroprogenitor cell populations are found in nonhuman primates and humans in amounts inversely proportional to age (41). This age-related relationship may explain why these relatively young animals (3 years of age at the time of radiation, which correlates to roughly a 9- to 13-year-old human) developed GBMs with such frequency and why children undergoing low-dose scalp irradiation (for tinea capitis) have a statistically significant increase in glioma formation later in life (43). Second, the rapid and widespread distribution of implanted neural stem cells is similar to that of infiltrative glioma cells (1, 2, 15). Thus, increased understanding of the mechanisms involved in the migration of neuroprogenitor cells could result in a better understanding of glioma cell infiltration, and vice versa. Third, if neuroprogenitor cells are the precursor cells in gliomagenesis, then irradiation of these cellular populations with an appropriate dosing scheme could provide a means for developing a reliable lower-animal model of high-grade invasive glioma formation.

CONCLUSIONS

We found that a high percentage (82%) of animals developed radiation-induced GBMs in the late delayed period after irradiation (latency, 2.9–8.3 years), suggesting that induction of high-grade glial neoplasms in irradiated primate CNS tissue may not be an infrequent late complication of this therapy. The clinical, serial MR imaging, histologic, and molecular analyses in these primates give unique insights regarding the nature and development of GBMs.

REFERENCES

1. Aboody KS, Brown A, Rainov NG, et al.: From the cover: Neural stem cells display extensive tropism for pathology in adult brain: evidence from intracranial gliomas. **Proc Natl Acad Sci U S A** 97:12846–12851, 2000.
2. Benedetti S, Pirola B, Pollo B, et al.: Gene therapy of experimental brain tumors using neural progenitor cells. **Nat Med** 6:447–450, 2000.
3. Bigner SH, Mark J, Burger PC, et al.: Specific chromosomal abnormalities in malignant human gliomas. **Cancer Res** 48:405–411, 1988.
4. Bobo RH, Laske DW, Akbasak A, et al.: Convection-enhanced delivery of macromolecules in the brain. **Proc Natl Acad Sci U S A** 91:2076–2080, 1994.

5. Boultwood J, Fidler C, Lewis S, et al.: Allelic loss of IRF1 in myelodysplasia and acute myeloid leukemia: Retention of IRF1 on the 5q-chromosome in some patients with the 5q-syndrome. **Blood** 82:2611–2616, 1993.
6. Brat DJ, James CD, Jedlicka AE, et al.: Molecular genetic alterations in radiation-induced astrocytomas. **Am J Pathol** 154:1431–1438, 1999.
7. Cahan WG, Woodard HQ, Higinbotham NL, et al.: Sarcoma arising in irradiated bone. **Cancer** 1:3–29, 1978.
8. Caveness WF: Pathology of radiation damage to the normal brain of the monkey. **Natl Cancer Inst Monogr** 46:57–76, 1977.
9. Cavin LW, Dalrymple GV, McGuire EL, et al.: CNS tumor induction by radiotherapy: A report of four new cases and estimate of dose required. **Int J Radiat Oncol Biol Phys** 18:399–406, 1990.
10. Chicoine MR, Silbergeld DL: Assessment of brain tumor cell motility in vivo and in vitro. **J Neurosurg** 82:615–622, 1995.
11. Chicoine MR, Silbergeld DL: The in vitro motility of human gliomas increases with increasing grade of malignancy. **Cancer** 75:2904–2909, 1995.
12. Chretien F, Boche D, Lorin de la Grandmaison G, et al.: Progressive multifocal leukoencephalopathy and oligodendroglioma in a monkey coinfected by simian immunodeficiency virus and simian virus 40. **Acta Neuropathol (Berl)** 100:332–336, 2000.
13. Chung CK, Stryker JA, Cruse R, et al.: Glioblastoma multiforme following prophylactic cranial irradiation and intrathecal methotrexate in a child with acute lymphocytic leukemia. **Cancer** 47:2563–2566, 1981.
14. Dalrymple GV, Nagle WA, Moss AJ, et al.: The protons of space and brain tumors: I. Clinical and dosimetric considerations. In Restor AC (ed): *AIP Conference Proceedings.* New York: American Institute of Physics, 1989, pp 407–411.
15. Dirks PB: Glioma migration: Clues from the biology of neural progenitor cells and embryonic CNS cell migration. **J Neurooncol** 53:203–212, 2001.
16. Fairbrother RW, Hurst EW: Spontaneous diseases observed in 600 monkeys. **J Path Bact** 35:867–873, 1932.
17. Fontana M, Stanton C, Pompili A, et al.: Late multifocal gliomas in adolescents previously treated for acute lymphoblastic leukemia. **Cancer** 60:1510–1518, 1987.
18. Friedlander DR, Zagzag D, Shiff B, et al.: Migration of brain tumor cells on extracellular matrix proteins in vitro correlates with tumor type and grade and involves αV and β1 integrins. **Cancer Res** 56:1939–1947, 1996.
19. Fujimoto M, Fults DW, Thomas GA, et al.: Loss of heterozygosity on chromosome 10 in human glioblastoma multiforme. **Genomics** 4:210–214, 1989.
20. Haymaker W, Rubinstein LJ, Miquel J: Brain tumors in irradiated monkeys. **Acta Neuropath (Berl)** 20:267–277, 1972.
21. Holland EC, Celestino J, Dai C, et al.: Combined activation of Ras and Akt in neural progenitors induces glioblastoma formation in mice. **Nat Genet** 25:55–57, 2000.
22. Hurley JP, Ilyinskii PO, Horvath CJ, et al.: A malignant astrocytoma containing simian virus 40 DNA in a macaque infected with simian immunodeficiency virus. **J Med Primatol** 26:172–180, 1997.
23. Kaido T, Hoshida T, Uranishi R, et al.: Radiosurgery-induced brain tumor. **J Neurosurg** 95:710–713, 2001.
24. Kallioniemi A, Kallioniemi O-P, Sudar D, et al.: Comparative genomic hybridization for molecular cytogenetic analysis of solid tumors. **Science** 258:818–821, 1992.
25. Karim ABMF: Radiation therapy and radiosurgery for brain tumors. In Kaye AH, Laws ER (eds): *Brain Tumors.* Edinburgh: Churchill Livingstone, 1995, pp 331–348.

26. Kaschten B, Flandroy P, Reznik M, et al.: Radiation-induced gliosarcoma: Case report and review of the literature. **J Neurosurg** 83:154–162, 1995.
27. Kennard MA: Abnormal findings in 246 consecutive autopsies on monkeys. **Yale J Biol Med** 13:701–712, 1941.
28. Kent SP, Pickering JE: Neoplasms in monkeys (*Macaca mulatta*): Spontaneous and irradiation induced. **Cancer** 11:138–147, 1958.
29. Kleihues P, Cavenee WK: *Pathology and Genetics of Tumors of the Nervous System*. Lyon: IARC Press, 2000.
30. Krupp JH: Nine-year mortality experience in proton-exposed *Macaca mulatta*. **Radiat Res** 67:244–251, 1976.
31. Laws ER Jr, Goldberg WJ, Bernstein JJ: Migration of human malignant astrocytoma cells in the mammalian brain: Scherer revisited. **Int J Dev Neurosci** 11:691–697, 1993.
32. Liwnicz BH, Berger TS, Liwnicz RG, et al.: Radiation-associated gliomas: A report of four cases and analysis of postradiation tumors of the central nervous system. **Neurosurgery** 17:436–445, 1985.
33. Lonser RR, Gogate N, Morrison PF, et al.: Direct convective delivery of macromolecules to the spinal cord. **J Neurosurg** 89:616–622, 1998.
34. Morrison PF, Laske DW, Bobo H, et al.: High-flow microinfusion: Tissue penetration and pharmacodynamics. **Am J Physiol** 266:R292–R305, 1994.
35. Nakagaki H, Brunhart G, Kemper TL, et al.: Monkey brain damage from radiation in the therapeutic range. **J Neurosurg** 44:3–11, 1976.
36. O'Connor GT: Cancer—A general review. **Primates in Medicine** 3:9–22, 1969.
37. Oldfield EH, Friedman R, Kinsella T, et al.: Pentobarbital and lidocaine reduce brain injury by ionizing radiation. **J Neurosurg** 72:737–744, 1990.
38. Olopade OI, Jenkins RB, Ransom DT, et al.: Molecular analysis of deletions of the short arm of chromosome 9 in human gliomas. **Cancer Res** 52:2523–2529, 1992.
39. Olson JJ, Friedman R, Orr K, et al.: Enhancement of the efficacy of x-irradiation by pentobarbital in a rodent brain tumor model. **J Neurosurg** 72:745–748, 1990.
40. Olson JJ, Shelley C, Orr K, et al.: The cerebral radioprotective effect of alternative barbiturates to pentobarbital. **Neurosurgery** 30:720–723, 1992.
41. Palmer TD, Schwartz PH, Taupin P, et al.: Progenitor cells from human brain after death. **Nature** 411:42–43, 2001.
42. Rimm IJ, Li FC, Tarbell NJ, et al.: Brain tumors after cranial radiation for childhood acute lymphoblastic leukemia: A 13-year experience from the Dana-Farber Cancer Institute and the Children's Hospital. **Cancer** 59:1506–1508, 1987.
43. Ron E, Modan B, Boice JD, et al.: Tumors of the brain and nervous system after radiotherapy in childhood. **N Engl J Med** 319:1033–1039, 1988.
44. Scherer HJ: The forms of growth in gliomas and their practical significance. **Brain** 63:1–35, 1940.
45. Schlegel J, Scherthan H, Arens N, et al.: Detection of complex genetic alterations in human glioblastoma multiforme using comparative genomic hybridization. **J Neuropathol Exp Neurol** 55:81–87, 1996.
46. Schrantz JL, Araoz CA: Radiation induced meningeal fibrosarcoma. **Arch Pathol** 93:26–31, 1972.
47. Shamisa A, Bance M, Nag S, et al.: Glioblastoma multiforme occurring in a patient treated with gamma knife surgery. Case report and review of the literature. **J Neurosurg** 94:816–821, 2001.
48. Simmons NE, Laws ER: Glioma occurrence after sellar irradiation: Case report and review. **Neurosurgery** 42:172–178, 1998.
49. Soffer D, Gomori JM, Pomeranz S, et al.: Gliomas following low-dose irradiation to the head report of three cases. **J Neurooncol** 8:67–72, 1990.

50. Thomsen J, Mirz F, Wetke R, et al.: Intracranial sarcoma in a patient with neurofibromatosis type 2 treated with gamma knife radiosurgery for vestibular schwannoma. **Am J Otol** 21:364–370, 2000.
51. Traynor JE, Casey HW: Five-year follow-up of primates exposed to 55 MeV protons. **Radiat Res** 47:143–148, 1971.
52. Tysnes BB, Mahesparan R: Biological mechanisms of glioma invasion and potential therapeutic targets. **J Neurooncol** 53:129–147, 2001.
53. Wakisaka S, O-Neill RR, Kemper TL, et al.: Delayed brain damage in adult monkeys from radiation in the therapeutic range. **Radiat Res** 80:277–291, 1979.
54. Wood DH: Long-term mortality and cancer risk in irradiated rhesus monkeys. **Radiat Res** 126:132–140, 1991.
55. Yu JS, Yong WH, Wilson D, et al.: Glioblastoma induction after radiosurgery for meningioma. **Lancet** 356:1576–1577, 2000.
56. Zuccarello M, Sawaya R, deCourten-Meyers G: Glioblastoma occurring after radiation therapy for meningioma: case report and review of literature. **Neurosurgery** 19:114–119, 1986.

CHAPTER

22

Synthes Award for Resident Research in Brain and Craniofacial Injury: Poloxamer 188 Volumetrically Decreases Neuron Loss in the Rat Model of Excitotoxicity in a Time-Dependent Manner

DANIEL J. CURRY, M.D., DAVID A. WRIGHT, Ph.D., RAFAEL C. LEE, M.D., UN J. KANG, M.D., Ph.D., AND DAVID M. FRIM, M.D., Ph.D.

INTRODUCTION

Excitotoxicity is a cellular process that has been associated with neuron death in central nervous system trauma, ischemia, and neurodegeneration. It is thought to be the process in which the neuron is overly stimulated by excitatory amino acids, causing a cascade of cellular reactions that include liberation of intracellular calcium, creation of reactive oxygen species, lipid peroxidation, and cell death from disruption of the cell's plasma membrane. Although the process is not entirely understood, the cascade of excitotoxicity has been interrupted in both in vitro and in vivo models. Despite many studies elucidating the intricate details of this mechanism, there have been no successful clinical trials of inhibitors of this process.

Excitotoxicity, depending upon the nature and intensity of the insult, can result in either apoptotic or necrotic cell death. Previous laboratory interventions have focused upon inhibiting various steps in the process, such as interference with the glutamate–*N*-methyl-D-aspartate (NMDA) receptor interaction, calcium concentration, and oxygen radical formation. Few studies have focused on repair of the plasma membrane. This study explores the utility of membrane repair with the surfactant, Poloxamer 188 (P-188), in the amelioration of excitotoxicity in the striatum of the rat.

A synthetic surfactant, P-188 is a multiblock copolymer. A P-188 molecule is composed of two blocks (38 moieties each) of hydrophilic polyoxyethylene flanking one block (29 moieties) of hydrophobic polyoxypropylene. It has a molecular weight of 8.4 kDa and, being 80% hydrophilic, is water soluble. Despite its large size, it has been known to cross the blood–brain barrier when injected into the peritoneum of the rat (9). It is excreted by the kidney unmetabolized (11).

There have been many proposed and attempted uses of poloxamers. Intravenous poloxamer has been shown to enhance drug delivery of antimycobacterials (14), antiparasitics (23, 24), and chemotherapeutics in multidrug-resistant cancer cells (5). They have been shown to reduce tissue injury in the rabbit model of frostbite (16, 32) and to protect against myocardial infarction in angioplasty (26). Poloxamer 188 has been shown to increase blood flow in the rabbit after ligation of the middle cerebral artery (10). It also reduces sludging in extracorporeal oxygenators (4). In excitable tissues, intravenous P-188 has been shown to reduce neurologic injury in a dog model of hypothermic circulatory arrest (22) and to reduce inflammation and seal electropermeabilized muscle tissue (17).

Poloxamer 188 is an amphiphilic copolymer that self-aggregates in an aqueous medium and has the ability to intercalate into the plasma membrane when in contact with living cells. The intercalation capacity of this surfactant has been found to seal the membranes of experimentally electroporated tissue (17) to seal membranes in in vitro models of excitotoxicity (18). We have previously obtained preliminary data that indicated P-188 reduces the lesion size and inflammation in an in vivo model of excitotoxicity in the rat striatum (Frim and Curry, unpublished results). This study attempts to confirm these preliminary results and begin to examine the clinical utility of poloxamer therapy by investigating the optimal timing of this intervention.

Materials and Methods

Twenty-eight Sprague-Dawley rats underwent stereotactic lesioning of the right striatum under ketamine cocktail anesthesia (ketamine, xylazine, acepromazine, and saline). A Kopf stereotactic frame was used to calculate the striatal target coordinates from the bregma as AP 1.6, L −2.5, and V −4.5 from dura. A 1-min infusion of 120 nmol of quinolinic acid in a 1-μL volume was performed through a Hamilton syringe, and the animal subsequently received 50 μL of either P-188 or vehicle (artificial cerebrospinal fluid [CSF]) by direct infusion into the CSF at the cisterna magna injection. Four groups of animals were studied: Group 1 ($n = 11$) served as a control, with injection of the vehicle only. Group 2 ($n = 5$) received P-188 ten minutes after surgery, while group 3 ($n = 5$) received P-188 four hours after surgery. Group 4 ($n = 7$) received surfactant injection at both points. Poloxamer dose was determined by the maximal achievable concentration of the surfactant and the maximal volume that could be safely delivered intracisternally. The animals were sacrificed 7 days after surgery under deep anesthesia and cardiac perfusion with PBS followed by 4% paraformaldehyde. Animal brains were postfixed in 4% paraformaldehyde for 12 hours and allowed to equilibrate in 30% sucrose for sectioning. Tissues were cut in section (thickness, 40 μm), and every sixth section was stained immunocytochemically for neurons with Neu-N, an antibody to a rat neuronal nucleus marker.

The brain sections that contained the lesions were digitally photographed at 10× magnification. The lesion perimeter was then drawn for each section, and the area was calculated with the Metamorph Image Analyzer. Using the areas of the lesions on each section and their known thickness, the volumes of the lesions were then calculated. The respective groups were then compared to the control group using ANOVA.

RESULTS

Animals that received P-188 at the early injection time were shown to have smaller lesion volumes (average volume, 8.16 ± 6.12 mm^3) than controls (average volume, 18.25 ± 11.42 mm^3) (*Figs. 22.1 and 22.2*). The animals that received both the early and the late injection

Lesion Volumes (mm3)

Control (n=11)	Early P-188 (n=5)	Late P-188 (n=5)	Early and Late P-188 (n=7)
18.25 +/- 11.42	8.16 +/- 6.12	14.86 +/- 7.95	10.57 +/- 9.00
ANOVA	Significant P=0.0015	Not Significant	Significant P=.0095

FIG. 22.1 Poloxamer 188 significantly reduced excitotoxic lesion volume in rats treated 10 minutes after injury (Early) and in rats treated 10 minutes and 4 hours after injury (Early and Late). Intrathecal Poloxamer failed to significantly reduce excitotoxic lesion volume if given 4 hours after injury (Late).

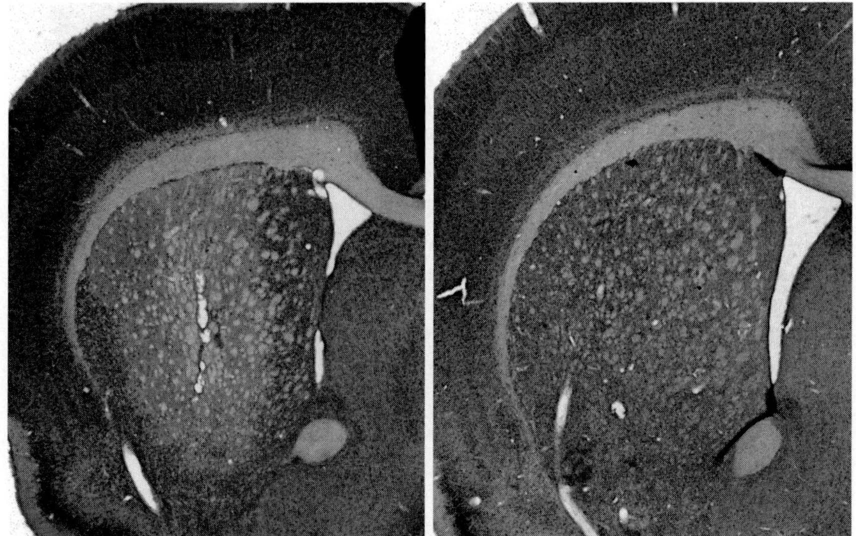

FIG. 22.2 Intrastriatal, quinolinic acid–induced excitotoxic lesions in the rat treated with intrathecal vehicle (*left*) and Poloxamer 188 (*right*) 10 minutes after injury.

of surfactant were also shown to have smaller lesion volumes (average volume, 10.57 ± 9.00 mm^3) than controls. The differences in lesion size when comparing controls to the early injected animals and to the early and late injected animals reached statistical significance (P = 0.0015 and 0.0095, respectively). The animals that received only the late injection of P-188 were shown to have smaller lesion volumes (average volume, 14.86 ± 7.95 mm^3) than controls, but this comparison failed to reach statistical significance.

DISCUSSION

Neuronal death is the permanent result of many neurologic disease processes, whether they are degenerative, traumatic or ischemic in nature. In situations of acute cell stress, glutamate, and glutamate-receptor agonists such as quinolinic acid (an NMDA-receptor agonist) may be toxic to the energy-depleted neuron and can serve as a model for traumatic, ischemic or degenerative cell death (25, 31). Regardless of the etiology, excitotoxicity is a multistep process that includes persistent depolarization of cell membrane, energy depletion from repolarization of the cell, deregulation of intracellular calcium, formation of reactive oxygen species, lipid peroxidation, rupture of cell membrane, loss of cellular ionic gradients, and nuclear DNA fragmentation. Many interventions have been attempted to interrupt this cascade, from receptor blockade, calcium antagonists, and antioxidants, with little efficacy in the treatment of trauma, stroke, or neurodegeneration. This is possibly because these are late interventions to an early element of the cascade of cell death. An intervention focused upon later stages of the cascade could be more effective. The restoration of membrane integrity is a potentially powerful technique in the treatment of disease processes involving neuronal death (7). Such a therapy could have significant impact on the current management of traumatic neurologic injury and stroke.

Although it has been the tradition to characterize neuron death in binomial terms of either necrotic or apoptotic, it has been recently revealed that both forms of neuron death can coexist in both in vivo and in vitro models (19). The acute cell swelling seen in excitotoxicity associated with necrotic cell death is sodium dependent and has an onset of minutes to hours (8). Defects in membrane permeability and depletion of high-energy phosphates are known to be causal in necrosis (12). In contrast, apoptosis is characterized by little inflammatory infiltration, and the mitochondria remain intact until late in the process (19). Where any one neuron's death falls on this necrosis–apoptosis continuum depend to some degree on the etiology of the fatal insult. Ischemic insults in the adult brain tend to create necrosis, whereas target deprivation and neurodegeneration tends to create apoptosis (19). The maturity of the tissue also influences the cell death pathway, with neonate brains exhibiting apoptosis from a wide variety of insults (29, 30). Lastly, the subtype of glutamate receptor also influences the mechanism of cell death, with non-NMDA receptors tending to induce apoptosis and NMDA receptors tending to induce necrosis (19). Our NMDA receptor agonist–induced lesion would therefore be expected to exhibit more necrotic cell death than apoptotic cell death.

Excitotoxicity is known to have a variable time course, depending on the nature of the insult. More intense excitotoxic lesions tend produce necrosis, and the greater the intensity of the insult, the more rapid the progression of neuronal injury. This phenomenon is termed *maturation phenomenon* (15). Most studies of in vivo excitotoxicity show necrosis occurring within 24 hours (13, 20, 27, 29, 30). In in vitro studies, necrotic cell death has been detected 1 to 3 hours after excitotoxic insult (3, 6). The time course of cell death by apoptosis does not vary drastically from that of necrosis, with the exception of a delay in onset that depends upon tissue type and experimental conditions. In in vivo models, cell death by apoptosis occurs over 24 hours (2, 29, 30) but can be delayed up to 7 days in some models (2). In vitro models of apoptosis show progression to cell death over 1 to 2 days, with the majority if the changes occurring over 6 to 18 hours, depending upon the severity of the insult (28). Our experiment analyzed the resultant excitotoxic damage after 7 days, far beyond the time at which the features of apoptosis and necrosis are distinct. The different intervention times, however, allow the detection of an effect of the poloxamer on either the early necrotic or the later apoptotic stages of excitotoxicity.

Our data show that poloxamer was more effective if given early, before 4 hours, after lesioning. This is consistent with the conclusion that surfactant therapy is more effective against necrosis than apoptosis. This is in agreement with in vitro data showing that poloxamers decrease excitotoxic cell death by interfering with the membrane rupture of necrosis and, to a much lesser degree, decreasing cell death in apoptosis (18). This is also in agreement with the time course of the necrotic phase of excitoxicity of up to 3 hours (8). It disagrees, however, with the results of the in vitro study that showed neuroprotective effect of poloxamer 188, even if given 8 hours after insult. The in vitro result implies that poloxamer intervention in excitotoxicity could have some effect on apoptosis not readily detectable in this in vivo model.

This study shows that P-188 can reduce neuron loss from excitotoxicity if given within 4 hours of injury. Poloxamer has already been approved for human use with minimal side effects (RheothRx) (1, 21). If given intrathecally, bleeding complications can be avoided. More subtle untoward effects of poloxamer are possible with continued infusion. Surfactants intercalate into the cell membrane and, therefore, affect the membrane fluidity. This can remedy situations of pathological membrane fluidity, but in high doses, it can rigidify the membrane and reduce the ability of membrane-bound receptors to modulate their shape in the lipid matrix. This process is known as molecular freezing (9) and is thought to be the pathophysiology of diabetes and atherosclerosis. Poloxamer 188 could be a direct treatment for traumatic or excitotoxic brain injury and could be delivered, either intraoperatively or via ventriculostomy, safely and easily.

REFERENCES

1. Adams-Graves P, Kedar A, et al.: RheothRx (poloxamer 188) injection for the acute painful episode of sickle cell disease: A pilot study. **Blood** 90(5):2041–2046, 1997.
2. Al-Abdulla NA, Portera-Cailliau C, et al. Occipital cortex ablation in the adult rat causes retrograde neuronal death in the lateral geniculate. **Neuroscience** 86(1):191–209, 1998.
3. Ankarcrona M, Dypbukt JM, et al. Glutamate-induced neuron death: A succession of necrosis or apoptosis depending on mitochondrial function. **Neuron** 15:961–973, 1995.

4. Armstrong JK, Meiselman HJ, et al. Inhibition of red blood cell-induced platelet aggregation in whole blood by a nonionic surfactant, poloxamer 188 (RheothRx injection). **Thromb Res** 79(5–6):437–450, 1995.
5. Batrakova EV, Lee S, et al. Fundamental relationship between the composition of pluronic block polymers and their hypersensitization effect in MDR cancer cells. **Pharmacol Res** 16:1317–1379, 1999.
6. Bonofoco E, Krainc D, et al.: Apoptosis and necrosis: Two distinct events induced, respectively, by mild and intense insults with *N*-methyl-D-aspartate or nitric oxide/superoxide in cortical cell cultures. **Proc Natl Acad Sci U S A** 92:7162–7166, 1995.
7. Borgens RB: Cellular engineering molecular repair of membranes to rescue cells of the damaged nervous system. **Neurosurgery** 49(2):370–378, 2001.
8. Choi DW: Ionic dependence of glutamate neurotoxicity. **J Neurosci** 7(2):369–379, 1987.
9. Clarke MSF, Prendergast MA, et al.: Plasma membrane ordering agent pluronic F-68 (PF-68) reduces neurotransmitter uptake and release and produces learning and memory deficits in rats. **Learning and Memory** 6:634–649, 1999.
10. Colbassani HJ, Barrow DL, et al.: Modification of acute focal ischemia in rabbits by poloxamer 188. **Stroke** 20(9):1241–1246, 1989.
11. Corporation BW: *Pluronic Polyols: Toxicity and Irritation Studies and Data.* Wyandotte, MI: Central Research and Development, 1975.
12. Farber JL, Chien KR, et al. Myocardial ischemia: The pathogenesis of irreversible cell injury in ischemia. **Am J Pathol** 102(2):271–281, 1981.
13. Ferrer I, Martin F, et al. Both apoptosis and necrosis occur following intrastriatal administration of excitotoxin. **Acta Neuropathol** 90:504–510, 1995.
14. Hunter RL, Jagannath C, et al. Enhancement of antibiotic susceptibility and suppression of *Mycobacterium avium* complex growth by poloxamer 331. **Antimicrob Agents Chemother** 39(2):435–439, 1995.
15. Ito U, Spatz M, et al. Experimental cerebral ischemia in mongolian gerbils. I. Light microscopic observations. **Acta Neuropathol** 32:209–223, 1975.
16. Knize DM, Weatherley-White RCA, et al. Use of antisludging agents in experimental cold injuries. **Surg Gynecol Obstet** 129:1019–1026, 1969.
17. Lee RC, River LP, et al.: Surfactant-induced sealing of electropermeabilized skeletal muscle membranes in vivo. **Proc Natl Acad Sci U S A** 89(10):4524–4528, 1992.
18. Marks JD, Pan CY, et al. Amphiphilic, triblock copolymers provide potent, membrane-targeted neuroprotection. **FASEB J** 15(6):1107–1109, 2001.
19. Martin LJ, Al-Abdulla NA, et al.: Neurodegeneration in excitotoxicity, global cerebral ischemia, and target deprivation: A perspective on the contributions of apoptosis. **Brain Res Bull** 4:281–309, 1998.
20. Martin LJ, Brambrink AM, et al.: Hypoxia-ischemia causes abnormalities in glutamate transporters and death of astroglia and neurons in newborn striatum. **Ann Neurol** 42:335–48, 1997.
21. Maynard C, Swenson R, et al.: Randomized, controlled trial of RheothRx (poloxamer 188) in patients with suspected acute myocardial infarction. RheothRx in Myocardial Infarction Study Group. **Am Heart J** 135(5 Pt 1):797–804, 1998.
22. Mezrow CK, Mazzoni M, et al.: Poloxamer 188 improves neurologic outcome after hypothermic circulatory arrest. **J Thorac Cardiovasc Surg** 103(6):1143–1146, 1992.
23. Moghimi SM, Hunter AC: Poloxamers and poloxamines in nanoparticle engineering and experimental medicine. **Trends Biotechnol** 18:412–420, 2000.

24. Moghimi SM, Murray C: Poloxamer 188 revisited: A potentially valuable immune modulator? **J Natl Cancer Inst** 88(11):766–768, 1996.
25. Novelli A, Reilly JA, et al.: Glutamate becomes neurotoxic via the *N*-methyl-D-aspartate receptor when intracellular energy levels are reduced. **Brain Res** 451:205–212, 1988.
26. O'Keefe JH, Grines CL, et al.: Poloxamer-188 as an adjunct to primary percutaneous transluminal coronary angioplasty for acute myocardial infarction. **Am J Cardiol** 78(7):747–750, 1996.
27. Petito CK, Pulsinelli WA: Sequential development if reversible and irreversible neuronal damage following cerebral ischemia. **J Neuropathol Exp Neurol** 43:141–153, 1984.
28. Pittman RN, Wang S, et al.: A system for characterizing cellular and molecular events in programmed neuronal death. **J Neurosci** 13:3669–3680, 1993.
29. Portera-Cailliau C, Price DL, et al.: Excitotoxic neuronal death in the immature brain is an apoptosis-necrosis morphological continuum. **J Comp Neurol** 378:70–87, 1997.
30. Portera-Cailliau C, Price DL, et al.: Non-NMDA and NMDA receptor mediated excitotoxic neuronal deaths in adult brain are morphologically distinct: Further evidence for a apoptosis-necrosis continuum. **J Comp Neurol** 378:88–104, 1997.
31. Uhler TA, Frim DM, et al.: The effects of megadose methylprednisolone and U-78517F on toxicity mediated by glutamate receptors in the rat neostriatum. **Neurosurgery** 34(1):122–128, 1995.
32. Weatherley-White RCA, Knize DM, et al.: Experimental studies in cold injury. **Surgery** 66:208–214, 1969.

CHAPTER

23

Ronald Tasker Award: A Novel Model of Neuroma Pain

MICHAEL J. DORSI, B.A., LUN CHEN, M.D., RICHARD A. MEYER, M.S., ESTHER POGATZKI, Ph.D., AND ALLAN J. BELZBERG, M.D., F.R.C.S.C.

INTRODUCTION

Peripheral nerve injury may lead to the formation of a painful neuroma. Patients present with symptoms and signs of neuropathic pain, including tenderness to palpation of the skin overlying the neuroma, spontaneous burning pain, and allodynia and hyperalgesia in the distribution of the injured nerve.

The structural and electrophysiological changes that characterize a neuroma have been well described (3). Microscopic examination of the neuroma reveals a loss of normal fascicular organization and an increase in connective tissue. The nerve fibers trapped in the neuroma develop aberrant activity, such as spontaneous activity, cross-talk, and hypersensitivity to mechanical, chemical, and metabolic stimuli.

Several animal models have been developed to study pain following nerve injury (1, 2, 3, 4, 6). In general, such models involve interruption of a peripheral or spinal nerve by transaction, ligation, or crush. Pain is measured by quantifying the behavioral responses evoked by applying mechanical or thermal stimuli to the distribution of the injured nerve. These behavioral models do not involve direct mechanical stimulation of the neuroma.

Although current animal models of nerve injury pain have succeeded in producing a reliable behavioral change, several lines of evidence question their validity as models of human painful neuroma. For example, the hyperalgesia following spinal nerve ligation and cut can develop and persist independent of input from the neuroma (5). Furthermore, the same behavioral change (i.e., mechanical hyperalgesia) can be produced following lesions that do not lead to the formation of a neuroma, such as dorsal root ganglionectomy (7). Finally, the behavioral responses characteristic of the current models are evoked by applying stimuli at a site that is distant from the neuroma. Currently, no model measures the behavioral effect of directly applying stimuli to the neuroma.

The aim of the present investigation was to design a new model of neuroma pain. An ideal model would involve the formation of a neuroma that demonstrated the characteristic pathological and electrophysiological changes. In addition, such a model would produce consistent, severe, and lasting behavioral changes that modeled those seen in human patients following nerve injury (i.e., pain evoked by palpation of the skin overlying the neuroma).

METHODS

Male Sprague-Dawley rats were used in the study. Following habituation and baseline testing, the animals were randomly divided into four surgical groups.

Group 1 (*Fig. 23.1*) represents the neuroma model group. To produce a neuroma, the posterior tibial nerve of the rat was exposed in the region of the division into lateral and medial plantar branches, tightly ligated with silk suture just proximal to the branching, and transected. To allow for easy application of mechanical stimuli as well as to avoid the confounding hyperalgesia observed in the distribution of the injured nerve, the ligated nerve stump was tunneled subcutaneously across the anterior aspect of the leg to a position just superior to the lateral malleolus. This placed the neuroma well outside of the innervation territory of the tibial nerve.

Three control groups were included to account for various aspects of the surgical manipulation. To control for the subcutaneous passage of the posterior tibial nerve, surgery was performed as described above for group 2, but following tunneling, the nerve was ligated and transected a second time at the entrance to the subcutaneous tunnel. This led to formation of a neuroma at the entrance of the tunnel as opposed to the lateral aspect of the leg. To control for the effect of ligating and cutting the tibial nerve and forming a subcutaneous tunnel, animals in group 3 underwent posterior tibial nerve ligation and transection, but the nerve stump was left in place. A small piece of connective tissue was dissected, ligated, and passed through the subcutaneous tunnel. Finally, to control for exposure of the posterior tibial nerve and tunnel formation, animals in group 4 had the posterior tibial nerve dissected free but left intact. Again, connective tissue was passed through the subcutaneous tunnel as described above for group 3.

Behavioral testing was performed in a blinded fashion, with the different surgical groups being tested concurrently. The suture tied around the rotated nerve or connective tissue was visualized through the skin and served as the target for application of mechanical stimuli. An analogous site served as the target on the contralateral

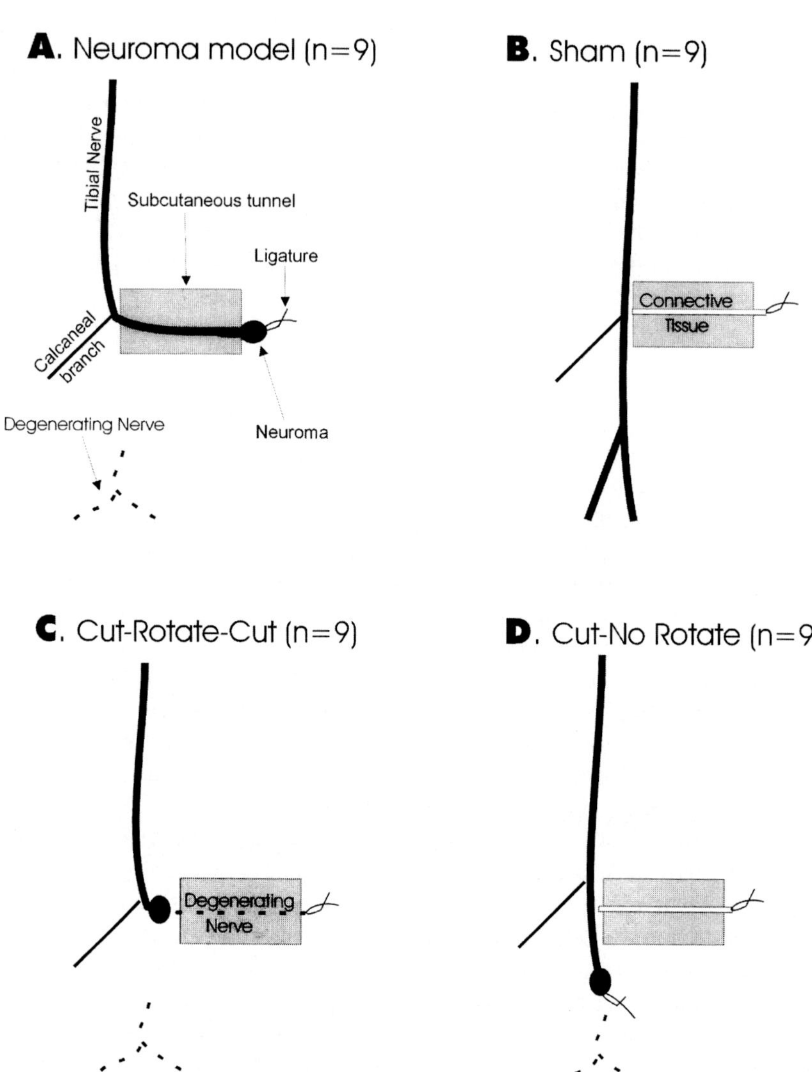

FIG. 23.1 Schematic representation of the experimental groups. For all experimental groups, the left tibial nerve was dissected free in the medial aspect of the hindlimb. A subcutaneous tunnel was formed, passing from medial incision anteriorly across the ankle to just above the lateral malleolus. (*A*) The neuroma-model operation involved ligation and transection of the tibial nerve. The distal end of the tibial nerve was passed through the subcutaneous tunnel (n = 9). (*B*) The sham operation involved dissection of the tibial nerve, but the nerve was left intact. Adjacent connective tissue was ligated, transected, and passed through the subcutaneous tunnel (n = 9). (*C*) The cut-rotate-cut group underwent the same procedure as described for the neuroma-model group, but once the tibial nerve was passed through the tunnel, it was transected proximally at the entrance to the tunnel (n = 9). (*D*) In the cut–no rotate group, the tibial nerve was ligated and transected as described above but was then left in place. Adjacent connective tissue was ligated, cut, and passed through the tunnel as described above for the sham group (n = 9).

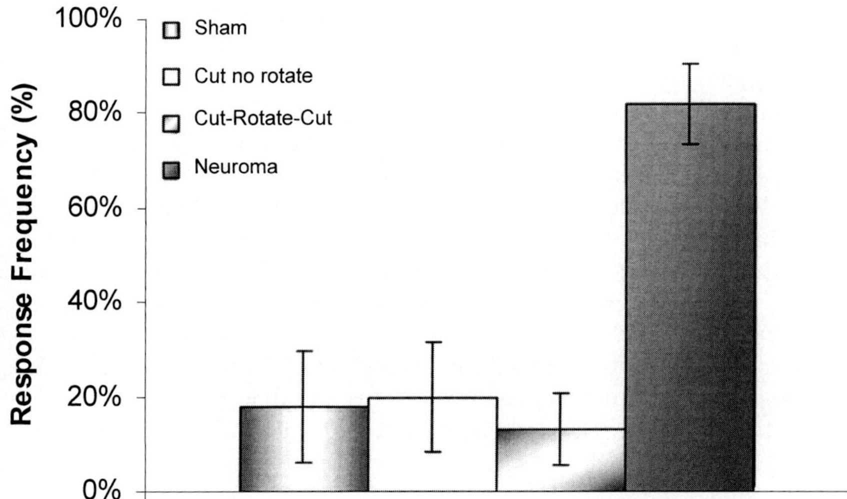

FIG. 23.2 Behavior response to mechanical stimulation. Paw withdrawal response frequency to the application of a 150-mN von Frey hair on Postoperative Day 87 is plotted for the four experimental groups. The response frequency was significantly lower for the three control groups compared to the neuroma-model group. There was no difference among control groups. $P < 0.001$, Student's t-test.

hindlimb. Von Frey filaments (150 and 250 mN) were applied to the target test site for 2 sec. A positive response was defined as a rapid withdrawal of the hindpaw or a slow withdrawal with licking or shaking of the hindpaw. The frequency of response to five applications of the von Frey probe was determined. Testing began 3 days postoperatively and continued for 3 mo.

At the conclusion of the behavioral testing, several animals were selected for electrophysiological and histological evaluation. Teased fiber techniques were used to record from single A fibers and C fibers in the tibial nerve of the anesthetized rat. Mechanical stimuli were applied to the skin overlaying the neuroma. The nerve fibers were assessed for spontaneous activity, mechanical sensitivity, and electrical coupling. For histological evaluation, the tibial nerve was harvested.

RESULTS AND DISCUSSION

Application of the von Frey probe to the test site near the lateral malleous led to behavioral signs of pain only for animals in the neuroma-model group. A significant increase in the behavioral response frequency was initially evident on Postoperative Day 3 and persisted throughout the duration of the study (94 days). In contrast, none of the three control groups exhibited a significant change in behavioral response frequency, either with respect to baseline or each other. The response frequency of the neuroma-model group was significantly increased compared to that of all control groups (*Fig. 23.2*). There was no change in behavior response frequency for any of the groups following application of stimuli to the contralateral paw.

Von Frey stimulation of the neuroma led to an evoked response in some A fiber and C fiber afferents. Some A fiber and C fiber afferents also exhibited spontaneous activity. Coupling between nerve fibers was also observed, suggesting the possibility of backward regeneration of fibers from the neuroma.

Microscopic examination of the sections cut through the neuromas demonstrated findings typical for a neuroma: disordered distribution of myelinated fibers, multiple fibers cut longitudinally, and dense connective tissue.

CONCLUSIONS

We have developed a novel animal model of neuroma pain. Unique to this model is the ability to study behavior in response to stimulation applied to the neuroma as opposed to an anatomic region supplied by injured nerve.

REFERENCES

1. Bennett GJ, Xie Y-K: A peripheral mononeuropathy in rat that produces disorders of pain sensation like those seen in man. **Pain** 33:87–107, 1988.
2. Decosterd I, Woolf CJ: Spared nerve injury: an animal model of persistent peripheral neuropathic pain. **Pain** 87:149–158, 2000.
3. Devor M, Seltzer Z: Pathophysiology of damaged nerves in relation to chronic pain. In Wall PD, Melzak R (eds): *Textbook of Pain,* 4th ed. Edinburgh: Churchill Livingstone, 1999, pp 129–164.
4. Kim SH, Chung JM: An experimental model for peripheral neuropathy produced by segmental spinal nerve ligation in the rat. **Pain** 50:355–363, 1992.
5. Li Y, Dorsi MJ, Meyer RA, Belzberg AJ: Mechanical hyperalgesia after an L5 spinal nerve lesion in the rat is not dependent on input from injured nerve fibers. **Pain** 85:493–502, 2000.
6. Seltzer Z, Dubner R, Shir Y: A novel behavioral model of neuropathic pain disorders produced in rats by partial sciatic nerve injury. **Pain** 43:205–218, 1990.
7. Sheth RN, Dorsi MJ, Li Y, et al.: Mechanical hyperalgesia after an L5 ventral rhizotomy or an L5 ganglionectomy in the rat. **Pain** 96:63–72, 2002.

CHAPTER

24

CSNS Resident Award: The Economics of Trigeminal Neuralgia Surgery

ROBERT D. ECKER, M.D., AND BRUCE E. POLLOCK, M.D.

INTRODUCTION

Trigeminal neuralgia (tic touloureux) is the most common facial pain syndrome. Although Arateus, in the first century AD, is credited with a depiction of facial pain consistent with trigeminal neuralgia, John Locke, in 1677, was the first physician to describe the condition (18). Based on population studies from Olmsted County, the incidence rate of trigeminal neuralgia is 4.3 per 100,000 per year, translating into 15,000 new patients each year in the United States (19, 35). The incidence of trigeminal neuralgia increases with age, and women are more commonly affected. Focal demyelination secondary to vascular compression at the trigeminal root entry zone, where the central oligodendroglia meets the peripheral Schwann cells, is believed to be the etiology in the majority of patients (11, 16). The demyelinated nerve fibers become hyperexcitable, and innocuous stimuli can lead to ephaptic transmission between pain fibers and paroxysms of facial pain. Mass lesions, such as tumors and aneurysms, along with more widespread demyelinating disorders, such as multiple sclerosis, cause trigeminal neuralgia in a minority of patients (10, 14, 15).

Medical therapy with drugs like carbamazepine and phenytoin is considered to be the initial treatment and can eliminate or reduce symptoms in as many as 75% of patients (13). However, medication side effects and tachyphylaxis occur. More than 50% of newly diagnosed patients eventually undergo surgical treatment (18). Microvascular decompression (MVD) (4, 6, 9), radiofrequency rhizotomy (17, 32), glycerol rhizotomy (25, 30), balloon compression (7, 31), and stereotactic radiosurgery (SR) (5, 20, 23, 26, 28) are all currently used operations for intractable trigeminal neuralgia. Only MVD directly addresses the vascular compression on the nerve; all other surgical treatments rely on damage to the trigeminal nerve to relieve pain. Facial numbness is traded for pain relief. In our practice, MVD is advised as the best treatment for a medically fit patient. Stereotactic radiosurgery and the percutaneous procedures are reserved for patients who are elderly, suffer from significant medical comorbidities, have recurrent pain after previous MVD, or do not choose to undergo open surgery.

Approximately 7,700 patients undergo surgical treatment of trigeminal neuralgia in the United States each year at an estimated cost of \$100 million (1, 2) (*Fig. 24.1*). Although accounting for only a small fraction of the \$1.4 trillion annually spent on health care in the United States, surgical treatment of trigeminal neuralgia provides a uniquely clear model of a surgical cost-effectiveness analysis. The outcome is well defined: The patient is pain free (either on or off medication) or has continued pain. The latency to effect of treatment is short; radiosurgery is the longest, at 6 weeks. The procedures have detailed historical benchmarks for success and complications. Finally, the unique aspect of the American health care system, in which patient choice can trump cost and treatment efficacy, is reflected in the care of trigeminal neuralgia. A healthy, 40-year-old woman may choose to have SR over MVD despite a greater chance for failure and need for further treatment. With these issues in mind, we undertook a cost-effective-

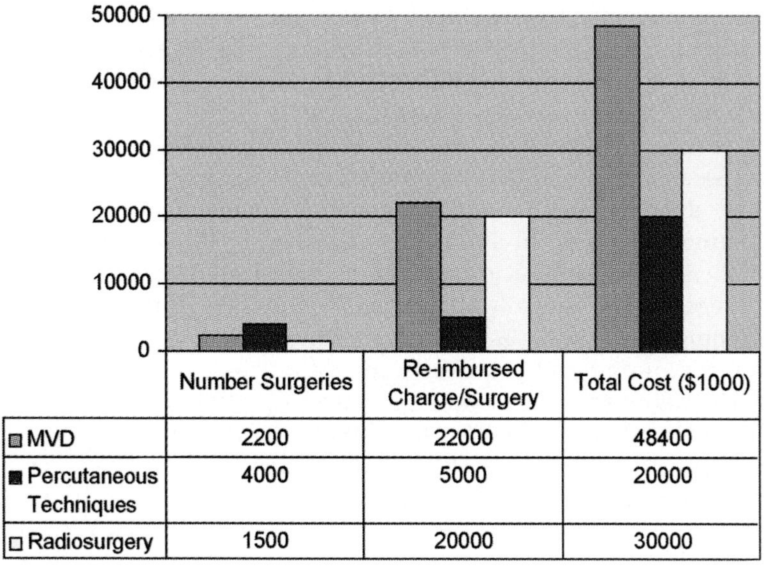

	Number Surgeries	Re-imbursed Charge/Surgery	Total Cost ($1000)
MVD	2200	22000	48400
Percutaneous Techniques	4000	5000	20000
Radiosurgery	1500	20000	30000

FIG. 24.1 Annual cost to third-party payers for trigeminal neuralgia surgery in the United States.

ness analysis comparing three commonly performed procedures for trigeminal neuralgia.

MATERIALS AND METHODS

Patients

The Institutional Review Board of the Mayo Clinic and Foundation in Rochester, Minnesota, approved all aspects of this study. Patients undergoing surgery for idiopathic trigeminal neuralgia by the senior author (BEP) between July 1999 and December 2001 were eligible for enrollment in the study. Every patient had persistent pain despite medical therapy and suffered episodic, shock-like pain within the trigeminal distribution. Twenty-three patients had atypical trigeminal neuralgia characterized by a more constant pain between paroxysms of facial pain. The decision as to which surgery was performed for individual patients was based on the patient's age, medical condition, surgical history, severity of pain, and patient preference. Six patients did not have sufficient follow-up after surgery to be included. The remaining 126 patients underwent 153 separate operations for trigeminal neuralgia.

Surgical Technique

The operative techniques have been described previously: MVD (24), percutaneous glycerol rhizotomy (PRGR) (22), and SR (26). Specific details for each are as follows: During posterior fossa exploration, the superior cerebellar artery compressed the trigeminal nerve either alone or in conjunction with other vessels in 22 cases (67%), the anterior interior cerebellar artery in 2 cases (6%), and veins in 4 cases (12%). In five cases (15%), no evidence of neurovascular compression was detected, and nerve manipulation or partial nerve section was performed (12, 21, 27). The mean operating time for MVD was 198 minutes (range, 85–290 minutes); the mean hospital length of stay (LOS) was 3.2 days (range, 2–8 days). Percutaneous glycerol rhizotomy was performed with local anesthesia and intravenous sedation. In three cases (6%), the trigeminal cistern was not adequately visualized, and no glycerol was injected. In the other 48 cases, the mean volume of glycerol injected was 0.29 mL (range, 0.19–0.40 mL). The mean operating time of PRGR was 44 minutes (range, 10–115 minutes). Thirty-eight patients (74%) were taken to the postanesthesia recovery unit after PRGR; 13 patients were returned directly to the outpatient floor. Stereotactic radiosurgery was performed using the Gamma Knife (Elekta Instruments, Norcross, GA). The mean radiation dose delivered to the trigeminal nerve was 83.5 Gy (range, 70–90 Gy). All patients were discharged on the day of surgery after PRGR and SR.

Outcomes and Statistical Analysis

Preoperative, surgical, and postoperative follow-up information were placed into a prospectively maintained database. Facial pain outcomes were classified as excellent (absence of lancinating facial pain without medications for trigeminal neuralgia), good (complete pain relief but still requiring a low dosage of medications), fair (continued facial pain but reduced more than 50% compared to before surgery), and poor. Patients were contacted 1 mo after surgery and then yearly thereafter to assess their facial pain outcome. Patient follow-up was censored at last contact (n = 112), time of subsequent surgery (n = 37), or death (n = 4).

Kaplan-Meier curves were calculated to determine the percentage of patients achieving and maintaining an excellent facial pain outcome after surgery. Differences in facial pain outcomes between the surgical groups were tested by log rank methods. Univariate comparisons of continuous variables were compared using Student's *t*-test; proportional differences were compared by the chi-squared test.

Cost-Effectiveness Analysis

The outcome measure used in the cost-effectiveness analysis (CEA) was quality-adjusted, pain-free years (QAPFYs). This measure was determined by multiplying the length of follow-up after each operation by the adjusted facial pain outcome. Facial pain outcomes were adjusted as follows: excellent (1.0), good (0.7), fair (0.5), and poor (0.1). Costs were estimated from a societal viewpoint. Uncomplicated procedure costs, cost of complications, and costs of additional surgery were determined using our center's administrative decision support system (Eclipsys Corporation, Boca Raton, FL). This software assembles costs for each encounter and factors in both physician and hospital-based expenses. The calculation of cost per procedure included the uncomplicated procedure cost plus the average cost of complications plus the costs associated with additional procedures performed for persistent or recurrent facial pain. The costs associated with continuing medications were not factored in because of the wide range of drugs used and the relatively small amount compared with the cost of the surgeries themselves. Numbers were adjusted to Year 2000 dollars using the medical care component of the Consumer Price Index. Discounting of costs was not performed, because this would have little impact due to the short follow-up interval.

RESULTS

Patients having PRGR (mean age, 72.2 years) were older compared to the MVD group (mean age, 55.9 years; $P < 0.01$) and SR group (mean age, 67.8 years; $P < 0.05$). Fewer patients in the PRGR (45%) group had undergone previous surgery compared to the SR group (67%; $P < 0.05$). In addition, of those patients having had previous surgery, the PRGR group (mean, 0.6) underwent a lower number of operations compared to the MVD and SR groups (MVD mean, 1.5; SR mean, 1.1; $P < 0.01$).

Thirty-seven patients underwent later operations at a mean of 9.3 mo (range, 1 day to 32 mo). Four patients died of unrelated causes at 6, 12, 15, and 17 mo, respectively. The mean follow-up of the remaining 112 patients was 24.3 mo (range, 6–42 mo). The mean overall follow-up after surgery was 20.4 mo.

Immediate facial pain outcomes after MVD were excellent (n = 30, 91%), good (n = 1, 3%), and fair (n = 2, 6%). Five patients (15%) experienced recurrent pain; three patients (9%) have undergone additional surgery (PRGR, n = 1; SR, n = 2). Initial facial pain outcomes after PRGR were excellent (n = 35, 68%), good (n = 5, 10%), fair (n = 4, 8%), and poor (n = 7, 14%). Ten patients (19%) had recurrent pain; 16 patients (31%) required additional surgery (MVD, n = 1; PRGR, n = 7; SR, n = 8). Early facial pain outcomes after SR were excellent (n = 45, 65%), good (n = 5, 7%), fair (n = 9, 13%), and poor (n = 10, 15%). Eight patients (12%) had recurrent pain; 18 patients (26%) have undergone additional surgery (MVD, n = 6; PRGR, n = 8; SR, n = 3; balloon compression, n = 1). Patients having MVD more commonly achieved and maintained an excellent outcome (85% and 79% at 6 and 24 mo, respectively) compared to those having PRGR (61% and 55%, respectively; $P = 0.01$) and SR (60% and 52%, respectively, $P < 0.01$). No difference was detected between PRGR and SR ($P = 0.61$) (*Fig. 25.1*).

Postoperative complications in the MVD group included superior cerebellar artery infarct (n = 1), symptomatic transverse sinus injury (n = 2), cerebrospinal fluid leak (n = 2), wound infection (n = 1), and ipsilateral deafness (n = 1). Two of these patients required surgery. One patient underwent bilateral optic nerve fenestration for visual decline secondary to a transverse sinus occlusion. The other patient underwent wound reexploration and cranioplasty removal before initiation of antibiotics for a wound infection. Complications after PRGR included aseptic meningitis (n = 1). No procedure-related complications occurred after SR.

The cost per QAPFY was $6,041, $8,098, and $8,138 for PRGR, MVD, and SR, respectively. Threshold analyses were performed to determine the amount of change required in the key variables that would result in equalization of the cost-effectiveness between PRGR and the other procedures. Reduction in the cost of morbidity and additional surgeries to zero did not make either MVD or SR more cost-effective than PRGR. Both MVD and SR would be more cost-effective than PRGR if the cost of additional surgeries after PRGR doubled.

DISCUSSION

Clinical CEAs are designed to measure the economic efficiency of comparable treatments for a health problem that are intended to produce the same end result. By design, a CEA is constrained by the historical and economic context in which it is created and the perspective from which it is written. A CEA from a country with a national health care system is not easily applicable to our more economically diverse health system. A CEA of treatment strategies today is not relevant if a new "cure" is discovered tomorrow or if the pathogenesis of a disease is further refined and diseases once lumped are regrouped. A CEA written from the perspective of a third-party payer is not readily relevant to the individual. However, unlike its cousins, cost-benefit analysis and cost analysis, a CEA compares the economic efficiency of a competing set of treatments measured in clinically relevant terms.

What have we learned about the economic efficiency of trigeminal neuralgia treatment? In the short term, PRGR is more cost-effective than MVD and SR in the treatment of medically refractory trigeminal neuralgia. The cost of an uncomplicated PRGR would have to increase 50% or, conversely, SR and MVD would have to decrease approximately 30% to surpass PRGR. Focusing on mean morbidity cost, the complication rate of PRGR would have to increase more than 4,000% to make the operation less cost-effective than SR and MVD. However, the historical failure rate of PRGR is 50% at 2 to 3 years, and patients often require further surgery. In the long-term, MVD, with its durability and low pain recurrence rate, likely is the most cost-effective treatment of trigeminal neuralgia. These data support our general treatment algorithm in which healthy patients are counseled for MVD while patients with medical comorbidity and surgical failure are treated with PRGR and SR.

Importantly, in our CEA regarding the surgical treatment of trigeminal neuralgia, the success rates of MVD and PRGR performed by the senior author (BEP) are comparable to those of historical controls. Excellent immediate facial pain outcomes occurred in 91% of patients undergoing MVD, 68% of patients undergoing PRGR, and 65% of patients undergoing SR. Fifteen percent of patients undergoing MVD had recurrent pain, compared with 19% of patients undergoing PRGR and 12% of patients undergoing SR. Large series of more than 1,000 patients undergoing MVD have suggested that 10-year pain-free rates are approximately 70% (4, 34). Published pain recurrence rates for PRGR, from studies with designs similar to the short follow-up of our study, are on the order of 50% at 18 to 35 months (8, 25). Long-term follow-up for SR is not available, but our figures are similar to those in the published literature (23). Complications rates were low, with three major complications in the MVD group, two of which required reoperation. One patient with PRGR developed aseptic meningitis; no complications occurred secondary to SR. Large series of patients undergoing MVD have found major complication rates form zero to 2.5% (3, 6, 9, 33, 34).

Three critiques of our study impact the widespread application of our findings. First, indirect costs, such as those associated with loss of work, were not calculated. Patients undergoing MVD would have greater indirect costs in the short term than those patients undergoing percutaneous and stereotactic treatments. However, the indirect costs would likely be outweighed by the durability of the procedure and the low rate of recurrence. Second, the estimated cost of SR was calculated at a center performing more than 275 radiosurgical cases annually. Therefore, the per-case sharing of fixed indirect costs for equipment, construction, and personnel would be higher at a center performing only 150 cases a year. Finally, the study follow-up time was short. However, with the similarity of our patient population, outcomes, and complications to those of historical controls, we have no reason to believe that pain recurrence and complication rates will be different in future surgeries.

The direct applicability of CEAs in the American health care system is limited by patient choice and concepts of distributive justice. Independent of efficacy and clinical appropriateness, a patient may choose to have a less effective treatment. In our series, 17 patients younger than age 70 underwent radiosurgery as an initial treatment. The less invasive draw of radiosurgery is powerful, despite lack of long-term follow-up. Patients perceive little risk in trying SR as a “first” surgery. To limit patient choice by codifying a treatment paradigm would be perceived as inequitable, because there is always an avenue for patients willing to pay a higher price to receive the treatment of their choice. Despite their shortcomings, well-designed CEAs, from a societal perspective, provide useful data to leaders on a national level as health care expenditures, now 14.1% of the U.S. gross domestic product, continue to rise. In 1996, the Panel on Cost-Effectiveness in Health and Medicine concluded, “Although CEA does not reflect every element of importance in health care decisions, the information it provides is critical to informing decisions about the allocation of health care resources” (29).

REFERENCES

1. *Leksell Gamma Knife Treatment Statistics.* Norcross, GA: Elekta Instruments, Inc., 2000.
2. *National Neurosurgical Statistics: 1999 Procedural Statistics.* Rolling Meadow, IL: American Association of Neurological Surgeons, 2000.
3. Apfelbaum RI: Neurovascular decompression: The procedure of choice? **Clin Neurosurg** 46:473–498, 2000.
4. Barker FG II, Jannetta PJ, Bissonette DJ, et al.: The long-term outcome of microvascular decompression for trigeminal neuralgia. **N Engl J Med** 334:1077–1083, 1996.
5. Brisman R, Khandji AG, Mooij RB: Trigeminal nerve-blood vessel relationship as revealed by high-resolution magnetic resonance imaging and its effect on pain relief after gamma knife radiosurgery for trigeminal neuralgia. **Neurosurgery** 50:1261–1267, 2002.
6. Broggi G, Ferroli P, Franzini A, et al.: Microvascular decompression for trigeminal neuralgia: comments on a series of 250 cases, including 10 patients with multiple sclerosis. **J Neurol Neurosurg Psychiatry** 68:59–64, 2000.
7. Brown JA, McDaniel MD, Weaver MT: Percutaneous trigeminal nerve compression for treatment of trigeminal neuralgia: Results in 50 patients. **Neurosurgery** 32:570–573, 1993.
8. Burchiel KJ: Percutaneous retrogasserian glycerol rhizolysis in the management of trigeminal neuralgia. **J Neurosurg** 69:361–366, 1988.
9. Burchiel KJ, Clarke H, Haglund M, et al.: Long-term efficacy of microvascular decompression in trigeminal neuralgia. **J Neurosurg** 69:35–38, 1988.
10. Cheng TM, Cascino TL, Onofrio BM: Comprehensive study of diagnosis and treatment of trigeminal neuralgia secondary to tumors. **Neurology** 43:2298–2302, 1993.
11. Dandy W: Concerning the cause of trigeminal neuralgia. **Am J Surg** 24:447–455, 1934.
12. Delitala A, Brunori A, Chiappetta F: Microsurgical posterior fossa exploration for trigeminal neuralgia: A study on 48 cases. **Minim Invasive Neurosurg** 44:152–156, 2001.
13. Fields H: Treatment of trigeminal neuralgia. **N Engl J Med** 334:1125–1126, 1996.
14. Hooge JP, Redekop WK: Trigeminal neuralgia in multiple sclerosis. **Neurology** 45:1294–1296, 1995.
15. Ildan F, Gocer AI, Bagdatoglu H, et al.: Isolated trigeminal neuralgia secondary to distal anterior inferior cerebellar artery aneurysm. **Neurosurg Rev** 19:43–46, 1996.
16. Jannetta PJ: Arterial compression of the trigeminal nerve at the pons in patients with trigeminal neuralgia. **J Neurosurg** 26(suppl):159–162, 1967.
17. Kanpolat Y, Savas A, Bekar A, et al.: Percutaneous controlled radiofrequency trigeminal rhizotomy for the treatment of idiopathic trigeminal neuralgia: 25-Year experience with 1,600 patients. **Neurosurgery** 48:524–534, 2001.

18. Katusic S, Beard CM, Bergstralh E, et al.: Incidence and clinical features of trigeminal neuralgia, Rochester, Minnesota, 1945–1984. **Ann Neurol** 27:89–95, 1990.
19. Katusic S, Williams DB, Beard CM, et al.: Epidemiology and clinical features of idiopathic trigeminal neuralgia and glossopharyngeal neuralgia: Similarities and differences, Rochester, Minnesota, 1945–1984. **Neuroepidemiology** 10:276–281, 1991.
20. Kondziolka D, Lunsford LD, Flickinger JC, et al.: Stereotactic radiosurgery for trigeminal neuralgia: A multi-institutional study using the gamma unit. **J Neurosurg** 84:940–945, 1996.
21. Kureshi SA, Wilkins RH: Posterior fossa reexploration for persistent or recurrent trigeminal neuralgia or hemifacial spasm: surgical findings and therapeutic implications. **Neurosurgery** 43:1111–1117, 1998.
22. Lunsford LD, Bennett MH: Percutaneous retrogasserian glycerol rhizotomy for tic douloureux: Part 1. Technique and results in 112 patients. **Neurosurgery** 14:424–430, 1984.
23. Maesawa S, Salame C, Flickinger JC, et al.: Clinical outcomes after stereotactic radiosurgery for idiopathic trigeminal neuralgia. **J Neurosurg** 94:14–20, 2001.
24. McLaughlin MR, Jannetta PJ, Clyde BL, et al.: Microvascular decompression of cranial nerves: Lessons learned after 4400 operations. **J Neurosurg** 90:1–8, 1999.
25. North RB, Kidd DH, Piantadosi S, et al.: Percutaneous retrogasserian glycerol rhizotomy. Predictors of success and failure in treatment of trigeminal neuralgia. **J Neurosurg** 72:851–856, 1990.
26. Pollock BE, Phuong LK, Gorman DA, et al.: Stereotactic radiosurgery for idiopathic trigeminal neuralgia. **J Neurosurg** 97:347–353, 2002.
27. Rath SA, Klein HJ, Richter HP: Findings and long-term results of subsequent operations after failed microvascular decompression for trigeminal neuralgia. **Neurosurgery** 39:933–940, 1996.
28. Rogers CL, Shetter AG, Fiedler JA, et al.: Gamma knife radiosurgery for trigeminal neuralgia: The initial experience of the Barrow Neurological Institute. **Int J Radiat Oncol Biol Phys** 47:1013–1019, 2000.
29. Russell LB, Gold MR, Siegel JE, et al.: The role of cost-effectiveness analysis in health and medicine. Panel on Cost-Effectiveness in Health and Medicine. **JAMA** 276:1172–1177, 1996.
30. Saini SS: Reterogasserian anhydrous glycerol injection therapy in trigeminal neuralgia: observations in 552 patients. **J Neurol Neurosurg Psychiatry** 50:1536–1538, 1987.
31. Skirving DJ, Dan NG: A 20-year review of percutaneous balloon compression of the trigeminal ganglion. **J Neurosurg** 94:913–917, 2001.
32. Taha JM, Tew JM Jr: Comparison of surgical treatments for trigeminal neuralgia: reevaluation of radiofrequency rhizotomy. **Neurosurgery** 38:865–871, 1996.
33. Theodosopoulos PV, Marco E, Applebury C, et al.: Predictive model for pain recurrence after posterior fossa surgery for trigeminal neuralgia. **Arch Neurol** 59: 1297–1302, 2002.
34. Tronnier VM, Rasche D, Hamer J, et al.: Treatment of idiopathic trigeminal neuralgia: comparison of long-term outcome after radiofrequency rhizotomy and microvascular decompression. **Neurosurgery** 48:1261–1268, 2001.
35. Yoshimasu F, Kurland LT, Elveback LR: Tic douloureux in Rochester, Minnesota, 1945–1969. **Neurology** 22:952–956, 1972.

CHAPTER

25

CSNS Young Neurosurgeon Award: Is It Appropriate to Treat Complex Cerebrovascular Pathology in Nonacademic Medical Centers?

DONGWOO JOHN CHANG, M.D., F.R.C.S.(C.)

Selective referral to high-volume hospitals has been demonstrated to reduce the mortality for certain high-risk diagnoses (1).

It has been traditionally accepted that complex neurosurgical problems can and should be managed in academic medical centers. The management of intracranial vascular disease has become increasingly multidisciplinary with the advent of refined methods in surgical technique, neuroprotective strategies, endovascular technology, and further development in the cognitive understanding of cerebrovascular disease. Concurrently, the overall level of neurosurgical care in all sectors has improved. The unanswered questions are: How much sophisticated care can be provided by nontertiary centers, and what is an appropriate level of care in various settings?

Therefore, it is timely to entertain the question: Is it appropriate to treat complex cerebrovascular pathology in nonacademic medical centers?

This paper is written from the perspective from the experience of a single cerebrovascular/skull base surgery fellowship–trained neurosurgeon at a well-respected, 600-bed, freestanding regional resource level I trauma center (Lehigh Valley Hospital) in Allentown, Pennsylvania. There is a nominal academic affiliation with the Penn State/Hershey College of Medicine, approximately 75 miles away. This paper does not necessarily represent the opinions of any other physicians or institutions.

It is a direct, subjective comparison of different clinical environments in which the author worked, from residency training at McGill University/Montreal Neurological Institute to cerebrovascular/skull base fellowship experience at the University of Florida, Gainesville, to a community-based referral practice at Lehigh Valley Hospital, Allentown, Pennsylvania, and presently to a full-time academic practice at The Ohio State University, Columbus, Ohio.

TABLE 25.1
Aneurysm Locations

Location	N	Location	n
Acomm	17	Pcomm	9
Ophthalmic	3	ACA/A1	2
Distal ACA	1	Basilar	2
MCA	7	Vert-PICA	1
MCA/Lenticulostriate	1	ICA bifurcation	3
		Total	46

The author's initial experience with cerebrovascular neurosurgery was retrospectively analyzed from practice data over a 22-mo consecutive period. Forty-eight total intracranial vascular cases were treated with surgery, of which 46 aneurysms were clipped (33 ruptured and 13 unruptured). One cerebellar AVM and one temporal lobe cavernous malformation were also resected during this time interval. Patient ages ranged from 30 to 86 years. There were 32 female and 14 male patients. All surgeries were performed by the author (DJC). Aneurysm location, aneurysm size, clinical grade, and clinical outcome based on the Glasgow Outcome Scale are enumerated in *Tables 25.1, 25.2, 25.3,* and *25.4*, respectively.

All patients who present with subarachnoid hemorrhage are directly admitted to the medical intensive care unit (ICU), with a medicine PGY1 resident on first call for medical management. A medical critical care attending is on backup call for these medical residents. The neurosurgery attending is on call for all neurosurgical issues as perceived and defined by house staff. There are no neurosurgery residents, fellows, or house physicians at Lehigh Valley Hospital. The ICU itself is a general ICU with no particular inclination among the nursing staff toward "neuro" care.

There is a neurosurgical operating room (OR) team at Lehigh Valley Hospital that is quite comfortable with routine general neuro-

TABLE 25.2
Aneurysm Sizes

Size (mm)	n
2–5	10 (all with SAH)
6–9	19
10–14	7
15–24	7
≥25	3

TABLE 25.3
Clinical Grades (Hunt and Hess)

Grade	n
0	13
1	4
2	7
3	12
4	10
5	0 (none treated surgically)

surgery, trauma craniotomies, and ventriculostomies. All surgery in this series was performed by a single neurosurgeon (DJC). Technical adjuncts such as skull base approaches, temporary clipping, evoked potentials, and intraoperative ventriculostomy were liberally utilized in this clinical series.

The reflections of the author, based on the 22-mo consecutive data and 46 surgically clipped aneurysms, are presented. Potential endovascular candidates numbered 28% (13/46). The point is not so much that they would necessarily have been coiled or that others would agree that they should be coiled. The thought, however, crossed the author's mind that these cases represented an opportunity to entertain alternative management options on behalf of the patient. There is no neuroendovascular capability at Lehigh Valley Hospital. To allow maximum treatment choice, all patients and families were given the option to seek treatment elsewhere.

Fifty-five percent (18/33) of the patients with ruptured aneurysms experienced cerebral vasospasm. Empiric triple-H therapy and continuous ventricular drainage was employed (typically placed intraoperatively) until Day 10 to Day 12 postsubarachnoid hemorrhage. Angiograms were usually not performed. (What would I do with the results anyway?) Therefore, in most cases, the diagnosis was clinical (head CT-negative for blood or hydrocephalus) and, in some cases, of CT-demonstrated hypodensities that later were found to be irre-

TABLE 25.4
Clinical Outcome (Glasgow Outcome Scale)

Grade	n
5	33
4	2
3	6
2	0
1	5 (4/5 deaths in Hunt-Hess grade 4)

versible. There is no routine capability of transcranial Doppler at Lehigh Valley Hospital.

Delay in surgical treatment, typically of 2 to 3 days, was experienced by 52% (17/33) of the patients. The reasons for the delay were, first, the availability of angiography ("Are you going to the OR tonight?") and, second, the availability of an appropriate OR team and anesthesia as well as appropriate neurosurgical backup for level I trauma coverage and in case of a catastrophic intraoperative rupture. One attending neurosurgeon was on call for a 600-bed, level I trauma center that admits more than 500 total head injuries per year without midlevel providers after hours and on weekends.

A delay in detection and treatment of medical/neurological complications occurred in 28% (13/46). Some potential reasons for this issue include, medical interns being on first call, most of the medical/critical care attending staff not being particularly comfortable caring for patients with aneurysm, nursing staff not being attuned to neuro-critical care, and the need for neurosurgeons to attend to competitive mandates, such as the development of an elective neurosurgical practice, level I neurotrauma call, and weekend school (one colleague obtained an executive MBA on the weekends during this same time interval). However, there was one extremely enthusiastic and interested director of the medical ICU with several colleagues who shared the similar vision of interest and support for these sick patients.

It is difficult to make sweeping generalizations on the issue of appropriate care for neurovascular patients. The ideal situation for patients with aneurysms and AVMs, in the author's opinion, includes the following: a tertiary university hospital; dedicated neurosurgeons with special interest, training, and experience in cerebrovascular neurosurgery; a vigorous program incorporating neurosurgical education and research in cerebrovascular disease; active endovascular capability; TCD expertise and routine availability; intraoperative monitoring; critical care medical/nursing interest and expertise; adequate OR support for high-risk cases; adequate equipment; 24/7 neurosurgical house staff coverage; and an institutional commitment to the highest levels of care in this particular subspecialty area. Life is not perfect, however, and one cannot necessarily have everything all at once. Academic medical centers are being eroded by strong political and economic forces that make it difficult to carry out the traditional mandates of tertiary care, education, and research in a manner that does justice to this mission.

Important questions to ponder are: What is best for the patient (honestly . . .), and what would you do if the index patient was yourself or a family member?

Questions and dilemmas include the role of the neurosurgical house staff coverage in relation to clinical outcome, university hospitals with low cerebrovascular volumes, university hospitals without endovascular capability or TCD expertise, community hospitals with high cerebrovascular volumes, community hospitals with endovascular capabilities and TCD expertise, the role of cerebrovascular fellowship training or special experience in clinical outcome, resource allocation in a competitive health care environment, liability issues related to perception of patients and referring physicians ("Am I getting the best available care?"), and institutional priorities.

It has been well established that high-volume hospitals have a lower mortality rate than low-volume hospitals for certain conditions (2). That higher volume results in decreased mortality for cerebral aneurysms was well demonstrated in a review of New York State data (3) and in the an older patient population (4). It has also been well established that the availability of endovascular services in a hospital reduces the mortality rate of patients treated for cerebral aneurysms (5). The role of neurovascular surgical results as related to special training and experienced was elucidated by Dr. Lawton at UCSF in a review of his initial experience (6). The sole paper relating the neurovascular outcomes in a community-based setting was addressed in a recent article (7).

A review of the published articles demonstrates that they are generally from large, tertiary institutions that have neurosurgical residency training programs and experienced neurovascular surgeons. Multidisciplinary teams, consisting of neurology, neuropathology, neuroanesthesia, critical care, nursing, and the OR team, are typically present to varying degrees. University hospital referrals are typically most complex in that they are of higher-grade SAH, dominant hemisphere location, posterior circulation location, fusiform dissections, large or giant aneurysms, and AVMs in eloquent locations; require extensive skull base approaches (basilar, ophthalmic); are associated with concurrent medical illnesses; and are often exploration/treatment failures. Therefore, a direct comparison of outcomes may not be accurate even if there were many published articles from the private, nontertiary sector.

Is centralization of neurovascular care to academic medical centers appropriate? This intuitively appears to be true, as it happens elsewhere around the globe (Canada, Japan, Scandinavia, England, Australia, etc.). It promotes better resource allocation and utilization instead of everyone trying to do everything in every setting. There may be some issues of risk involved in transferring patients to tertiary care facilities, however. Centralization would promote optimal patient care, because the most experienced, knowledgeable individuals and institutions are treating the most complex and involved problems. It promotes the goals of neurosurgical education, because future neurosurgeons are exposed to the most complex problems during the formative years of residency and fellowship, thereby promoting the development of a keen sense of clinical judgment based on experience. The goals of neurosurgical research are promoted, because community cases generally do not become part of a clinical series from which knowledge can be gained. Centralization could decrease litigious activity ("I want the best care for my brain . . . "). Clearly, there are many technically excellent neurosurgeons in all venues and many excellent hospitals of all sizes and outlooks, including the index hospital, Lehigh Valley Hospital. Ultimately, however, there is the surgeon comfort level in feeling that he or she is, in fact, providing the best state-of-the-art care with diagnoses in which small differences can translate into big differences in overall clinical outcome.

Are there exceptions? Always, of course, but the important question remains: What pathway would increase the access to the best average level of care to the largest number of patients with these resource-exhaustive diagnoses?

We, as a neurosurgical community, have an obligation to attempt, to the best of our abilities, to provide the highest level of care to *all* patients with cerebrovascular disease by optimally utilizing all available resources, both institutional and human.

Arguably the greatest technical neurosurgeon of our time, Professor M. Gazi Yasargil remarked in his publication, *A Legacy of Microneurosurgery*:

> This development (hypothermic cardiac standstill) has proved the importance of another fact, that successful accomplishments in neurosurgery, particularly in neurovascular surgery, demand and are dependent on optimal conditions for the neurosurgeon and his team (neuroradiologist, neuroanesthesiologist, neuro-scrub nurses, neurointensive care unit, and adequate hospital infrastructure). A surgical procedure first must develop and reach maturity to secure its application in a given hospital. Cardiovascular centers have become well established worldwide within the last 50 years. This, however, is still not the case in the field of neurosurgery, not because the mechanical aspects of surgery are below standard, but because the much higher complexity of dynamic homeostasis of the CNS organs in the pre-, peri-, and postoperative phases requires more advances in science and technology to achieve effective and optimal treatment of these patients.

REFERENCES

1. Dudley RA, Johansen KL, Brand R, Rennie DJ, Milstein A: Selective referral to high-volume hospitals—Estimating potentially avoidable deaths. **JAMA** 283:1159–1166, 2000.
2. Dudley RA, Johansen KL, Brand R, Rennie DJ, Milstein A: Selective referral to high-volume hospitals—Estimating potentially avoidable deaths. **JAMA** 283:1159–1166, 2000.
3. Solomon RA, Mayer SA, Tarmey JJ: Relationship between the volume of craniotomies for cerebral aneurysms performed at New York State hospitals and in-hospital mortality. **Stroke** 27:13–17, 1996.
4. Taylor CL, Yuan Z, Selman WR, Ratcheson RA Rimm A: Mortality rates, hospital length of stay, and the cost of treating subarachnoid hemorrhage in older patients: Institutional and geographic differences. **J Neurosurg** 86: 583–588, 1997.
5. Johnston SC: Effect of endovascular services and hospital volume on cerebral aneurysm treatment outcomes. **Stroke** 31:111–117, 2000.
6. Lawton MT. Basilar apex aneurysms: Surgical results and perspective from an initial experience. **Neurosurgery** 50:1–10, 2002.
7. Naso WB, Rhea AH, Poole A: Management and outcomes in a low-volume cerebral aneurysm practice. **Neurosurgery** 48:91–100, 2001.

Author Index

Subject Index